Epithelial Cell Culture Protocols

METHODS IN MOLECULAR BIOLOGY™

John M. Walker, SERIES EDITOR

204. **Molecular Cytogenetics:** *Methods and Protocols,* edited by *Yao-Shan Fan, 2002*

203. **In Situ Detection of DNA Damage:** *Methods and Protocols,* edited by *Vladimir V. Didenko, 2002*

202. **Thyroid Hormone Receptors:** *Methods and Protocols,* edited by *Aria Baniahmad, 2002*

201. **Combinatorial Library Methods and Protocols,** edited by *Lisa B. English, 2002*

200. **DNA Methylation Protocols,** edited by *Ken I. Mills and Bernie H, Ramsahoye, 2002*

199. **Liposome Methods and Protocols,** edited by *Subhash C. Basu and Manju Basu, 2002*

198. **Neural Stem Cells:** *Methods and Protocols,* edited by *Tanja Zigova, Juan R. Sanchez-Ramos, and Paul R. Sanberg, 2002*

197. **Mitochondrial DNA:** *Methods and Protocols,* edited by *William C. Copeland, 2002*

196. **Oxidants and Antioxidants:** *Ultrastructural and Molecular Biology Protocols,* edited by *Donald Armstrong, 2002*

195. **Quantitative Trait Loci:** *Methods and Protocols,* edited by *Nicola J. Camp and Angela Cox, 2002*

194. **Post-translational Modification Reactions,** edited by *Christoph Kannicht, 2002*

193. **RT-PCR Protocols,** edited by *Joseph O'Connell, 2002*

192. **PCR Cloning Protocols, 2nd ed.,** edited by *Bing-Yuan Chen and Harry W. Janes, 2002*

191. **Telomeres and Telomerase:** *Methods and Protocols,* edited by *John A. Double and Michael J. Thompson, 2002*

190. **High Throughput Screening:** *Methods and Protocols,* edited by *William P. Janzen, 2002*

189. **GTPase Protocols:** *The RAS Superfamily,* edited by *Edward J. Manser and Thomas Leung, 2002*

188. **Epithelial Cell Culture Protocols,** edited by *Clare Wise, 2002*

187. **PCR Mutation Detection Protocols,** edited by *Bimal D. M. Theophilus and Ralph Rapley, 2002*

186. **Oxidative Stress and Antioxidant Protocols,** edited by *Donald Armstrong, 2002*

185. **Embryonic Stem Cells:** *Methods and Protocols,* edited by *Kursad Turksen, 2002*

184. **Biostatistical Methods,** edited by *Stephen W. Looney, 2002*

183. **Green Fluorescent Protein:** *Applications and Protocols,* edited by *Barry W. Hicks, 2002*

182. **In Vitro Mutagenesis Protocols, 2nd ed.,** edited by *Jeff Braman, 2002*

181. **Genomic Imprinting:** *Methods and Protocols,* edited by *Andrew Ward, 2002*

180. **Transgenesis Techniques, 2nd ed.:** *Principles and Protocols,* edited by *Alan R. Clarke, 2002*

179. **Gene Probes:** *Principles and Protocols,* edited by *Marilena Aquino de Muro and Ralph Rapley, 2002*

178. `Antibody Phage Display:` *Methods and Protocols,* edited by *Philippa M. O'Brien and Robert Aitken, 2001*

177. **Two-Hybrid Systems:** *Methods and Protocols,* edited by *Paul N. MacDonald, 2001*

176. **Steroid Receptor Methods:** *Protocols and Assays,* edited by *Benjamin A. Lieberman, 2001*

175. **Genomics Protocols,** edited by *Michael P. Starkey and Ramnath Elaswarapu, 2001*

174. **Epstein-Barr Virus Protocols,** edited by *Joanna B. Wilson and Gerhard H. W. May, 2001*

173. **Calcium-Binding Protein Protocols, Volume 2:** *Methods and Techniques,* edited by *Hans J. Vogel, 2001*

172. **Calcium-Binding Protein Protocols, Volume 1:** *Reviews and Case Histories,* edited by *Hans J. Vogel, 2001*

171. **Proteoglycan Protocols,** edited by *Renato V. Iozzo, 2001*

170. **DNA Arrays:** *Methods and Protocols,* edited by *Jang B. Rampal, 2001*

169. **Neurotrophin Protocols,** edited by *Robert A. Rush, 2001*

168. **Protein Structure, Stability, and Folding,** edited by *Kenneth P. Murphy, 2001*

167. **DNA Sequencing Protocols,** *Second Edition,* edited by *Colin A. Graham and Alison J. M. Hill, 2001*

166. **Immunotoxin Methods and Protocols,** edited by *Walter A. Hall, 2001*

165. **SV40 Protocols,** edited by *Leda Raptis, 2001*

164. **Kinesin Protocols,** edited by *Isabelle Vernos, 2001*

163. **Capillary Electrophoresis of Nucleic Acids, Volume 2:** *Practical Applications of Capillary Electrophoresis,* edited by *Keith R. Mitchelson and Jing Cheng, 2001*

162. **Capillary Electrophoresis of Nucleic Acids, Volume 1:** *Introduction to the Capillary Electrophoresis of Nucleic Acids,* edited by *Keith R. Mitchelson and Jing Cheng, 2001*

161. **Cytoskeleton Methods and Protocols,** edited by *Ray H. Gavin, 2001*

160. **Nuclease Methods and Protocols,** edited by *Catherine H. Schein, 2001*

159. **Amino Acid Analysis Protocols,** edited by *Catherine Cooper, Nicole Packer, and Keith Williams, 2001*

158. **Gene Knockout Protocols,** edited by *Martin J. Tymms and Ismail Kola, 2001*

157. **Mycotoxin Protocols,** edited by *Mary W. Trucksess and Albert E. Pohland, 2001*

156. **Antigen Processing and Presentation Protocols,** edited by *Joyce C. Solheim, 2001*

155. **Adipose Tissue Protocols,** edited by *Gérard Ailhaud, 2000*

154. **Connexin Methods and Protocols,** edited by *Roberto Bruzzone and Christian Giaume, 2001*

153. **Neuropeptide Y Protocols,** edited by *Ambikaipakan Balasubramaniam, 2000*

152. **DNA Repair Protocols:** *Prokaryotic Systems,* edited by *Patrick Vaughan, 2000*

151. **Matrix Metalloproteinase Protocols,** edited by *Ian M. Clark, 2001*

150. **Complement Methods and Protocols,** edited by *B. Paul Morgan, 2000*

149. **The ELISA Guidebook,** edited by *John R. Crowther, 2000*

148. **DNA–Protein Interactions:** *Principles and Protocols* (**2nd ed.),** edited by *Tom Moss, 2001*

147. **Affinity Chromatography:** *Methods and Protocols,* edited by *Pascal Bailon, George K. Ehrlich, Wen-Jian Fung, and Wolfgang Berthold, 2000*

METHODS IN MOLECULAR BIOLOGY™

Epithelial Cell Culture Protocols

Edited by

Clare Wise

Medical Research Council,
National Institute for Medical Research,
London, UK

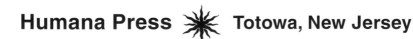

Humana Press ✳ Totowa, New Jersey

©2002 Humana Press Inc.
999 Riverview Drive, Suite 208
Totowa, New Jersey 07512

www.humanapress.com

This publication is printed on acid-free paper. ∞
ANSI Z39.48-1984 (American Standards Institute)
Permanence of Paper for Printed Library Materials.

Cover illustration: Scanning electron micrograph of conventionally fixed and processed differentiated human airway epithelia grown on a semipermeable membrane filter. *See* Fig. 1 on page 117.

Cover design by Patricia F. Cleary.

Production Editor: Mark J. Breaugh.

For additional copies, pricing for bulk purchases, and/or information about other Humana titles, contact Humana at the above address or at any of the following numbers: Tel.: 973-256-1699; Fax: 973-256-8341; E-mail: humana@humanapr.com or visit our Website: http://humanapress.com

Printed in the United States of America. 10 9 8 7 6 5 4 3 2 1

Library of Congress Cataloging in Publication Data

Epithelial cell culture protocols / edited by Clare Wise.
     p. cm. -- (Methods in molecular biology ; 188)
  Includes bibliographical references and index.
  ISBN 0-89603-893-9 (alk. paper)
   1. Epithelial cells--Laboratory manuals. 2. Epithelium--Cultures and culture
media--Laboratory manuals. 3. Cell culture--Laboratory manuals. I. Wise, Clare. II.
Series.

QP88.4 .E625 2002
611'.0181--dc21

                                                           2001039554

Preface

There have been significant advances in research involving the isolation and culture of epithelial cells in the past decade, and many new techniques have been developed. Monolayer cultures can be used to evaluate the nature and behavior of cells, while the use of epithelial cells in model systems has allowed a deeper understanding of cellular and molecular mechanisms and interactions. The aim of this book is to provide a comprehensive, step-by-step guide to many techniques for epithelial cell culture, combining in one volume the more commonly used protocols along with many that are more specialized. *Epithelial Cell Culture Protocols* should help those who are new to this field and want to learn the basic culture techniques, as well as those needing to use more wide ranging and specific protocols. It should be a useful resource on its own, and also complement the other volumes that have been written about cell culture in the *Methods in Molecular Biology* series.

Epithelial Cell Culture Protocols covers a wide variety of protocols, mostly aimed at the researcher, but also a few aimed at clinicians. The establishment and maintenance of primary cultures derived from many different tissues and different species is covered. Particular emphasis has been placed on protocols needed to further analyze and assess epithelial cells, for example, by looking at apoptosis and integrins and by measuring membrane capacitance and confluence. Using different co-culture techniques, it is possible also to develop models to investigate many different systems in vitro. There are chapters describing several of these, for example, models of the blood–brain barrier, systems to investigate the interaction of epithelial cells with bacteria, and models to investigate drug uptake. From a more clinical aspect, one of the most exciting advances in culturing epithelial cells has been the ability to use these cells in treating patients with burns and other skin disorders, and this area is also covered in this book.

I would like to thank everyone who helped me with the compilation of *Epithelial Cell Culture Protocols*, especially all of the authors who contributed to this book. Thank you for sharing your work and experience, and for the support you showed me. Thank you to John Walker for his help and amazingly rapid responses to my cries for help, and for having faith in me when he first asked me to edit this book. To the NIMR for allowing me the resources to complete this book, and to Robin Lovell-Badge for his encouragement and constant support. Finally, to Juan Pedro Martinez-Barbera, for his advice and for his patience during the many silent hours as I sat editing.

Clare Wise

Contents

Preface v

Contributors xi

1 Human Lens Epithelial Cell Culture
   Nobuhiro Ibaraki 1

2 Human Airway Epithelial Cell Culture
   **Mutsuo Yamaya, Masayoshi Hosoda, Tomoko Suzuki,
   Norihiro Yamada, and Hidetada Sasaki** 7

3 Rat Gastric Mucosal Epithelial Cell Culture
   Yoshitaka Konda and Tsutomu Chiba 17

4 Thymic Epithelial Cell Culture
   Carsten Röpke 27

5 Bile Duct Epithelial Cell Culture
   Alphonse E. Sirica 37

6 Liver Epithelial Cell Culture
   Rolf Gebhardt 53

7 Pulmonary Epithelial Cell Culture
   Ben Forbes 65

8 Prostate Epithelial Cell Isolation and Culture
   David L. Hudson 77

9 A Bovine Mammary Endothelial/Epithelial Cell Culture Model
   of the Blood/Milk Barrier
   Albert Guidry and Celia O'Brien 85

10 The Blood–CSF Barrier in Culture: *Development of a Primary Culture
   and Transepithelial Transport Model for Choroidal Epithelial Cells*
   Wei Zheng and Qiuqu Zhao 99

11 An In Vitro Model of Differentiated Human Airway Epithelia:
   Methods for Establishing Primary Cultures
   **Philip H. Karp, Thomas O. Moninger, S. Pary Weber,
   Tamara S. Nesselhauf, Janice L. Launspach,
   Joseph Zabner, and Michael J. Welsh** 115

12 Primary Mouse Keratinocyte Culture
   Kairbaan Hodivala-Dilke 139

13 Analyzing Apoptosis in Cultured Epithelial Cells
   Andrew P. Gilmore and Charles H. Streuli 145

14 Keratins as Markers of Epithelial Cells
   David L. Hudson *157*
15 Epithelial Cell Integrins
   Joachim Rychly *169*
16 Isolation, Cultivation, and Differentiation of Normal Human Epidermal
   Keratinocytes in Serum-Free Medium
   Sebastian Zellmer and Dieter Reissig *179*
17 Clinical Application of Autologous Cultured Epithelia
   for the Treatment of Burns and Disfigurement of Skin Surfaces
   Norio Kumagai *185*
18 Transplantation of Cultured Epithelial Cells
   Minoru Ueda, Yukio Sumi, Yoshitaka Hibino,
   and Ken-Ichiro Hata *197*
19 An Outgrowth Culture System of Normal Human Epithelium:
   An In Vitro Model to Study the Coordination
   of Cellular Migration and Proliferation
   Tohru Masui *213*
20 Application of Epithelial Cell Culture in Drug Transport
   in the Respiratory Tract
   Jie Shen and Vincent H. L. Lee *217*
21 Applications of Epithelial Cell Culture in Studies of Drug Transport
   Staffan Tavelin, Johan Gråsjö, Jan Taipalensuu,
   Göran Ocklind, and Per Artursson *233*
22 X-Ray Microanalysis of Epithelial Cells in Culture
   Godfried M. Roomans *273*
23 ENU Mutagenesis of Rat Mammary Epithelial Cells
   George Stoica *291*
24 ENU-Induced Ovarian Cancer
   George Stoica *305*
25 Measurement of Membrane Capacitance in Epithelial Monolayers
   Carol A. Bertrand and Ulrich Hopfer *315*
26 Assessing Epithelial Cell Confluence by Spectroscopy
   Simon A. Lewis *329*
27 Co-Cultivation of Liver Epithelial Cells with Hepatocytes
   Rolf Gebhardt *337*
28 Co-Culture and Crosstalk between Endothelial Cells and Vascular
   Smooth Muscle Cells Mediated by Intracellular Calcium
   Wee Soo Shin, Chieko Hemmi, and Teruhiko Toyo-oka *347*

Contents   *ix*

29 Establishing Epithelial–Immune Cell Co-Cultures:
      Effects on Epithelial Ion Transport and Permeability
      Derek M. McKay and Mary H. Perdue 359
30 Explant Cultures of Embryonic Epithelium:
      Analysis of Mesenchymal Signals
      Carin Sahlberg, Tuija Mustonen, and Irma Thesleff 373
31 Bacterial Interactions with Host Epithelium In Vitro
      **Nicola Jones, Mary H. Perdue, Philip M. Sherman,
        and Derek M. McKay** 383
Index 401

Contributors

PER ARTURSSON • *Division of Pharmaceutics, Uppsala University, Uppsala, Sweden*

CAROL A. BERTRAND • *Department of Cell Biology and Physiology, University of Pittsburgh School of Medicine, Pittsburgh, PA*

TSUTOMU CHIBA • *Department of Gastroenterology and Hepatology, Kyoto University Graduate School of Medicine, Kyoto, Japan*

BEN FORBES • *Department of Pharmacy, King's College London, London, UK*

ROLF GEBHARDT • *Institute of Biochemistry, Medical Faculty, University of Leipzig, Leipzig, Germany*

ANDREW P. GILMORE • *School of Biological Sciences, University of Manchester, Manchester, UK*

JOHAN GRÅSJÖ • *Division of Pharmaceutics, Uppsala University, Uppsala, Sweden*

ALBERT GUIDRY • *Immunology and Disease Resistance Laboratory, US Department of Agriculture, Beltsville, MD*

KEN-ICHIRO HATA • *Department of Tissue Engineering, Nagoya University School of Medicine, Nagoya City, Japan*

CHIEKO HEMMI • *Health Service Center, University of Tokyo, Tokyo, Japan*

YOSHITAKA HIBINO • *Department of Tissue Engineering, Nagoya University School of Medicine, Nagoya City, Japan*

KAIRBAAN HODIVALA-DILKE • *Cell Adhesion and Disease Laboratory, The Richard Dimbleby Department of Cancer Research/Imperial Cancer Research Fund, London, UK*

ULRICH HOPFER • *Department of Physiology and Biophysics, Case Western Reserve University, Cleveland, OH*

MASAYOSHI HOSODA • *Department of Geriatric and Respiratory Medicine, Tohoku University School of Medicine, Sendai, Japan*

DAVID L. HUDSON • *Institute of Urology, UCLH Medical School, London, UK*

NOBUHIRO IBARAKI • *Department of Ophthalmology, Chiba Hokusoh Hospital, Nippon Medical School, Chiba, Japan*

NICOLA JONES • *Division of Gastroenterology and Nutrition, Research Institute, Hospital for Sick Children, University of Toronto, Toronto, Ontario, Canada*

PHILIP H. KARP • *Howard Hughes Medical Institute, Department of Internal Medicine, University of Iowa College of Medicine, Iowa City, IA*

YOSHITAKA KONDA • *Department of Gastroenterology and Hepatology, Kyoto University Graduate School of Medicine, Kyoto, Japan*

NORIO KUMAGAI • *Department of Plastic and Reconstructive Surgery, St. Marianna University School of Medicine, Kawasaki, Japan*

JANICE L. LANSPACH • *Howard Hughes Medical Institute, Department of Internal Medicine, University of Iowa College of Medicine, Iowa City, IA*

VINCENT H. L. LEE • *Pharmaceutical Research, School of Pharmacy, University of Southern California, Los Angeles, CA*

SIMON A. LEWIS • *Department of Physiology and Biophysics, University of Texas Medical Branch, Galveston, TX*

TOHRU MASUI • *Division of Genetics and Mutagenesis, National Institute of Health Sciences, Tokyo, Japan*

DEREK M. MCKAY • *Intestinal Disease Research Programme, McMaster University, Hamilton, Ontario, Canada*

THOMAS O. MONINGER • *Central Electron Microscopy Facility, University of Iowa College of Medicine, Iowa City, IA*

TUIJA MUSTONEN • *Institute of Biotechnology, University of Helsinki, Helsinki, Finland*

TAMARA S. NESSELHAUF • *Department of Internal Medicine, University of Iowa College of Medicine, Iowa City, IA*

CELIA O'BRIEN • *Immunology and Disease Resistance Laboratory, US Department of Agriculture, Beltsville, MD*

GÖRAN OCKLIND • *Division of Pharmaceutics, Uppsala University, Uppsala, Sweden*

MARY H. PERDUE • *Intestinal Disease Research Programme, McMaster University, Hamilton, Ontario, Canada*

DIETER REISSIG • *Institute of Anatomy, Medical Faculty, University of Leipzig, Leipzig, Germany*

GODFRIED M. ROOMANS • *Department of Medical Cell Biology, Uppsala University, Uppsala, Sweden*

CARSTEN RÖPKE • *Institute of Medical Anatomy, The Panum Institute, Copenhagen, Denmark*

JOACHIM RYCHLY • *Department of Internal Medicine, University of Rostock, Rostock, Germany*

CARIN SAHLBERG • *Institute of Dentistry, University of Helsinki, Helsinki, Finland*

HIDETAKA SASAKI • *Department of Geriatric and Respiratory Medicine, Tohoku University School of Medicine, Sendai, Japan*

JIE SHEN • *Pharmacokinetics and Drug Metabolism, Allergan, Inc., Irvine, CA*

PHILLIP M. SHERMAN • *Division of Gastroenterology, Hospital for Sick Children, University of Toronto, Toronto, Ontario, Canada*

WEE SOO SHIN • *Health Service Center, University of Tokyo, Tokyo, Japan*

ALPHONSE E. SIRICA • *Department of Pathology, Division of Cellular and Molecular Pathogenesis, Medical College of Virginia Campus, Virginia Commonwealth University, Richmond, VA*

GEORGE STOICA • *Department of Veterinary Pathobiology, Texas A&M University, College Station, TX*

CHARLES H. STREULI • *School of Biological Sciences, University of Manchester, Manchester, UK*

YUKIO SUMI • *Department of Dentistry and Oral & Maxillofacial Surgery, Nagoya Daini Red Cross Hospital, Nagoya City, Japan*

TOMOKO SUZUKI • *Department of Geriatric and Respiratory Medicine, Tohoku University School of Medicine, Sendai, Japan*

JAN TAIPALENSUU • *Division of Pharmaceutics, Uppsala University, Uppsala, Sweden*

STAFFAN TAVELIN • *Division of Pharmaceutics, Uppsala University, Uppsala, Sweden*

IRMA THESLEFF • *Institute of Biotechnology, University of Helsinki, Helsinki, Finland*

TERUHIKO TOYO-OKA • *Department of Organ Pathophysiology and Internal Medicine, Health Service Center, Graduate School of Medicine, University of Tokyo, Tokyo, Japan*

MINORU UEDA • *Department of Oral and Maxillofacial Surgery, Nagoya University Graduate School of Medicine, Nagoya City, Japan*

S. PARY WEBER • *Howard Hughes Medical Institute, Department of Internal Medicine, University of Iowa College of Medicine, Iowa City, IA*

MICHAEL J. WELSH • *Howard Hughes Medical Institute, Department of Internal Medicine, University of Iowa College of Medicine, Iowa City, IA*

NORIHIRO YAMADA • *Department of Geriatric and Respiratory Medicine, Tohoku University School of Medicine, Sendai, Japan*

MUTSUO YAMAYA • *Department of Geriatric and Respiratory Medicine, Tohoku University School of Medicine, Sendai, Japan*

JOSEPH ZABNER • *Department of Internal Medicine, University of Iowa College of Medicine, Iowa City, IA*

SEBASTIAN ZELLMER • *Institute of Biochemistry, Medical Faculty, University of Leipzig, Leipzig, Germany*

QIUQU ZHAO • *Division of Environmental Health Sciences, School of Public Health, Columbia University, New York, NY*

WEI ZHENG • *Division of Environmental Health Sciences, School of Public Health, Columbia University, New York, NY*

1

Human Lens Epithelial Cell Culture

Nobuhiro Ibaraki

1. Introduction

Crystalline lens consists of epithelial cells, fiber cells, and a capsule. They originate from lens epithelial cells. Epithelial cells differentiate into fiber cells and produce collagen, which is the major compound of the capsule. The lens epithelial cells maintain normal physiology and homeostasis of the lens, so the cultures of human lens epithelial (HLE) cells provide important information concerning the role of epithelium in normal and cataract formation.

The difficulty of HLE cell culture is due to limited sources of the cells and a low viability and delicacy of the cells. HLE cells are easily damaged, resulting in the failure of the culture by mechanical injury, contamination, toxicity of reagents, and freezing for storage.

This chapter describes the procedures of HLE cell culture, so that scientists who are unfamiliar with this culture may carry it out successfully. The sources of HLE cells, explant culture, harvest, subculture, storage, and shipment are explained. The critical points for HLE cell culture are also stated in the note section.

2. Materials

1. Dulbecco's modified Eagle medium (DMEM).
2. Fetal bovine serum (FBS), qualified (*see* **Note 2**).
3. Gentamicin reagent solution.
4. Growth medium: DMEM supplemented with FBS is used as a standard medium. As the viability of HLE cells is very low (*see* **Note 3**), neither antibiotic nor antifungal agents should be used for HLE cell culture except cell line cell culture. Gentamicin reagent solution (10 µg/mL) can be used for HLE cell line cell

From: *Methods in Molecular Biology, vol. 188: Epithelial Cell Culture Protocols*
Edited by: C. Wise © Humana Press Inc., Totowa, NJ

culture. The concentration of serum should be at least 5%, and the best growth of HLE cells is observed in medium with 20% FBS *(1)*. Store the medium at 4°C.

5. Cell dissociation solution: 0.05% trypsin, 0.02% EDTA.
6. Dulbecco's phosphate-buffered saline (PBS–), Ca^{2+}-, Mg^{2+}-free.
7. Dimethylsulfoxide (DMSO).
8. 35-, 60-, 100-, and 150-mm Tissue culture grade petri dishes (all tissue culture plastic is from Falcon).
9. 25- and 75-cm^2 Tissue culture grade flasks.
10. 6-, 12-, and 24-well Tissue culture grade plates.
11. Equipment for freezing: Mr. Frosty (Nalgene).
12. 1.2-mL Cryovials.
13. 0.2-μm membrane filter.
14. Incubator (*see* **Note 1**).
15. HLE cells. There are five possible sources of human lens epithelial cells. As most countries do not allow the use of tissue obtained from fetuses, four alternative sources are available.

    a. HLE cells from infants. The infant HLE cells can be obtained from patients with retinopathy of prematurity or congenital cataracts. The small fragments of the anterior capsule of the lens, where the HLE cells attach, can be collected during pars plana lensectomy. However, as these cases are not common, it is very hard to get HLE cells from infants *(2)*.

    b. HLE cells from eye bank eyes. It is easiest to get HLE cells from eye bank eyes, if they are available for research purposes (some countries only allow use of eye bank eyes for keratoplasty). Take out the whole lens by cutting the zinn zonule, wash once in DMEM containing 50 μg/mL gentamicin, and dip into the growth medium. Peal off the posterior portion of the lens and remove the cortex and nucleous of the lens. HLE cells attached to the large anterior capsular flap are ready for explant culture.

    c. HLE cells from senile cataract patients. During senile cataract operations, the center part of the anterior capsule with HLE cells can be obtained. The capsular flap can be used for explant culture (usually HLE cells from elder patients over 60 yr do not proliferate when the cells are dissociated from the capsule) *(3)*.

    d. HLE cell line cells. There are two HLE cell line cells. B3 cells are immortalized by infecting cells with adenovirus 12 containing an immortalizing gene derived from simian virus 40 (SV40) *(4)*. The other cell line, SRA 01/04, is immortalized by transfecting cells with a plasmid vector containing a large T antigen (the immortalizing gene) of SV40 *(5)*. Both cell lines have characteristics of human origin, normal epithelial cell morphology, and normal expression of lens epithelial cell specific proteins, α- and/or β-crystallin. These cell lines have a high proliferative potency, and thus a large number of cells are readily available to undertake a wide range of lens studies. When HLE cell lines are not commercially available, they are provided by each investigator.

3. Methods

3.1. Explant Culture

1. Culture HLE cells. If HLE cells attached to the anterior capsule of the lens are dissociated, the cells will not attach well to the culture vessels, because the cell number is very low, approx 1×10^5 per one large anterior flap, and the cell concentration does not reach a level at which the cells can survive.
2. Put the anterior capsular flap, with HLE cells on, onto a 60-mm culture petri dish and add growth medium to just cover the anterior capsular flap (*see* **Note 7**).
3. Put the petri dish in the incubator. After 1 d, increase the volume of growth media to 1 mL and incubate for a further 2 to 3 d. During this time, it is not necessary to change the medium (*see* **Note 4**).
4. After 2 or 3 d of culture, an outgrowth of HLE cells should be observed around the anterior capsule.
5. To obtain the maximum number of cells from the anterior capsular flap, the following procedure is followed (*see* **Note 5**).
6. Remove the growth medium from the culture.
7. Wash the culture with PBS– once.
8. Add 0.5 mL of trypsin-EDTA solution to the dish (*see* **Note 6**).
9. After a 5-min incubation in the incubator, shake the dish gently to dissociate the cells from the culture vessel.
10. Add growth medium to the dish without removing the trypsin-EDTA solution and put the dish back into the incubator (*see* **Note 7**).
11. Change the growth medium every other day. After 4 d in culture, HLE cells from infants or eye bank eyes of young donors will proliferate and cover the whole surface of the dish (confluence).

3.2. Harvesting

Once the explant culture is confluent, harvest the HLE cells for the next step, which is either subculture or cell storage.

1. Remove the growth medium from the culture.
2. Wash the cells with 1 mL of PBS–
3. Incubate the culture at 37°C with 1 mL of trypsin-EDTA solution for 5 min. Almost all the cells should be dissociated from the culture vessel.
4. To remove all the cells, pipet up and down gently 3 to 5 times.
5. Transfer these cells to a centrifuge tube.
6. Stop the action of the trypsin-EDTA by adding 3 mL of growth medium.
7. Pipet up and down gently 2 to 3 times.
8. Count the cells in a hemocytometer and dilute with growth medium to an appropriate number of cells/mL, as determined by trypan blue exclusion. This cell suspension can be used for subculture or cell storage.

3.3. Subculture (see Note 8)

HLE cells (7000 ± 500 cells/cm^2) should be used for the initial seeding.

1. Centrifuge the cell suspension from the harvest at 1000g for 5 min.
2. Discard the supernatant and resuspend in growth medium.
3. Seed the cells out and incubate (*see* **Note 7**).
4. Change medium every other day.
5. When the culture becomes confluent, repeat the harvest, and subculture.

3.4. Storage (see Note 9)

The appropriate cell number for storage is 1×10^6 cells per mL.

1. Centrifuge the cell suspension from the harvest at 1000g for 5 min.
2. Discard the supernatant and resuspend in 1 mL of FBS containing 5% DMSO.
3. Transfer the suspension to a cryovial and put the vial into the freezing container (Mr. Frosty).
4. Store this at –70°C for 8 h. The temperature of the freezing container decreases 1°C/min automatically, when it is in the freezer.
5. Transfer the vial quickly to liquid nitrogen for storage in the liquid phase (–196°C).
6. To thaw the cells, warm the cryotube rapidly in a waterbath at 37°C to avoid cell damage by ice crystals.

3.5. Shipment

Shipment of frozen vials and monolayer cell cultures is possible. Frozen vials of cell cultures may be shipped in the package with dry ice. They do, however, require special handling. After delivery the vials must be placed in fresh dry ice or liquid nitrogen until they are thawed. If stored in a refrigerator (–4°C) or regular freezer (–20°C), the cells will be damaged.

The procedure for shipment of monolayer culture is as follows.

1. Subculture HLE cells onto a 25-cm^2 culture flask with a plug seal cap.
2. When the culture reaches confluency, remove the medium, and fill the flask completely with fresh growth medium.
3. Tape the screw cap in place and ship by mail at room temperature.
4. After delivery, the flask should be placed in the incubator overnight to permit recovery from trauma and shaking that may have dissociated some of the cells during the shipment.
5. The next day, open the flask and change the medium, or harvest and subculture the cells.

4. Notes

1. A CO$_2$ incubator is used for HLE cell culture. Five percent CO$_2$ and 100% humidity at 37°C are required. As antibiotic and antifungal reagents are not usually added to the medium, the culture is easily contaminated if the incubator is poorly

maintained. To avoid contamination, use the incubator only for HLE cells and clean it once a month by sterilizing the trays, wiping the inside with ethanol, and changing the water.

2. Cell attachment and proliferation are dependent on the serum condition. Batch testing should be performed before the purchase of the serum. If the serum tested is good, 80% of primary or secondary subculture of HLE cells from infants or eye bank eyes of young donors (below 40 yr) should attach to the culture vessels after a 3-h incubation. Also, FBS is a possible source of contamination. Filter the FBS before adding it to the DMEM.

3. HLE cells have a low proliferative potency and are very delicate. Usually antibiotic or antifungal reagents cannot be used for HLE cells, because they damage the cells. Keep the working area clean and use good aseptic technique.

4. For the first few days, especially on the first day of the explant culture, frequent observation of the culture should be avoided. The anterior capsular flap detaches easily from the surface of the culture dish if moved, and if the flap detaches, the cells cannot attach and outgrow on the dish.

5. Once the HLE cells outgrow on the dish in explant culture, the cells have the ability to attach and proliferate. Cell dissociation during explant culture, which is for loosening the contact inhibition of the cells around the capsular flap, is useful to get a large number of HLE cells.

6. Do not expose the cells to trypsin-EDTA solution for too long. This cell dissociation solution also damages the cells.

7. For at least 3 h after seeding HLE cells, do not move the culture vessel. The cells attach to the surface of the vessel during this 3-hour incubation.

8. The proliferative potency of HLE cells depends on their donor age. HLE cells from senile cataract patients, who are mostly aged around 60 yr, can be cultured with the anterior capsular flap (explant culture) and not be subcultured. HLE cells from donors aged between 20 and 50 yr can be subcultured once; under 20 yr, they can be passaged twice. Although HLE cells from infants can be subcultured through several passages, their proliferative potency is limited, and cytomegalic cells and cell degeneration in a long-term culture are observed.

9. During freezing and storage, damage of HLE cells is caused by mechanical injury by ice crystals, dehydration, pH changes, denaturation of proteins and other factors. These lethal effects can be minimized by: (*i*) adding DMSO, which lowers the freezing point; (*ii*) a slow cooling, which lets water move out of the cells before it freezes; (*iii*) storage in the liquid nitrogen ($-196°C$), which inhibits the growth of ice crystals; and (*iv*) rapid warming at the time of recovery, so that the frozen cells can pass rapidly through the temperature zone between $-50°$ and $0°C$, in which most cell damage is believed to occur.

References

1. Reddy, V. N., Lin, L. R., Giblin, F. J., Lou, M., Kador, P., and Kinoshita, J. H. (1992) The efficacy of aldose reductase inhibitors on polyol accumulation in human lens and retinal pigment epithelium in tissue culture. *J. Ocul. Pharmacol.* **8,** 43–52.

2. Reddy, V. N., Lin, L. R., Arita, T., Zigler, J. S., Jr., and Huang, Q. L. (1988) Crystallins and their synthesis in human lens epithelial cells in tissue culture. *Exp. Eye Res.* **47,** 465–478.
3. Ibaraki, N., Ohara, K., and Shimizu, H. (1993) Explant culture of human lens epithelial cells from senile cataract patients. *Jpn. J. Ophthalmol.* **37,** 310–317.
4. Andley, U. P., Rhim, J. S., Chylack, L. T., Jr., and Fleming, T. P. (1994) Propagation and immortalization of human lens epithelial cells in culture. *Invest. Ophthalmol. Vis. Sci.* **35,** 3094–3102.
5. Ibaraki, N., Chen, S. C., Lin, L. R., Okamoto, H., Reddy, V. N., and Pipas, J. M. (1998) Human lens epithelial cell line. *Exp. Eye Res.* **67,** 577–585.

2

Human Airway Epithelial Cell Culture

Mutsuo Yamaya, Masayoshi Hosoda, Tomoko Suzuki, Norihiro Yamada, and Hidetada Sasaki

1. Introduction

Development of methods to culture airway epithelial cells has been needed to carry out research into various lung diseases, such as cancer, cystic fibrosis, and bronchial asthma. However, the culture of airway epithelial cells remained difficult. We have improved the culture conditions of these cells, so that these cells can now be used to better understand the mechanisms underlying cystic fibrosis (1–4), for characterizing viral infections (5–7), and for advancing our knowledge of airway inflammation.

In order to improve the conditions under which cultured human tracheal epithelial cells can retain their ion transport properties and ultrastructure of the original tissue, we have developed the following protocol. Briefly, human tracheal epithelial cells are isolated by digestion with protease overnight (1,2,8,9). The isolated epithelial cells are plated on vitrogen gel-coated porous-bottomed inserts in media containing Ultroser G serum substitute (USG). Cells are grown with an air interface (i.e., no medium added to the mucosal surface). These culture conditions, the vitrogen gel, USG-supplemented medium, and the air interface, lead to the appearance of cilia, an increase in the depth of the cell sheets (50 µm), longer and more frequent apical microvilli, and increased interdigitations of the basolateral membrane (**Fig. 1**). Protein and DNA content are also significantly increased. Secretory granules are present, which stain with antibody to goblet cells, but serous or mucous gland cells are not seen (**Fig. 2**) (1).

Acini of human tracheal submucosal glands are isolated by digestion with various enzymes (5–7,10). The isolated gland acini are incubated in flasks coated with human placental collagen in media containing USG and a variety of growth factors. The attached gland acini make confluent cell sheets after

From: *Methods in Molecular Biology, vol. 188: Epithelial Cell Culture Protocols*
Edited by: C. Wise © Humana Press Inc., Totowa, NJ

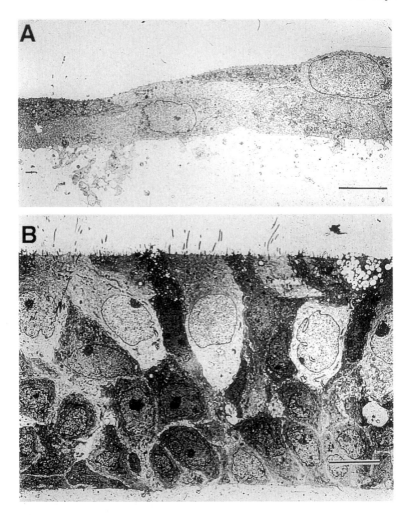

Fig. 1. Low power electron micrographs of cultured human tracheal epithelial cells. (**A**) human placental collagen, FCS-medium, immersed feeding. (**B**) vitrogen gel, USG medium, air interface feeding. Cells are multilayered, and the luminal surface contains cilia and secretory granules. Scale bars = 10 μm.

14–21 d *(5–7,10)*. The cells are then isolated by trypsinization and replated in media containing USG and growth factors on porous-bottomed inserts coated with human placental collagen and grown with an air interface *(5–7)*. Cells cultured under these conditions have high transepithelial electrical resistance and high short-circuit current. The human tracheal epithelial cells and gland cells can secrete chloride ions in response to bradykinin, α- and β-adrenergic and cholinergic agents, and ATP.

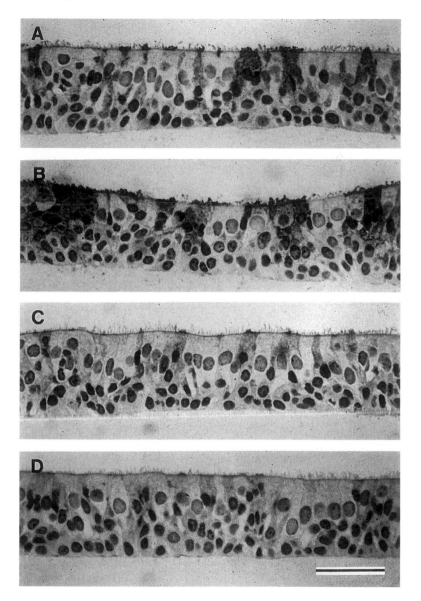

Fig. 2. Expression of goblet cell antigens by cultured human tracheal epithelial cells. Glycomethacrylate secretions were incubated with monoclonal antibodies and stained using an avidin-biotin-peroxidase procedure. (**A**) antibody A3G11 and (**B**) antibody B6E8. Both antibodies recognize tracheobronchial goblet epithelial and mucous gland cell antigens and stain cells throughout the cultured tracheal epithelial cells. (**C**) antibody A8E4. This antibody recognizes a tracheobronchial mucous gland cell antigen. Staining is absent. (**D**) antibody B1D8. This antibody recognizes a tracheo-bronchial serous gland cell antigen. Staining is absent. Scale bar = 50 μm.

Human tracheal epithelial cells and submucosal gland cells can be cultured in glass tubes, coverslips, slide glasses, and culture dishes as well as filter membranes. Cells cultured under these conditions can be used for studies on ion transport, intracellular calcium concentration, epithelial permeability, repair of epithelial cells after injury, and production of various enzymes and proteins, such as cytokines and intercellular adhesion molecules *(1–10)*.

2. Materials

2.1. Coating of Culture Vessels

2.1.1. Vitrogen Gels

1. Minimal essential media (MEM) (GIBCO BRL Life Technologies).
2. 0.1 mol/L Sodium hydroxide (NaOH).
3. Vitrogen solution (Collagen).
4. Millicell-CM or Millicell-HM inserts (Millipore): 0.45 μm pore size, 0.6 cm² area.

2.1.2. Collagen

1. Human placental collagen (Sigma).
2. 0.2% Glacial acetic acid in double-distilled water.
3. 12-well Tissue culture plates (Falcon).
4. Millipore-CM inserts with 0.45 μm pore size, 0.6 cm² area.
5. Transwell inserts (Corning Costar): 0.4 μm pore size.
6. Phosphate-buffered saline (PBS) (GIBCO BRL Life Technologies) supplemented with 10^5 U/L penicillin, 100 mg/L streptomycin, 50 mg/L gentamicin, and 2.5 mg/L amphotericin B (all from Sigma).

2.2. Human Tracheal Epithelial Cell Culture

1. Dissection kit.
2. Dissection tray.
3. PBS.
4. 5 mol/L Dithiothreitol (DTT) (Sigma) in PBS.
5. Protease solution: 0.4 mg/mL protease Sigma type XIV (Sigma), 10^5 U/L penicillin, 100 mg/L streptomycin, 50 mg/L gentamicin, and 2.5 mg/L amphotericin B in PBS.

    Dissolve 20 mg protease in 40 mL PBS, which already contains the penicillin, streptomycin, and gentamicin, in a 50-mL tube. Shake by hand until dissolved. Sterilize by passing through a 0.45-μm filter and then add the amphotericin B.
6. Fetal calf serum (FCS) (GIBCO BRL Life Technologies).
7. F-12-DMEM-FCS Mix I: Dulbecco's modified Eagle's medium (DMEM) (GIBCO BRL Life Technologies) mixed 1:1 with Ham's F-12 medium (GIBCO BRL Life Technologies) and supplemented with 5% FCS.
8. 0.4% Trypan blue (Sigma).

9. Ultroser G serum substitute (USG) medium: 1:1 DMEM:Ham's F12 supplemented with 2% USG (BioSepra), 10^5 U/L penicillin, 100 mg/L streptomycin, 50 mg/L gentamicin, and 2.5 mg/L amphotericin B.

   Dissolve the USG in distilled water to make a stock solution according to the manufacturer's instructions. Mix 10 mL of the USG stock solution with 480 mL DMEM:Ham's F-12, to give a final concentration of 2% USG. The medium should then be supplemented with the antibiotics *(1)*.
10. Vitrogen gel-coated Millicell inserts.
11. Collagen-coated Transwell inserts.
12. Millipore-CM inserts with 0.45 µm pore size, 0.6 cm² area.
13. Hemocytometer.
14. 50-mL Conical centrifuge tubes (Corning Costar).
15. T_{25} Tissue culture flasks (Corning Costar).
16. Glass tubes with round bottoms, 15 mm in diameter, 105 mm long (Iwaki Glass), coated with human placental collagen. To coat the tubes, add 1 mL of collagen working stock solution to the tubes. Keep the tubes stationary at a slant of 5° and incubate for at least 2 h. Remove the collagen solution and air-dry the tubes.
17. Roller culture incubator (HDR-6-T; Hirasawa, Tokyo, Japan).

2.3. Human Tracheal Submucosal Gland Culture

1. PBS.
2. Enzyme Solution: Hanks' buffered salt solution (HBSS) (GIBCO BRL Life Technologies) supplemented with 20 m*M* HEPES buffer, pH 7.4 (Sigma), 500 U/mL collagenase type IV (Sigma), 6 U/mL pancreatic porcine elastase (Sigma), 200 U/mL hyaluronidase (Sigma), 10 U/mL deoxyribonuclease (Sigma).

   Dissolve collagenase, pancreatic porcine elastase, hyaluronidase and deoxyribonuclease in 50 mL HBSS, containing 20 m*M* HEPES , penicillin, streptomycin and gentamicin. Sterilize by passing through a 0.45-µm filter and then add the amphotericin B *(5)*.
3. F-12-DMEM-FCS Mix II: 40% Ham's F12, 40% DMEM, 20% FCS.
4. Growth medium: 1:1 DMEM:Ham's F12 supplemented with 0.1% USG, 10 µg/mL insulin (Becton Dickinson), 5 µg/mL transferrin (Becton Dickinson), 20 ng/mL triiodothyronine (Becton Dickinson), 0.36 µg/mL hydrocortisone (water soluble) (Sigma), 7.5 µg/mL endothelial cell growth supplement (Becton Dickinson), 25 ng/mL epidermal growth factor (Becton Dickinson), 0.1 mol/L retinoic acid (Sigma), 20 ng/mL cholera toxin (Sigma), 10^5 U/L penicillin, 100 mg/L streptomycin, 50 mg/L gentamicin, and 2.5 mg/L amphotericin B.

   Stock solutions of growth factors:
   a. Insulin: 20 mg in 4 mL distilled water.
   b. Transferrin: 10 mg in 4 mL distilled water.
   c. Triiodothyronine: 20 mg in 10 mL distilled water.
   d. Hydrocortisone: 10 mg in 10 mL distilled water.
   e. Endothelial cell growth supplement: 15 mg in 4 mL distilled water.

    f. Epidermal growth factor: 100 µg in 10 mL distilled water.

    g. Retinoic acid: Dissolve in 100% ethanol to give a stock solution of 1 mM. Dilute to 10 µM in distilled water.

    h. Cholera toxin: 0.5 mg in 5 mL distilled water.

To make up growth medium (500 mL): mix 484 mL 1:1 DMEM:Ham's F12 (242 mL of each), 1 mL insulin stock solution, 1 mL distilled water containing 5 µL triiodothyronine stock solution, 1 mL distilled water containing 35 µL hydrocortisone stock solution, 1.25 mL epidermal growth factor stock solution, 5 mL 10 µM retinoic acid. Sterilize by passing the solution through a 0.45-µm filter. Then add 1 mL transferrin stock solution, 1 mL endothelial cell growth supplement stock solution. Add 10^5 U/L penicillin, 100 mg/L streptomycin, 50 mg/L gentamicin, and 2.5 mg/L amphotericin B, and 0.5 mL USG stock solution.

Because retinoic acid is photosensitive, the growth medium and stock solution of retinoic acid should be made up in the dark, as much as possible. Wrap the bottle of growth factor medium in foil and store at 4°C.

 5. 0.25% trypsin-EDTA solution (Sigma).

3. Methods

3.1. Coating of Culture Vessels

3.1.1. Vitrogen Gels

1. Mix 10% 10X MEM with 10% 0.1 M NaOH and 80% vitrogen solution, at 4°C (v/v/v).
2. The solution will be yellow.
3. Add 0.1 M NaOH until the color changes to red.
4. Add 0.15 mL/cm^2 of this solution to the Millicell inserts.
5. Place these at 37°C for 1 h.
6. Use within 2 h of manufacture.

3.1.2. Collagen

1. Make a stock solution of human placental collagen by dissolving 50 mg collagen in 100 mL 0.2% glacial acetic acid, using a magnetic stirrer.
2. Sterilize by passing the solution through a 0.45-µm filter.
3. Dilute the stock solution 1:5 with double-distilled water. This will give a working concentration of 20 µg of collagen per cm^2 of surface area, when added to the culture vessels.
4. Coat 35-mm dishes, wells, or coverslips in 6-well plates with 2 mL of working stock solution, 12-well plates with 1 mL/well, Millicell or Transwell inserts with 0.5 mL or glass tubes with 1 mL.
5. Incubate for at least 2 h, or preferably overnight, at room temperature.
6. Remove the collagen solution and allow to air-dry.
7. Prior to use, rinse dishes, plates or inserts with PBS containing antibiotics, and allow to dry.

3.2. Human Tracheal Epithelial Cell Culture

1. Open tracheas for cell culture longitudinally along the anterior surface.
2. Mount in a stretched position, with the epithelium uppermost, in a dissection tray.
3. Score the surface of the epithelium in longitudinal strips.
4. Clamp the end of one of these mucosal strips and pull off the entire length from the submucosa *(1,11)*.
5. Rinse the tissue strips 4× in 5 m*M* DTT in PBS. The DTT is important to prevent the formation of mucus globs.
6. Rinse the strips twice in PBS alone.
7. Incubate at 4°C overnight in 40 mL of protease solution in a 50 mL conical centrifuge tube.
8. The following day, add FCS to a final concentration of 2.5%, to stop the action of the protease solution.
9. Remove 20 mL of the solution and add the same volume of F-12-DMEM-FCS Mix I.
10. Dislodge the smaller sheets of cells from the epithelial strips by vigorous agitation.
11. Remove the denuded strips.
12. Disperse the remaining sheets of cells by repeated aspiration using a 10-mL pipet.
13. Pellet cells at 200*g* for 10 min.
14. Resuspend the pellet in F-12-DMEM-FCS.
15. Count the cells using a hemocytometer and estimate viability using trypan blue, counting cells with blue-stained nuclei as dead *(1,11)*.

3.2.1. Preparation of Cells for Further Analyses

1. To measure the electrical properties or enzyme production of epithelial cell sheets or transepithelial permeability, plate cells at 10^6 viable cells/cm^2 onto Millicell-CM or Millicell-HA inserts coated with Vitrogen gel (*see* **Subheading 3.1.**) *(1,2)*.
2. One day after plating the cells out, replace medium with USG medium.
3. The cells should be grown with an air interface by removal of fluid on the mucosal side.
4. Culture cells at 37°C in 5% CO_2-95% air incubator, and change the media every day for the first 7 d, and then every 2 d thereafter.
5. The epithelial cells will form a confluent cell sheet about 5 d after plating. At this point, the cells can be used for experiments.
6. To measure the intracellular calcium concentrations $[Ca^{2+}]i$ of the human tracheal epithelial cells, plate cells onto collagen-coated membranes and culture as above (*see* **Subheading 3.2.**) *(2)*.
7. To examine the repair and proliferation of epithelial cells, plate cells onto Millicell-CM inserts at 10^6 viable cells/cm^2, or plate onto 6-well culture dishes or T_{25} flasks at 1 to 2×10^5 viable cells/cm^2, and culture as above *(3)*.
8. To examine the repair of epithelial cells in T_{25} flasks touch the epithelial cells with a pipet tip to introduce defects in focal contacts.
9. Observe cell growth every day.

10. To examine cell proliferation, culture cells in medium supplemented with [³H] thymidine for 24 h and then measure radioactivity.
11. To examine the effects of virus infection on the production of inflammatory cytokines and intercellular adhesion molecules by the human tracheal epithelial cells, plate cells at 5×10^5 viable cells/mL (2×10^5 cells/cm²) in glass tubes with round bottoms coated with human placental collagen *(8,9)*.
12. Seal the glass tubes with rubber plugs, keep stationary at a slant of approximately 5°, and culture at 37°C.
13. When the epithelial cells have formed confluent sheets, infect the cells with rhinovirus, and culture at 33°C in a roller culture incubator.

3.3. Human Tracheal Submucosal Gland Cell Culture

1. Score the tracheal surface epithelium in longitudinal strips and pull away from the submucosa.
2. Dissect the gland-rich submucosal tissue away from the cartilage and the adventitia.
3. Immerse in fresh PBS.
4. Rinse the submucosal tissue 4 times in PBS.
5. Mince with scissors.
6. Centrifuge the tissue fragments at 200*g* for 10 min.
7. Resuspend the fragments in enzyme solution *(5,6,10)*.
8. Place in a flask on an orbital shake (set to 240 rpm) and leave to disaggregate for 12–16 h at room temperature.
9. Decant the fluid, which should contain the disaggregated tissue.
10. Centrifuge at 200*g* for 10 min.
11. Wash once in a mixture of F-12-DMEM-FCS Mix II.
12. Wash twice in PBS.
13. Resuspend the disaggregated tissue in F-12-DMEM-FCS Mix II.
14. Plate acini out onto two T_{25} tissue culture flasks and incubate for 24 h at 37°C in 5% CO_2-95% air. These are both the attached and the unattached acini.
15. The fragments of submucosal tissue remaining in the trypsinizing flask should be exposed again to enzymatic digestion as above.
16. The cells collected from the second digestion are dispersed gland acini.
17 Combine both the unattached acini from the two T_{25} flasks with the dispersed gland acini.
18. Spin the combined acini from these two sources at 200*g* for 10 min.
19. Resuspend in fresh F-12-DMEM-FCS Mix II and plate in the two T_{25} flasks containing the attached acini from the first plating.
20. The following morning, replace the medium with growth medium *(5–7,10)*.
21. It takes 14–21 d to achieve confluency, at which point the cells should be collected by trypsinization.
22. To trypsinize, wash twice with PBS and then add 5 mL trypsin.
23. Incubate for 10–20 min or until all the cells have detached.
24. Pellet the cells at 200*g* for 10 min.
25. Resuspended in F-12-DMEM-FCS Mix II.

26. Count cells using a hemocytometer and estimate the viability with trypan blue.

3.3.1. Preparation of Cells for Further Analyses

1. To measure the electrical properties of the human tracheal submucosal gland cells, plate the cells out in F12-DMEM-FCS Mix II at 10^6 cells/cm^2 on Millicell-CM inserts.
2. Cells will appear confluent after 24 h and should then be grown in growth media.
3. Culture the cells for 7–9 d, at which point they can be used in experiments.
4. Cells should be grown with an air interface; so no media is added to the mucosal surface.
5. To measure the intracellular calcium concentrations [Ca^{2+}]i of the human tracheal submucosal gland cells, plate cells onto either collagen-coated Transwell membranes *(2)* or collagen-coated coverslips *(see* **Subheading 3.1.**) *(7)*.
6. Culture the cells for 7–10 d before measurement of [Ca^{2+}]i.
7. To examine the effects of virus infection on the production of inflammatory cytokines and intercellular adhesion molecules by the human tracheal submucosal gland cells, plate the cells at 5×10^5 viable cells/mL (2×10^5 cells/cm^2) in glass tubes with round bottoms coated with human placental collagen *(10)*.
8. When the submucosal gland cells have formed confluent sheets, infect the cells with rhinovirus, and culture at 33°C in a roller culture incubator.

Acknowledgments

We thank Mr. Grant Crittenden for the English correction.

References

1. Yamaya, M., Finkbeiner, W. E., Chun, S. Y., and Widdicombe, J. H. (1992) Differentiated structure and function of cultures from human tracheal epithelium. *Am. J. Physiol.* **262,** L713–L724.
2. Yamaya, M., Ohrui, T., Finkbeiner, W. E., and Widdicombe, J. H. (1993) Calcium-dependent chloride secretion across cultures of human tracheal surface epithelium and glands. *Am. J. Physiol.* **265,** L170–L177.
3. Yamaya, M., Sekizawa, K., Masuda, T., Morikawa, M., Sawai, T., and Sasaki, H. (1995) Oxidants affect permeability and repair of the cultured human tracheal epithelium. *Am. J. Physiol.* **268,** L284–L293.
4. Yamaya, M., Sekizawa, K., Yamauchi, K., Hoshi, H., Sawai, T., and Sasaki, H. (1995) Epithelial modulation of leukotriene-C4-induced human tracheal smooth muscle contraction. *Am. J. Respir. Crit. Care Med.* **151,** 892–894.
5. Yamaya, M., Finkbeiner, W. E., and Widdicombe, J. H. (1991) Ion transport by cultures of human tracheobronchial submucosal glands. *Am. J. Physiol.* **261,** L485–L490.
6. Yamaya, M., Finkbeiner, W. E., and Widdicombe, J. H. (1991) Altered ion transport by tracheal glands in cystic fibrosis. *Am. J. Physiol.* **261,** L491–L494.
7. Yamaya, M., Sekizawa, K., Kakuta, Y., Ohrui, T., Sawai, T., and Sasaki, H. (1996) P2u-purinoceptor regulation of chloride secretion in cultured human tracheal submucosal glands. *Am. J. Physiol.* **270,** L979–L984.

8. Terajima, M., Yamaya, M., Sekizawa, K., et al. (1997) Rhinovirus infection of primary cultures of human tracheal epithelium: role of ICAM-1 and IL-1β. *Am. J. Physiol.* **273,** L749–L759.
9. Suzuki, T., Yamaya, M., Sekizawa, K., et al. (2000) Effects of dexamethasone on rhinovirus infection in cultured human tracheal epithelial cells. *Am. J. Physiol.* **278,** L560—L571.
10. Yamaya, M., Sekizawa, K., Suzuki, T., et al. (1999) Infection of human respiratory submucosal glands with rhinovirus: effects on cytokine and ICAM-1 production. *Am. J. Physiol.* **277,** L362–L371.
11. Widdicombe, J. H. (1988) Culture of tracheal epithelial cells, p. 291–302, in *Methods in bronchial mucology* (Braga P. C. and Allegra, L., eds.), Raven Press, New York.

3

Rat Gastric Mucosal Epithelial Cell Culture

Yoshitaka Konda and Tsutomu Chiba

1. Introduction

The stomach consists of many types of cells, including smooth muscle cells, mesenchymal cells, vessel forming cells, nerve cells, blood cells, including immune cells and gastric gland cells. Gastric epithelial cells can be further subdivided into at least 11 different cell types, ranging from highly differentiated cells to actively proliferating undifferentiated cells (1). Chief cells are characterized by production and secretion of pepsinogen, parietal cells have a specialized function as acid secreting cells, and neck cells and pit cells (surface mucous cells) are recognized as mucous producing cells. In addition, there are several kinds of endocrine cells producing gastrin, somatostatin, and histamine. These cells are considered to be terminally differentiated. On the other hand, premature forms of these cells such as pre-pit cells and pre-parietal cells also exist in the gastric gland. Interestingly and importantly, all of these different cell types are known to be originated from a single "stem cell".

When researchers try to culture gastric epithelial cells, they are faced with at least two major problems. First, is the problem of the "purity" of the cells. As mentioned above, the stomach or gastric gland consists many different cell types. Therefore, it is difficult to get a highly purified culture, consisting only of a single cell type. Soll et al. (2) first solved this problem. They made isolated cell suspensions from canine fundic mucosa and fractionated the cells by their size, using a counterflow elutriation technique followed by a Percoll density gradient. Using this method, our knowledge of parietal cells, ECL cells, D cells, G cells, and chief cells has been greatly enhanced. Cell purity obtained by this method is sufficient for certain experiments such as acid output and gastrin or somatostatin secretion.

From: *Methods in Molecular Biology, vol. 188: Epithelial Cell Culture Protocols*
Edited by: C. Wise © Humana Press Inc., Totowa, NJ

However, for more precise experiments such as elucidation of intracellular signal transduction mechanisms, contamination of the culture by other cell types is a critical problem. Kinoshita et al. succeeded in culturing primary pit (surface epithelial) cells based on this method *(3)*. Fortunately, in the case of primary culture of gastric pit cells, they are present in high numbers and attach and grow on a culture plate relatively faster than other types of gastric gland cells *(4)*. The methods we describe here finely utilize these characteristics of gastric pit cells.

Secondly, is the problem of "differentiation". Immediately after gastric cells are separated and inoculated onto plastic plates, they start to de-differentiate and rapidly lose or decrease their terminally differentiated characteristics. Although culture conditions, such as cell density in culture medium, additives in the culture medium, and plate coating materials, can modify the tendency towards de-differentiation, careful observation of cultured cells and close comparison with in vivo models are indispensable.

Here, we introduce two methods of primary culture of rat gastric epithelial cells and two cell lines derived from nontransformed rat or mouse gastric glands.

1.1. Primary Culture of Gastric Epithelial Cells from Newborn Rat Stomach

There have been a number of attempts to establish primary cultures of gastric epithelial cells *(5–7)*, but the methods developed by Terano et al. *(8)* have been most widely adopted. Using this method, over 90% of the cultured cells have the characteristics of epithelial cells. Although previous researchers tried to reduce the number of fibroblasts by 20% by administration of pentagastrin *(7)*, this method using newborn rat stomach is more efficient. Even using this method, however, fibroblast overgrowth can be observed after subculturing on d 4. This overgrowth can be prevented by collagenase treatment or using F-12 medium containing D-valine. The mitotic index is maximum on d 2 (2.0%).

After the success of primary culture of gastric epithelial cells from newborn rat stomach, many attempts were made to obtain a large number of cells from a single procedure from adult rat stomach. Gastric epithelial cell culture systems from adult rat *(9)*, rabbit *(10,11)*, and guinea pig *(12)* were reported. Generally, epithelial cultures from adult stomach contain more fibroblasts than those from newborn stomach. To prevent contamination with a large number of fibroblasts, Matsuoka et al. *(10)* inverted the stomach to expose the mucosa to proteinase E to digest only surface epithelial cells efficiently and then scraped off the mucous layer before enzymatic digestion with collagenase *(12)*.

2. Materials

2.1. Primary Culture of Gastric Epithelial Cells from Newborn Rat Stomach

1. 1- to 2-wk-old Sprague-Dawley rats.
2. Hank's balanced salt solution (HBSS) containing 100 U/mL of penicillin and 100 µg/mL of streptomycin.
3. Enzyme solution: HBSS supplemented with 0.1% collagenase and 0.05% hyaluronidase (both from Sigma).
4. Nylon mesh 200 (Nakarai Tesque, Japan).
5. Growth medium: Coon's modified Ham's F-12 medium supplemented with 10% fetal bovine serum (FBS), 15 mol/L HEPES, 100 U/mL fibronectin, 100 U/mL penicillin, 100 µg/mL streptomycin, 100 µg/mL gentamycin.
6. Sodium pentobarbitol: 5 mg/mL stock; use 10 µL/g bodyweight.

2.2. Primary Culture of Gastric Epithelial Cells from Adult Rat Stomach

1. 8-wk-old Wistar rats.
2. Perfusion solution: calcium- and magnesium-free HBSS supplemented with 50 mM EDTA.
3. Digestion solution: HBSS supplemented with 0.75% type IV collagenase, 0.1% hyaluronidase.

3. Methods

3.1. Primary Culture of Gastric Epithelial Cells from Newborn Rat Stomach

1. Sacrifice the rats by anethestizing with an ip injection of diluted sodium pentobarbital (5 mg/mL stock; 10 µL/bodyweight g).
2. Resect the stomachs from the rats (*see* **Note 1**).
3. Place in HBSS containing penicillin and streptomycin in a 10-cm plastic plate at room temperature.
4. Excise the fundic area (this is usually recognized as the area with folds) with fine scissors from the stomach.
5. Cut the fundic tissue into strips.
6. Rinse the strips 3 times with HBSS and then mince into 2- to 3-mm³ pieces (*see* **Note 2**).
7. Place the minced tissue into enzyme solution.
8. Incubate this suspension at 37°C in a shaking water bath for 60 min (*see* **Note 3**)
9. Pipet the tissues up and down several times to complete dispersion of the cells.
10. Incubate for a further 15 min and then pipet again.
11. Filter through nylon mesh.
12. Centrifuge the filtrate, containing cell clumps, at 1000g for 5 min.
13. Wash the pellet in growth medium and centrifuge as before.

14. Resuspend the pellet in growth medium.
15. Maintain the cultures at 37°C with 5% CO_2 in air in a humidified atmosphere. When cells are cultured on a plastic plate coated with type I collagen, they attach and grow better than on a noncoated plate. Generally, culture medium (Dulbecco's modified Eagle medium [DMEM]/F12 with 10% FBS) is changed every other day. Commercial trypsin-EDTA solution can be used when subculturing these cells. However, in comparison with other cultured cells, these cells need more time to detach completely. After 4 to 5 passages, most cells lose their growth activity and die.

3.2. Primary Culture of Gastric Epithelial Cells from Adult Rat Stomach

Even using the methods described in **Subheading 3.1.**, contamination of the epithelial cell cultures with fibroblasts is still a major problem (*see* **Note 4**). Ichinose and his group partially solved this problem *(13,14)* using the following protocol. This method makes it possible *(i)* to obtain epithelial cultures with less fibroblast contamination, and consequently *(ii)* to observe in detail the relationship between gastric epithelial cells and mesenchymal cells.

They also investigated the role of substratum (type I collagen, type IV collagen, fibronectin, and laminin) on epithelial cell attachment and proliferation. They reported that gastric epithelial cells obtained by this method were able to form a monolayer and proliferate on plastic plates coated with those substratum when cultured with Ham's F-12 medium supplemented with only 0.1% of bovine serum together with epidermal growth factor (EGF), cholera toxin, hydrocortisone, and insulin. Unlike intestinal epithelial cells obtained by the same method *(15)*, response to transferrin was not significant in gastric epithelial culture.

1. Anesthetize the rats with pentobarbital.
2. Cut the abdomen with scissors in the middle to upper left upper region.
3. Insert a needle (18 or 16 G) connected to a silicon-coated tube into the right atrium of the heart.
4. Cut 5 mm from the left ventricle.
5. Perfuse the rat using ice-cold perfusion solution, using a perfusion pump (5 mL/min or slower) until the whole liver looks pale.
6. After perfusion, the stomach can easily be separated into epithelium and mesenchyme under a dissecting microscope.
7. Add digestion solution to the stomach epithelium.
8. Shake the epithelium and digestion solution in a flask in a water bath (100 cycle/min) at 37°C for 15 min (this time will vary depending on the experiment).
9. Check small samples of epithelium under light microscopy while shaking, until digestion is seen to be complete.
10. After removing the digestion solution by centrifugation, culture cells on type I collagen-coated plastic plates in DMEM/F-12 with 10% FBS.

3.3. An Epithelial Cell Line Derived from Nontransformed Rat Stomach (see Note 5)

Although the methods were improved, primary cell culture of gastric mucosal cells is time-consuming, and the resulting cells cannot reach 100% purity. In many cases, these cells are not suitable for DNA transfection. Furthermore, because these cells have begun apoptosis as soon as they have lost the physiological 3-dimensional relationship that they have within a tissue, they are basically not suitable for experiments that examine apoptotic events.

Matsui has established a cell line derived from normal rat gastric mucosa, RGM1 *(16)*. The stomach was harvested from an anesthetized 4-wk-old Wistar rat and inverted so that it was inside-out. After washing the mucosa with phosphate-buffered saline (PBS) at 4°C, the inverted pouch was immersed in a 0.2% pronase E solution at 37°C. The solution was then changed every 15 min and centrifuged to collect the exfoliated gastric cells. Thereafter, the cells were washed twice with PBS and cultivated in a 1:1 mixture of DMEM and Ham's F-12 medium supplemented with 20% FBS (RGM1 could be cultured with 10% fetal calf serum [FCS]). When the cells were at the tenth passage, the cell line was named RGM1.

They examined characteristics of RGM1 using cells at passage 30-40. RGM1 cells are homogeneous epithelial-like cells with large oval nuclei and a polygonal shape. They grow as a monolayer with a doubling time of 15.7 h and a saturation density of $1.97 \pm 0.38 \times 10^5$ cells/cm^2. They stop proliferating when they become confluent and do not grow in multiple layers. RGM1 cells do not form colonies and form single cells in soft agarose. Notably, RGM1 DNA was found to have diploid pattern by flow cytometry. These features are the characteristics of untransformed cells. Prostaglandins, ICAM1, insulin-like growth factor (IGF)-II, des-1-IGF-II, IGF binding protein-2, SPARC, and β2-microgloblin are produced in RGM1 cells.

During the past few years, RGM1 has been used as the standard nontransformed epithelial culture model and precise characteristics of RGM1 have been reported. For example, Miyazaki showed that heparin-binding EGF-like growth factor is an autocrine growth factor for rat gastric epithelial cells *(17)*. Hassan found that prostaglandin (PG) E2 plays a role on mucin synthesis through PG EP4 receptor, not EP1 and EP3 *(18)*. Jones investigated the expression of COX-2 in RGM1 and the stimulatory effect of hybridoma growth factor (HGF) on COX-2 expression *(19)*. Pai reported effects of *Helicobacter pylori* vacuolating cytotoxin (VacA) on re-epithelialization of wounded gastric epithelial monolayers *(20)*.

RGM1 is registered at RIKEN cell bank in Japan (RCB0876). The RIKEN home page is (http://www.rtc.riken.go.jp), and the fax number is +81–298–36–9130.

3.4. Epithelial Cell Line Derived from Nontransformed
Mouse Stomach (see Notes 7 and 8)

Although this chapter is on "rat" gastric epithelial cell culture, we would like to describe GSM06 cell line, a nontransformed epithelial cell line derived from mouse stomach. Many investigators have suggested that immortalization of cells by a temperature-sensitive simian virus 40 (stSV40) large T-antigen gene retains more or less stable cell type specific function of the original cells and that the oncogene products are rapidly degraded at nonpermissive temperature but functions at the permissive temperature. Obinata and his group had established transgenic mice harboring a tsSV40 large T-antigen gene, and Tabuchi had established a surface mucous cell line GSM06 from the stomachs of these transgenic mice (21,22).

Gastric fundic mucosal cells from the transgenic mouse were isolated as a modification of a method for rats described by Schepp (23). The isolated gastric fundic mucosal cells were suspended in DMEM/F12 medium supplemented with 2% FBS, 1% ITES, 10 ng/mL EGF, and antibiotics (100 U/mL penicillin, 100 µg/mL streptomycin, 25 µg/mL amphotericin B), and seeded onto a collagen-coated plastic culture dish and incubated at 37°C for 24 h in a humidified incubator in a 5% CO_2 atmosphere. The cells were then cultured under similar conditions except for a temperature change to 33°C. When the cells were used for experiments, they were cultured in DMEM/F12 medium supplemented with 10% FBS, 1% ITES, and 10 ng/mL EGF in a humidified atmosphere. Like RGM1, GSM06 forms a confluent monolayer and shows characteristics of untransformed pit cells (see Note 6). GSM06 cells grown at 33°C (permissive temperature) and 37°C (intermediate temperature) having a doubling time of about 29 h and a saturation density of $2.76 \pm 0.19 \times 10^5$ cells/cm². In contrast, at the nonpermissive temperature (39°C), GSM06 cells did not grow, but when the temperature of the culture was lowered to 33°C, cell growth was restored. Chromosome analysis showed that the chromosome number in GSM06 cells was distributed widely (2n = 35 – 102). In contrast, primary culture cells from the gastric mucosa of normal mice or transgenic mice had 38–43 or 38–42 chromosomes, respectively (for mouse, 2n = 40).

By modifying culture conditions, a wide variety of different types of pit cells can be simulated using GSM06. When cells were cultured in a tightly confluent monolayer or at 39°C, GSM06 shows more differentiated features. On the contrary, when they are at a nonconfluent cell density or at 33°C, the GSM06 are less differentiated (24–26). This change of differentiation is significant and reliable, however, compared to terminally differentiated pit cells in vivo mucous granules in GSM06 cultured in confluence or at 39°C are small in number. Like the primary cultured gastric epithelial cells, GSM06 contain periodic acid Schiff reaction (PAS)-positive granules and are able to synthesize and secrete glycoprotein. In spite of production of such glycoprotein, primary cultured cells usually do not produce a glycoprotein sheet as is seen in the case of the gastric surface mucosa in vivo *(8,10)*. However, GSM06 could produce mucous sheets.

Further information on GSM06 can be obtained at Exploratory Research Laboratories III, Daiichi Pharmaceutical Co. Ltd., 16–13, Kitakasai 1-chome, Edogawa-ku, Tokyo 134, Japan. Fax +81-3-5696-8334.

4. Notes

1. It is important to keep the cells at a low temperature during the whole procedure.
2. Do not allow the cells to dry out. Even while in the procedure of mincing, a small amount of culture medium should be added to the tissue.
3. When cells are treated with enzyme, the treatment period must be as short as possible.
4. Be careful to avoid fibroblast contamination. It takes more than 10 min for the cells mentioned above to attach to a plastic plate. Fibroblasts can attach more quickly, so cells can be preplated, the fibroblasts allowed to adhere, and then the epithelial cells removed and replated.
5. Neither primary cultured gastric pit cells nor the gastric pit cell line are sufficient material for investigating the physiological function of pit cells. Although they are derived from normal or nontransformed animals, once they start growing as cultured cells, many of their physiological functions will become different from normal pit cells in vivo.
6. It is important to note that primary pit cell cultures contain not only other types of epithelial cells, but also nonepithelial cells such as fibroblasts and blood cells, and the type and percentages of such contaminating cells can vary from experiment to experiment. This is especially important for sensitive experiments, such as polymerase chain reaction (PCR).
7. Gastric epithelial cells migrate upward rapidly and finish their life in 3 d *(27)*. On the other hand, RGM1 cells are more resistant to apoptotic stimulation than most of the cultured gastric cancer cell lines.
8. It should be emphasized that in the living stomach, epithelial cells are continuously affected by the signals from mesenchymal cells, extracellular matrix, and influencing luminal milieu. Experiments using cultured cells could exclude this "noise", although no epithelial cells can exist without them under physiological conditions.

References

1. Karam, S. M., Leblond, C. P. (1992) Identifying and counting epithelial cell types in the "corpus" of the mouse stomach. *Anat. Rec.* **232,** 231–246.
2. Soll, A. H., Grossman, M. I. (1978) Cellular mechanisms in acid secretion. *Annu. Rev. Med.* **29,** 495–507.

3. Kinoshita, Y., Hassan, S., Nakata, H. et al. (1995) Establishment of primary epithelial cell culture from elutriated rat gastric mucosal cells. *J. Gastroenterol.* **30,** 135–141.
4. Chew, C. S. (1994) Parietal cell culture: new models and directions. *Annu. Rev. Physiol.* **56,** 445–461.
5. Logsdon, C. D., Bisbee, C. A., Rutten, M. J. et al. (1982) Fetal rabbit gastric epithelial cells cultured on floating collagen gels. *In Vitro* **18,** 233–242.
6. Mardh, S., Norberg, L., Ljungstrom, M. et al. (1984) Preparation of cells from pig gastric mucosa: isolation by isopycnic centrifugation on linear density gradients of Percoll. *Acta Physiol. Scand.* **122,** 607–613.
7. Miller, L. R., Jacobson, E. D., and Johnson, L. R. (1973) Effect of pentagastrin on gastric mucosa cells grown in tissue culture. *Gastroenterology* **64,** 254–267.
8. Terano, A., Ivey, K. J., Stachura, J. et al. (1982) Cell culture of rat gastric fundic mucosa. *Gastroenterology* **83,** 1280–1291.
9. Ota, S., Razandi, M., Sekhon, S. et al. (1988) Salicylate effects on a monolayer culture of gastric mucous cells from adult rats. *Gut* **29,** 1705–1714.
10. Matsuoka, K., Tanaka, M., Mitsui, Y. et al. (1983) Cultured rabbit gastric epithelial cells producing prostaglandin I_2. *Gastroenterology* **84,** 498–505.
11. Watanabe, S., Hirose, M., Wang, X. E. et al. (1994) Hepatocyte growth factor accelerates the wound repair of cultured gastric mucosal cells. *Biochem. Biophys. Res. Commun.* **199,** 1453–1460.
12. Matsuda, K., Sakamoto, C., Konda, Y. et al. (1996) Effects of growth factors and gut hormones on proliferation of primary cultured gastric mucous cells of guinea pig. *J. Gastroenterol.* **31,** 498–504.
13. Matsubara, Y., Ichinose, M., Tatematsu, M. et al. (1996) Stage specific elevated expression of the genes for hepatocyte growth factor, keratinocyte growth factor and their receptors during the morphogenesis and differentiation of rat stomach mucosa. *Biochem. Biophys. Res. Commun.* **222,** 669–677.
14. Matsubara, Y., Ichinose, M., Yahagi, N. et al. (1998) Hepatocyte growth factor activator: a possible regulator of morphogenesis during the fetal development of rat gastrointestinal tract. *Biochem. Biophys. Res. Commun.* **253,** 477–484.
15. Fukamachi, H., Ichinose, M., Tsukada, S. et al. (1995) Hepatocyte growth factor region specifically stimulates gastro-intestinal epithelial growth in primary culture. *Biochem Biosphys Res. Commun.* **205,** 1445–51.
16. Kobayashi, I., Kawano, S., Tsuji, S. et al. (1995) RGM1, a cell line derived from normal gastric mucosa of rat. *In Vitro Cell. Dev. Biol.* **32,** 259–261.
17. Miyazaki, Y., Shinomura, Y., Higashiyama, S. et al. (1996) Heparin-binding EGF-like growth factor is an autocrine growth factor for rat gastric epithelial cells. *Biochem. Biophys. Res. Commun.* **223,** 36–41.
18. Hassan, S., Kinoshita, Y., Min, D. et al. (1996) Presence of prostaglandin EP4 receptor gene expression in a rat gastric mucosal cell line. *Digestion* **57,** 196–200.
19. Jones, M. K., Sasaki, E., Halter, F. et al. (1999) HGF triggers activation of the COX-2 gene in rat gastric epithelial cells: action mediated through the ERK2 signaling pathway. *FASEB J.* **13,** 2186–2194.

20. Pai, R., Sasaki, E., and Tarnawski, A. S. (2000) *Helicobacter pylori* vacuolating cytotoxin (VacA) alters cytoskeleton-associated proteins and interferes with re-epithelialization of wounded gastric epithelial monolayers. *Cell Biol. Int.* **24,** 291–301.
21. Sugiyama, N., Tabuchi, Y. Horiuchi, T. et al. (1993) Establishment of gastric surface mucous cell lines from transgenic mice harboring temperature-sensitive simian virus 40 large T-antigen gene. *Exp. Cell Res.* **209,** 382–387.
22. Tabuchi, Y., Sugiyama, N., Horiuchi, T. et al. (1996) Biological characterization of gastric surface mucous cell line GSM06 from transgenic mice harboring temperature-sensitive simian virus 40 large T-antigen gene. *Digestion* **57,** 141–148.
23. Schepp, W., Kath, D., Tatge, C. et al. (1989) Leukotrienes C4 and D4 potentiate acid production by isolated rat parietal cells. *Gastroenterology* **97,** 1420–1429.
24. Konda, Y., Yokota, H., Kayo, T. et al. (1997) Proprotein-processing endoprotease furin controls the growth and differentiation of gastric surface mucous cells. *J. Clin. Invest.* **99,** 1842–1851.
25. Tabuchi, Y., Sugiyama, N., Horiuchi, T. et al. (1997) Insulin stimulates production of glycoconjugate layers on the cell surface of gastric surface mucous cell line GSM06. *Digestion* **58,** 28–33.
26. Dohi, T., Nakasuji, M. Nakanishi, K. et al. (1996) Biochemical bases in differentiation of a mouse cell line GSM06 to gastric surface cells. *Biochim. Biophys. Acta* 1**289,** 71–78.
27. Karam, S. M., Leoblond, C. P. (1993) Dynamics of epithelial cells in the corpus of the mouse stomach. II. Outward migration of pit cells. *Anat. Rec.* **236,** 280–296.

4

Thymic Epithelial Cell Culture

Carsten Röpke

1. Introduction

Two dimensional monolayer culture of thymic epithelial cells has been used for more than two decades for evaluation of the nature of these cells. Both cells from infant thymi and from thymi from a variety of laboratory animals have been used. The main reason for the broad interest in culture of these epithelial cells is the documented importance of thymic stromal cells, and among them, especially, epithelial cells in the selection of T-lymphocyte precursors and their differentiation to functionally mature T lymphocytes *(1–4)*. However, differentiation of T-lymphocyte precursors, which is dependent on correct spatial organization of subtypes of epithelial and mesenchymal cells, may be better studied in murine fetal organ cultures or reaggregate cultures *(5,6)*, whereas the culture of thymic epithelial cells in 2-dimensional monolayer cultures, as described here, is useful for characterization of the epithelial cells *per se,* their morphology, subtypes, surface characteristics, secretion, antigen presentation, and direct interaction with T-lymphocyte precursors added to the cultures, as well as for establishment of epithelial cell lines.

Numerous methods have been developed for the culture of thymic epithelium in 2-dimensional monolayer cultures. The vast majority of these methods includes the use of fetal calf serum or human serum (for survey *see* **ref.** *7*). Serum addition has several disadvantages *(8,9)* and among these, especially, promotion of fibroblast growth, although this can be hampered *(10–15)*. Methods using serum-free medium are given in this chapter. The serum-free culture system allows for the definition of growth requirements for the cells and for the isolation of molecules released by the cells into the culture medium, as well as interpretation of the significance of biological activities executed by these molecules. Below, a culture method for newborn mouse epithelial cells is given

From: *Methods in Molecular Biology, vol. 188: Epithelial Cell Culture Protocols*
Edited by: C. Wise © Humana Press Inc., Totowa, NJ

as a basic protocol, and thereafter, modified methods for the culture of fetal mouse epithelial cells and of human epithelial cells from children are given.

2. Materials

2.1 Culture of Newborn Mouse Thymic Epithelial Cells in Serum-Free Medium

Primary cultures of thymic epithelial cells can be obtained without fibroblast or macrophage growth in serum-free medium supplemented with cholera toxin (CT), insulin (IN), hydrocortisone (HC), and epidermal growth factor (EGF). To avoid keratinization of cells, low calcium medium is used, containing 0.021 mg/mL Ca^{2+} as compared to the 0.155 mg/mL of the normal Dulbecco's modified Eagle's medium (DMEM)/F12 medium.

After collagenase/DNase treatment, thymic fragments are plated directly in serum-free medium with growth supplements in Vitrogen-coated plastic flasks or chamber slides. Monolayers of epithelial cells spread out from fragments for 2 to 3 wk. Secondary cultures are made by trypsinization of cultures. The phenotype of the cultured cells is predominantly medullary, the percentage of cells labeled with cortical markers is usually below 20, and nonepithelial cells constitute below 5% of the cultured cells. Class I antigen is presented by virtually all cells, while class II antigen expression is variable and usually weak *(7,16)*.

1. 2- to 5-day old mice.
2. Ether.
3. Corkplate.
4. Pins.
5. 70% ethanol.
6. Forceps, scissors, and surgical knives.
7. Glass dishes (7 cm).
8. Plastic dishes (9 cm).
9. Plastic tubes (12 mL).
10. 2- and 10-mL pipets.
11. Finnpipets and plastic tips.
12. Plastic culture flasks (25 mL).
13. Plastic chamber slides (2-chamber slides; NUNC).
14. Phosphate-buffered saline (PBS) without Ca^{2+} and Mg^{2+}.
15. DMEM/Ham's F12 medium 1:1 mixture. DMEM is prepared without calcium. The medium is supplemented with 2 mM glutamine, 250 U/mL penicillin, and 25 µg/mL streptomycin, and is stored at 4°C for up to 1 wk.
16. DNase (Sigma) 15,000 U are added to 10 mL of distilled water, sterilized, and kept at –20°C for months.
17. Collagenase/DNase solution: 15 mg collagenase IV (176 U/mg; Worthington), 10 mg collagenase/dispase (Boehringer Mannheim), 500 µL DNase solution are added to 10 mL medium and sterilized just prior to use.

18. Vitrogen 100 (3 mg/mL; Collagen Biomaterials), kept at 4°C for 1 yr. Dilute 1:30 in PBS before use.
19. Trypsin-EDTA (×1) (Life Technologies). Stored at –20°C for 1 yr.
20. Growth supplements to be added to medium immediately before use (*see* **Notes 1** and **2**)
    a. In (NOVO), 100 U/mL, kept 1:1 diluted in saline at –20°C for months. Stable at 4°C for 1 wk. Fifteen microliters are added to 10 mL of medium, giving a concentration of 0.075 IU or 3 μg/mL medium.
    b. CT (Sigma), one ampoule of 0.5 mg is diluted in 1 mL sterile water, and further diluted 1:50 in sterile water. To be stored at 4°C for 1 wk. Ten microliters are added to 10 mL of medium, giving a final concentration of 10 ng/mL medium.
    c. EGF (Collaborative Research), one ampoule of 100 μg EGF is dissolved in 5 mL sterile water and stored for a prolonged time at –20°C. Stable at 4°C for 1 wk. Ten μL are added to 10 mL of medium, giving a final concentration of 20 ng/mL medium.
    d. HC (Collaborative Research), 50 mg HC are added to 10 mL 96% ethanol and stored for a prolonged time at –20°C. Dilute further 1:10 in 96% ethanol. Stable at 4°C for 1 wk. Ten microliters are added to 10 mL of medium, giving a final concentration of 0.5 μg/mL medium (*see* **Note 3**).
18. 1% Soybean trypsin inhibitor.

2.2. Culture of Fetal Mouse Thymic Epithelial Cells in Serum-Free Medium

Primary cultures of thymic epithelial cells can be obtained from murine thymic lobes from fetuses (13–18 d old). The cells grow readily in the above-defined medium, and usually faster than cells obtained from baby mice. In addition, cell transfer to secondary cultures is performed with greater success with these cells than with cells derived from baby mice. As in cultures derived from baby mice, the majority of cells are of the medullary phenotype.

1. Time mated pregnant mice (vaginal plug = day 0).
2. Stereomicroscope.
3. Small scissors.
4. Needle pointed forceps.
5. 2.5-mL tubes.

Otherwise materials are the same as described in **Subheading 2.1.**

2.3. Culture of Human Thymic Epithelial Cells in Serum Free Medium

Human thymic tissue gives rise to primary thymic epithelial cell cultures after collagenase/DNase treatment and can be transferred to defined serum-free medium in Vitrogen coated culture chambers. Cell islets form by migrating–dividing epithelial cells and can reach confluence within 1 to 3 wk, and Hassall's bodies are formed. Cells are easily passaged 4 to 5 times. The majority of the cells (usually up to 80%) show a medullary phenotype, while the rest is of cortical phenotype *(17)*.

1. Thymic tissue obtained from children, aged 1 mo to 2 yr, undergoing cardiovascular surgery for congenital heart disease.
2. Screw-capped 50-mL tube containing PBS.

Otherwise, essentially as in **Subheading 2.1.**, although DMEM/Ham's F12 medium with normal Ca^{2+} concentration can be used in this method.

3. Methods

3.1. Culture of Newborn Mouse Thymic Epithelial Cells in Serum-Free Medium

1. The day before the initiation of cultures, flood the culture chambers with 1 mL of Vitrogen solution per chamber, or flood 25-mL flasks with 4 mL, and leave at 4°C till just before use (*see* **Note 4**). The chambers/flasks are ready to use after being washed twice with PBS (after addition of PBS, unused chambers/flasks can be kept for a month at 4°C).
2. Kill a litter (usually 6–10) of newborn mice (*see* **Note 5**) by the use of ether.
3. After washing with 70% ethanol, pin the mice to a paper-covered corkplate. Make a longitudinal incision through the skin of the upper part of abdomen and the thorax with scissors, and lift the front of the thoracic cage upwards with forceps, after making cuts with scissors through the rib cage towards the right and left axilla from the xiphoid process.
4. Locate the thymus on the back side of the elevated front part of the thoracic cage, and gently remove the gland from this using forceps (or sterile cottonwool-tipped wooden sticks). Carefully lift the gland from the other mediastinal organs by the use of a forceps, which are located below the thymus. With the aid of another pair of forceps, remove connective tissue and blood vessels between the thymus and the underlying mediastinum.
5. Place the gland in 5 mL DMEM/F12 in a glass dish and free from unwanted tissue.
6. Change the medium.
7. Cut, with the aid of surgical knives, all the collected glands into about 1-mm^3 pieces.
8. Transfer the pieces to a 12-mL tube using a finnpipet. Cut the plastic tip of the latter obliquely to allow entrance of the thymic pieces.
9. Wash the pieces twice with 10 mL medium. Allow 5 min between washes.
10. Aspirate the medium from the tube, and add 10 mL of sterile filtered collagenase/dispase/DNase solution.
11. Pour the content of the tube into a plastic dish, and place in an incubator at 37°C for 90 min. Shake the dish gently by hand every 5–10 min (or place on a mechanical shaker).

12. After this treatment, transfer the pieces with a finnpipet to a 12-mL tube once more, and wash the pieces twice with 10 mL medium. Allow about 5 min between washes (*see* **Note 6**).

13. Add the growth factors: IN, CT, EGF, and HC to the DMEM/F12 medium within the last hour before step 14.

14. Place the thymic pieces in culture using a finnpipet mounted with an obliquely cut tip. Place 5 or 6 pieces in each chamber of the 2-chamber slides, and add 1 mL of the complete medium to each chamber. About 30–40 pieces may be placed in a 25-mL flask and 5 mL of medium added.

15. Place the cultures in a humidified 5% CO_2/95% air incubator at 37°C.

16. Change the medium every second or third day. Pieces that do not adhere to the bottom after 3 d should be removed.

17. Monitor the progress of the cultures by observing them using an inverted microscope. After 2 to 3 d, epithelial cells should be seen expanding from the thymic pieces, forming islets with a few single cells between the islets. The islets expand and may grow to confluence within 2 to 3 wk. Thereafter, expansion usually stops, but cultures are viable for a few weeks more.

18. In the second or third week of culture, cells may be transferred to new Vitrogen-coated culture chambers by trypsinization.

19. Add 1 mL of trypsin-EDTA solution to chambers or 5 mL to flasks from which the medium has been removed.

20. Incubate the cultures at 37°C for 15–20 min. At this time, check that the cells are detached. If they are not, incubate for a few more minutes.

21. To stop the effects of trypsin, add 200 µL of 1% solution of soybean trypsin inhibitor/mL medium to the cultures. Serum-containing medium should not be used instead of trypsin inhibitor (*see* **Note 7**).

22. Pipet the cells into a tube, add medium, and wash the cells.

23. After removal of the medium, add complete medium, and transfer the cells to the culture chambers with a pipet.

24. The best transfer results are obtained by transferring about 10^5 cells to a 1-mL chamber or 10^6 cells to a 25 mL flask. If fewer cells are harvested, Vitrogen-coated Terasaki plates or 96-well microtiter plates are suitable (if cells are to be used in a functional assay in which the medium include serum, 5% serum is used in the washing medium instead of trypsin inhibitor).

3.2. Culture of Fetal Mouse Thymic Epithelial Cells in Serum-Free Medium

1. *See* **Subheading 3.1., step 1**.

2. Kill a pregnant mouse by cervical dislocation under ether anesthesia (*see* **Note 5**).

3. After washing with 70% ethanol, pin the mouse to a paper-covered corkplate. Make a longitudinal incision through the skin of the abdomen, pull the skin to the sides, and divide the muscles of the abdominal wall longitudinally in the midline.

4. Lift the uterine horns with forceps and, using scissors, free them from the underlying tissue.
5. Cut off with scissors below the swellings made by the fetuses and place in a plastic dish containing medium.
6. Cut the uterine horns longitudinally with scissors. Extract the fetuses and their placentas from the uterine cavity with forceps and place in a new plastic dish containing medium.
7. Using forceps, free the fetuses from the placenta, membranes, and umbilical cord, and decapitate the fetuses by gently squeezing the neck with forceps.
8. Transfer the fetuses to a new plastic dish with medium and place under a stereomicroscope. Place a fetus on its back, and keep in position by placing a leg of a pair of forceps in each of the axillas.
9. Open the front of the rib cage longitudinally with forceps, and keep it open with them, while using another pair of forceps to carefully remove the thymic lobes (about 1/2 mm in size), which are found just cranial to the heart.
10. Place the thymic lobes in 1 mL medium in a 3.5-cm plastic dish with a pipet.
11. If the fetuses are 17 to 18 d post coitum, cut the lobes a few times with surgical knives. Lobes from younger fetuses should be left unharmed.
12. Remove the medium and add 1 mL of sterile filtered collagenase/dispase/DNase solution.
13. Place the dish in an incubator at 37°C for 90 min. Shake the dish gently by hand every 5–10 min (or place on a mechanical shaker).
14. After this treatment, transfer the lobes/pieces with a finnpipet to a 2.5-mL tube and wash twice with 2 mL medium. Allow about 5 min between washes (*see* **Note 6**).
15. Add the growth factors: IN, CT, EGF, and HC to the DMEM/F12 medium within the last hour before step 14.
16. Place the thymic pieces in culture using a finnpipet mounted with an obliquely cut tip. Place 5 or 6 pieces in each chamber of the 2-chamber slides, and add 1 mL of the complete medium to each chamber. About 30–40 pieces may be placed in a 25-mL flask and 5 mL of medium added.
17. Place the cultures in a humidified 5% CO_2/95% air incubator at 37°C.
18. Change the medium every second or third day. Pieces which do not adhere to the bottom after 3 d should be removed.
19. Monitor the progress of the cultures by observing them using an inverted microscope. After 2–3 d, epithelial cells should be seen expanding from the thymic pieces, forming islets with a few single cells between the islets. The islets expand and may grow to confluence within 2–3 wk. Thereafter, expansion usually stops, but cultures are viable for a few weeks more.
20. In the second or third week of culture, cells may be transferred to new Vitrogen-coated culture chambers by trypsinization.
21. Add 1 mL of trypsin-EDTA solution to chambers or 5 mL to flasks from which the medium has been removed.
22. Incubate the cultures at 37°C for 15–20 min. At this time, check that the cells are detached. If they are not, incubate for a few more minutes.

23. To stop the effects of trypsin, add 200 μL of 1% solution of soybean trypsin inhibitor/mL medium to the cultures. Serum-containing medium should not be used instead of trypsin inhibitor (*see* **Note 7**).
24. Pipet the cells into a tube, add medium, and wash the cells.
25. After removal of the medium, add complete medium, and transfer the cells to the culture chambers with a pipet.
26. The best transfer results are obtained by transferring about 10^5 cells to a 1-mL chamber, or 10^6 cells to a 25-mL flask. If fewer cells are harvested, Vitrogen-coated Terasaki plates or 96-well microtiter plates are suitable (if cells are to be used in a functional assay in which the medium include serum, 5% serum is used in the washing medium instead of trypsin inhibitor).

3.2. Culture of Human Thymic Epithelial Cells in Serum Free Medium.

1. *See* **Subheading 3.1., step 1**.
2. Collect the tissue in the surgery room as soon as possible after removal and place into a 50-mL tube containing some PBS. Safety and ethical recommendations of the particular country must be heeded (*see* **Notes 5** and **8**).
3. In the sterile hood, transfer the tissue into a glass dish and wash several times by flooding with PBS.
4. Select suitable pieces free of connective tissue and blood and cut them off using surgical knives.
5. Transfer the pieces to another dish, cut them into 1–2-mm fragments, and transfer these into a 12-mL tube using a finnpipet. The plastic tip of the latter is cut obliquely to allow entrance of the thymic pieces.
6. Wash the pieces twice with 10 mL medium.
7. Aspirate the medium from the tube and add 10 mL of sterile filtered collagenase/dispase/DNase solution.
8. Pour the content of the tube into a plastic dish, and place in an incubator at 37°C for 90 min. Shake the dish gently by hand every 5–10 min (or place on a mechanical shaker).
9. After this treatment, transfer the pieces with a finnpipet to a 12-mL tube once more, and wash the pieces twice with 10 mL medium. Allow about 5 min between washes (*see* **Note 6**)
10. Add the growth factors: IN, CT, EGF, and HC to the DMEM/F12 medium within the last hour before step 11.
11. Place the thymic pieces in culture using a finnpipet mounted with an obliquely cut tip. Place 5 or 6 pieces in each chamber of the 2-chamber slides, and add 1 mL of the complete medium to each chamber. About 30–40 pieces may be placed in a 25-mL flask and 5 mL of medium added.
12. Place the cultures in a humidified 5% CO_2/95% air incubator at 37°C.
13. Change the medium every second or third day. Pieces which do not adhere to the bottom after 3 d should be removed.

14. Monitor the progress of the cultures using an inverted microscope. After 2 to 3 d, epithelial cells should be seen expanding from the thymic pieces, forming islets with rather few single cells between the islets. The islets expand and may grow to confluence within 1 to 2 wk. Hereafter, Hassall's corpuscles are formed, and cells are regularly shed while the adherent cells maintain their viability.
15. In the second or third week of culture, cells may be transferred to new Vitrogen-coated culture chambers by trypsinization.
16. Add 1 mL of trypsin-EDTA solution to chambers or 5 mL to flasks from which the medium has been removed.
17. Incubate the cultures at 37°C for 15–20 min. At this time, check that the cells are detached. If they are not, incubate for a few more minutes.
18. To stop the effects of trypsin, add 200 μL of 1% solution of soybean trypsin inhibitor/mL medium to the cultures. Serum-containing medium should not be used instead of trypsin inhibitor (*see* **Note 7**).
19. Pipet the cells into a tube, add medium, and wash the cells.
20. After removal of the medium, add complete medium, and transfer the cells to the culture chambers with a pipet (*see* **Note 9**).
21. The best transfer results are obtained by transferring about 10^5 cells to a 1-mL chamber or 10^6 cells to a 25-mL flask. If fewer cells are harvested, Vitrogen-coated Terasaki plates or 96-well microtiter plates are suitable (if cells are to be used in a functional assay in which the medium include serum, 5% serum is used in the washing medium instead of trypsin inhibitor).

4. Notes

1. It is essential for the cultures that water of the highest obtainable purity is used. If retarded growth is observed, fresh solutions of growth factors should be made. The factors should never be left for more than 1 wk at 4°C.
2. Transferrin (TF) was originally added to the medium (add 20 mg TF [stored for 1 yr at 4°C] to 10 mL distilled water. Stable at 4°C for 1 wk. Add 10 μL to 10 mL medium, giving a final concentration of 2 μg/mL). However, no harmful effects of omission have been detected, e.g., on interleukine secretion, and a better growth of cells is usually seen in TF-free cultures. This applies both to murine and human cultures *(16,17)*.
3. Omission of HC from the medium leads to a drift from proliferating towards more differentiated cells, and to a significantly increased secretion of some cytokines in cultures of human cells *(18)*. Cytokine secretion is generally also increasing by increased passage number *(19)*.
4. All three methods can usually be performed within 4 h. If necessary, the time for Vitrogen coating can be decreased to 2 h with acceptable results.
5. Mice of ages above 5 d may be used as donors, but the growth of the cultures is retarded as compared with younger mice. We have limited experience with human thymic tissue from donors older than 2 yr. However, already in late childhood, the amount of connective tissue and fat in the thymus increase considerably, making cutting and selection of tissue more difficult.

6. The adherence of thymic fragments may at times be affected by high numbers of thymocytes in the cultures. This situation may be prevented by some extra washes before plating. It is not usually a good idea to change medium in murine cultures the first day of the culture to get rid of the thymocytes. However, this can be done with success in human cultures, and the nonadherent fragments put back in the culture chamber.

7. The chance for getting adherent thymic fragments without Vitrogen coating of the plastic is very small, while the type of plastic container used is not critical. Initial addition of serum to the medium may improve the adherence of the fragments, but this is a bad idea. Although fibroblasts are few and dormant in the cultures, even a short exposure to serum will lead to proliferation of these cells for weeks, making precise evaluation of the functions of epithelial cells uncertain.

8. Human thymic fragments may be stored overnight in medium at 37°C or at 4°C before being put to culture, or they may be frozen in liquid nitrogen in medium containing 10% dimethyl sulfoxide (DMSO) and 10% serum. However, seeding efficiency will be inferior to the one obtained using fresh tissue.

9. After trypsinization, cultured human epithelial cells may be kept in liquid nitrogen in 10% DMSO plus 10% serum for a prolonged time and are easily brought to culture by seeding about 10^5 cells/mL. The cells are washed several times in serum-free medium before being recultured. We have no experience with the freezing of murine cells.

References

1. Ritter, M. A., and Boyd, R. L. (1993) Development in the thymus; it takes two to tango. *Immunol. Today* **14,** 462–469.
2. van Ewijk, W., Shores, E. W., and Singer, A. (1994) Crosstalk in the mouse thymus. *Immunol. Today* **15,** 214–217.
3. Res, P., and Spits, H. (1999) Developmental stages in the human thymus. *Sem. Immunol.* **11,** 39–46.
4. Shortman, K., and Wu, L. (1996) Early T lymphocyte progenitors. *Annu. Rev. Immunol.* **14,** 28–47.
5. Anderson, G., Jenkinson, E. J., Moore, N. C., and Owen, J. J. T. (1993) MHC class II-positive epithelium and mesenchyme cells are both required for T-cell development in the thymus. *Nature* **362,** 70–73.
6. Ernst, B. B., Surh, C. D., and Sprent, J. (1996) Bone marrow-derived cells fail to induce positive selection in thymus reaggregation cultures. *J. Exp. Med.* **183,** 1235–1240.
7. Ropke, C. (1997) Thymic epithelial cell culture. *Microsc. Res. Tech.* **38,** 276–286.
8. Barnes, D., and Sato, G. (1980) Methods for growth of cultured cells in serum-free medium. *Anal. Biochem.* **102,** 255–270.
9. Barnes, D. W., and Sato, G. H. (1980) Serum-free culture: a unifying approach. *Cell* **22,** 649–655.
10. Farr, A. G., Eisenhardt, D. J., and Anderson, S. K. (1986) Isolation of thymic epithelium and an improved method for its propagation *in vitro*. *Anat. Rec.* **216,** 85–94.

11. Galy, A. H. M., Hadden, E. M., Touraine, J.-L., and Hadden, J. W. (1989) Effects of cytokines on human thymic epithelial cells in culture: IL-1 induces thymic epithelial cell proliferation and change in morphology. *Cell. Immunol.* **124,** 13–27.

12. Singer, K. H., Harden, E. A., Robertson, A., Lobach, D. F., and Haynes, B. F. (1985) *In vitro* growth and phenotypic characterization of mesodermal-derived and epithelial components of normal and abnormal human thymus. *Hum. Immunol.* **13,** 161–176.

13. Sun, T.-T., Bonitz, P., and Burns, W. H. (1984) Cell culture of mammalian thymic epithelial cells: growth, structural, and antigenic properties. *Cell. Immunol.* **83,** 1–13.

14. Munoz-Blay, T., Benedict, C. V., Picciano, P. T., and Cohen, S. (1987) Substrate requirements for the isolation and purification of thymic epithelial cells. *J. Exp. Pathol.* **3,** 251–258.

15. Nieburgs, A. C., Picciano, P. T., Korn, J. H., MacAlister T., Allred, C., and Cohen, S. (1985) *In vitro* growth and maintainance of two morphologically distinct populations of thymic epithelial cells. *Cell. Immunol.* **90,** 439–450.

16. Röpke, C., Petersen, O. W., and van Deurs, B. (1990) Short-term cultivation of murine thymic epithelial cells in a growth factor defined serum-free medium. *In Vitro Cell. Dev. Biol.* **26,** 671–681.

17. Röpke, C., and Elbroend, J. (1992) Human thymic epithelial cells in serum-free culture: nature and effects on thymocyte cell lines. *Dev. Immunol.* **2,** 111–121.

18. Andersen, A., Pedersen, H., Bendtzen, K., and Röpke, C. (1993) Effects of growth factors on cytokine production in serum-free cultures of human thymic epithelial cells. *Scand. J. Immunol.* **38,** 233–238.

19. Petersen, H., Andersen, A., and Röpke, C. (1994) Human thymic epithelial cells in serum-free culture. Changes in cytokine production in primary and successive culture periods. *Immunol. Lett.* **41,** 43–48.

5

Bile Duct Epithelial Cell Culture

Alphonse E. Sirica

1. Introduction

In 1985, we first described a method for establishing primary cultures of nontransformed well differentiated hyperplastic biliary epithelium isolated in high purity and yield from the liver of bile duct-ligated rats *(1)*. Subsequently, numerous models for culturing biliary epithelial cell populations isolated from the livers of various experimental animal species, as well as the human, have been described. These include models of primary culture of intrahepatic biliary epithelial cells isolated from normal adult *(2–4)* and bile duct-ligated rats *(5–7)*, from normal adult *(8,9)* and bile duct-ligated mice *(10,11)*, from syrian golden hamster *(12)*, from guinea pig *(13)*, from pig *(14)*, from rainbow trout *(15)*, and from normal *(16,17)* and diseased human livers *(18)*. Primary culture models have also been established for extrahepatic bile duct and gallbladder epithelial cells, respectively, isolated from both experimental animals and man *(5,8,12,19,20)*. In addition, simian virus 40 (SV40) immortalized intrahepatic mouse *(21)* and human biliary *(22)* epithelial cell lines have been developed, which together with the establishment of a number of biliary cancer (cholangiocarcinoma) cell lines *(23)*, have each proven to be valuable in vitro systems for use in investigating important aspects of selected biliary functions and pathophysiology.

Not surprisingly, the significant advances made over the past decade and one-half in the isolation and culturing of normal, hyperplastic, and malignant neoplastic biliary epithelium have coincided with the remarkable progress that is now increasingly being made in our understanding of biliary ductal cell biology and physiology, pathobiology, and pathophysiology (for recent reviews of these advances, *see* refs. *24–26*). In this context, I will describe in this chapter three protocols currently in use in our laboratory, two of which were developed to isolate and culture from rat liver nontransformed well differentiated

From: *Methods in Molecular Biology, vol. 188: Epithelial Cell Culture Protocols*
Edited by: C. Wise © Humana Press Inc., Totowa, NJ

hyperplastic biliary epithelium *(27,28)*, and the third developed to establish a novel rat cholangiocarcinoma cell culture model *(29)*.

The first protocol that will be described represents a more recent modification developed by us *(27)* of our initial 1985 method *(1)* used to isolate and culture hyperplastic biliary epithelial cells from 6- to 15-wk bile duct-ligated rat liver. **Subheading 3.2.** details our method for isolating and culturing nontransformed hyperplastic biliary epithelial cells from the livers of 7-wk bile duct-ligated/6-wk furan-treated rats *(28)*. This latter animal model was first described by us in 1994, and represents a unique rat model of intrahepatic biliary hyperplasia, in which liver is almost totally replaced with well differentiated bile ducts/ductules *(30)*. **Subheading 3.3.** details our establishment of a novel rat cholangiocarcinoma cell line derived from a transplantable cholangiocarcinoma originally induced in the liver of a long-term furan-treated rat *(29)*. We are using these respective biliary epithelial cell culture models to identify potentially critical differences in molecular pathways regulating hyperplastic versus malignant neoplastic biliary cell growth and morphogenesis, as well as to test novel therapeutic strategies in vitro aimed at selectively inhibiting cholangiocarcinoma cell growth *(31)*. Additional information relating to the rationale behind the methods being described, as well as a schematic outline of the steps involved in each, is given below under Methods.

2. Materials

All of the reagents used in the protocols described in this chapter are of tissue culture grade or of the highest purity available. All reagents and tissue culture media preparations are made fresh and under aseptic or sterilized conditions.

2.1. Isolation and Culturing of Nontransformed Well-Differentiated Biliary Epithelium from the liver of Bile Duct-Ligated Rats

1. Adult Fischer 344 male rats 6–15 wk after surgery to ligate the bile duct.
2. Temperature-controlled water bath.
3. Peristaltic pump.
4. Dissection kit.
5. Plastic fine tooth comb. The combs we use are plastic "flea" combs that can be purchased at local Pet Supply Stores. Typical examples are shown in **Fig. 1**.
6. Perfusion medium: Swim's S77 Medium, pH 7.4 (Sigma), supplemented with 1 g/L bovine serum albumin (BSA) (Sigma), 26 mM NaHCO$_3$, 8.3 mM α-D (+)-glucose, 0.1 µM insulin (Sigma), 2000 U/L heparin (Sigma), 2 mmol/L L-glutamine, 85 µM L-cysteine, 100,000 U/L penicillin G (Sigma), and 100 mg/L streptomycin sulfate (Sigma).
7. Collagenase (type I) (Sigma).
8. 95% Oxygen/5% carbon dioxide.
9. DNase I (Sigma).

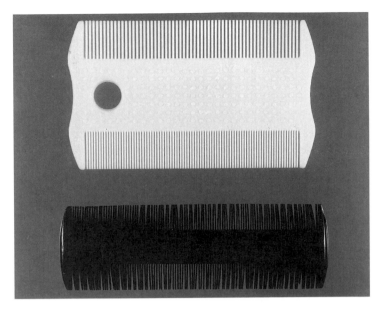

Fig. 1. Examples of fine-tooth combs used to effectively separate intact hyperplastic biliary tissue from hepatic parenchyma following perfusion of bile duct-ligated rat liver *in situ* with collagenase-type 1.

10. Enzyme solution: Leibowitz L-15 tissue culture medium, pH 7.4 (Sigma), supplemented with 1 g/L BSA, 36 mM 4-(2-hydroxyethyl)-1-piperazineethanesulfonic acid, 8.3 mM α-D-glucose, 0.1 µM insulin, 2 mM L-glutamine, 3% fetal bovine serum (FBS) (Sigma), 100,000 U/L penicillin G, and 100 mg/L streptomycin sulfate, 360,000 U/L collagenase (type I), 130,000 U/L DNase I, 700,000 U/L hyaluronidase (type III) (Sigma), and 100 mg/L soybean trypsin inhibitor (type I-S) (Sigma).
11. Nitex Swiss nylon monofilament screens: pore diameter ranging from 253–20 µm (TETKO, Elmford, NY).
12. 32% Isotonic Percoll (Amersham Pharmacia) in L-15 medium, pH 7.4, layered as 6-mL aliquots on top of a 4 mL cushion of 90% isotonic Percoll in 12-mL centrifuge tubes.
13. Density marker beads (Amersham Pharmacia). These are color-coded beads of predetermined densities that are used for calibration of Percoll gradients. They have specific banding patterns to permit rapid and precise determination of densities of cells separated in Percoll gradients. These beads are supplied as a kit from Amersham Pharmacia.
14. Trypan blue.
15. L-15 Medium. For the washes after Percoll gradients, we typically have used unsupplemented L-15 medium at pH 7.4, or L-15 medium supplemented with penicillin and streptomycin as described above.

16. Growth medium: Dulbecco's modified Eagle's medium (DMEM), pH 7.4 (Life Technologies), or L-15 medium supplemented with 5 μm/mL transferrin (Sigma), 0.1 μmol/L insulin, 100 U/mL penicillin, and 100 μg/mL streptomycin, plus 5 or 10% FBS. Typically, we use 10% FBS, and, also to obtain optimum cell proliferation, we include 25 ng epidermal growth factor/mL in the medium *(28)*. For some experiments aimed at elucidating select growth and differentiation properties of cultured rat cholangiocarcinoma cells compared to cultured rat hyperplastic bile ductular cells, we have varied the FBS concentrations to include 0, 1.0, 5.0, and 10.0% with and without the addition of specific growth factors, such as epidermal growth factor.

2.2. Substratum

1. Type I rat tail tendon collagen *(32,33)*. We prepare our own Type 1 collagen from tendons that we dissect from the tails of Fischer 344 male rats, as referenced previously *(32,33)*. Type I collagen can also be commercially obtained from suppliers such as Becton Dickinson/Collaborative Biomedical Products. In the past, we have coated the plastic ourselves, but presently we use Biocoat precoated plastic. Type 1 rat tail collagen is presently used by us to prepare collagen gel substrata *(27,28,32,33)*.
2. BioCoat® multiwell plastic cellware coated with Type I collagen (Becton Dickinson/Collaborative Biomedical Products).
3. Matrigel (Becton Dickinson/Collaborative Biomedical Products). We no longer use Matrigel, although we previously reported the development of cell growths that appeared to be organized in the form of distinct acinar-like structures when rat hyperplastic bile ductular epithelial cells were plated at low density within Matrigel *(27)*. Bile duct morphogenesis in vitro is, in our opinion, best investigated using Type I rat tail collagen gels as the substratum, as demonstrated in *(28)* and in **Figs. 2** and **3**. The use of different substrata is predicated by the specific cell property or function being investigated. For routine cell culture, we use Biocoat plastic wells precoated with Type I collagen. To investigate aspects of in vitro morphogenesis and cell proliferation, we use Type I rat tail tendon collagen gels.

2.3. Isolation and Culturing of Nontransformed Well-Differentiated Biliary Epithelium from the Liver of Bile Duct-Ligated/Furan-Treated Rats

1. Young adult male Fischer 344 rats.
2. Furan in corn oil (Sigma). One week after bile duct ligation, furan in corn oil is administered to the rats by gavage at a concentration of 45 mg/kg body weight, once a day (in the morning), 5 times a week, for 6 weeks. We prepare a stock solution twice a week that is based on the number of rats to be treated. The administered volume is 1.0% body weight. Thus, for rats weighing 200 g, (five 200 g rats to a kg) we prepare a stock of 45 mg furan in a final volume of 1.0 mL and give 0.2 mL per rat.

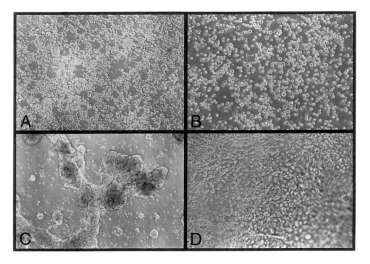

Fig. 2. (**A**) Phase contrast photomicrograph of nontransformed rat intrahepatic hyper-plastic biliary epithelial cells in 4-h primary culture on type 1 rat tail collagen gel (×33). (**B**) Phase contrast photomicrograph of rat cholangiocarcinoma cells in 4-h primary culture on type 1 rat tail collagen gel (×33). (**C**) Phase contrast photomicrograph depicting a 3-dimensional branching duct-like structure formed in 7-d-old primary gel culture of rat intrahepatic hyperplastic biliary epithelial cells (×13). (**D**) Phase contrast photomicrograph of primary rat cholangiocarcinoma epithelial cell culture maintained on type 1 collagen gel substratum. Note the apparent piling up of the cultured cholangiocarcinoma cells (×13).

3. Dissociation medium: Leibovitz L-15 medium, pH 7.4, supplemented with 1 mg/mL BSA, 36 mM 4-(2 hydroxyethyl)-1-piperazineethanesulfonic acid, 8.3 mM α-D-glucose, 0.1 μM insulin, 2 mM L-glutamine, 100 U/mL penicillin, 100 μg/mL streptomycin, 5 μg/mL transferrin, 10^{-8} M dexamethasone (Sigma), 3% FBS, 1,140 U/mL type I collagenase, 0.1 mg/mL DNase I, 1 mg/mL type III hyalu-ronidase, and 0.1 mg/mL type I-S soybean trypsin inhibitor.
4. Growth medium 2: Leibovitz L-15 or DMEM supplemented with 8.3 mM α-D-glucose, 0.1 μM insulin, 5 μg/mL transferrin, 100 U/mL penicillin, 100 μg/mL streptomycin, 10% FBS, and 25 ng/mL epidermal growth factor.
5. Rat tail tendon type I collagen gels. The procedure to make rat tail tendon type I collagen gels is described *(32,33)*. Briefly, to prepare the gelling solution, 0.34 M NaOH is added to 10× concentrated tissue culture medium (i.e., Waymouth MB 752/1 from Life Technologies) at a ratio of approx 1.15 to 2.7. To prepare a collagen gel in a 35-mm diameter plastic tissue culture well, first add 1.0 mL of rat tail tendon type I collagen solution and gently swirl to evenly cover the bot-tom of the well. Quickly add approx 0.3 mL of the gelling solution to the well, swirl to mix with the collagen, and then allow to gel. The final pH of the collagen gel is approx 7.4. Conditions for gelling are somewhat variable for different batches of type I collagen solutions, so obtaining optimum gelling conditions

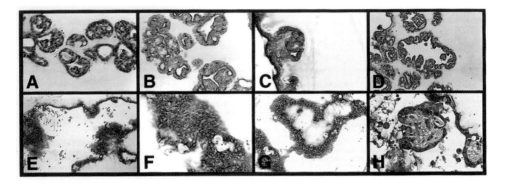

Fig. 3. (**A**) Light photomicrograph showing numerous ductal structures in a 7-d-old primary gel culture of nontransformed rat intrahepatic hyperplastic biliary epithelial cells (hematoxylin and eosin, ×132). (**B** and **C**) Immunohistochemical staining demonstrating strong immunoreactivity for cytokeratin 19 in the cytoplasm of rat hyperplastic biliary epithelium organized into ductal structures in primary gel culture (×132). (**D**) Negative histochemical staining reaction for mucin in ductal structures formed in primary gel culture of rat hyperplastic biliary epithelial cells (mucicarmine, ×132). (**E**) Light photomicrograph demonstrating rat cholangiocarcinoma cells in 4-d-old primary gel culture. Note the piling up of the malignant neoplastic epithelial cells at the medium surface and an adenocarcinomatous glandular or tubular structure formed inside the collagen gel (hematoxylin and eosin, ×33). (**F** and **G**) Primary rat cholangiocarcinoma cells showing strongly positive cytoplasmic immunoreactivity for cytokeratin 19. Note in panel **F**, the cholangiocarcinoma cells exhibit the more common piling up pattern, whereas in panel **G**, they have organized into an adenocarcinomatous glandular-like structure within the gel (×132). (**H**) Positive histochemical staining reaction for mucin (pink-red staining) exhibited by rat cholangiocarcinoma cells in primary gel culture (mucicarmine, ×132). **Fig. 3E**, **F**, and **H** reproduced from **ref.** *29* with permission from *Carcinogenesis* (Oxford University Press).

requires a bit of trial and error. Also, the collagen/NaOH gelling solution can first be mixed on ice, and the mixture can then be pipetted into the tissue culture well. This lower temperature will delay the gelling process, which is then accelerated by placing the gels at 37°C. Prior to cell plating, the collagen gels are covered with either 1.0 mL unsupplemented Leibovitz L-15 or DMEM medium, pH 7.4, and stored for up to 4 h at 37°C in a tissue culture incubator.

3. Methods

3.1 Isolation and Culturing of Nontransformed Well-Differentiated Biliary Epithelium from the Liver Of Bile Duct-Ligated Rats

In normal adult rat liver, the biliary epithelium account for 3–5% of the total nucleated intrahepatic cell population (*34*). However, bile duct ligation in rats

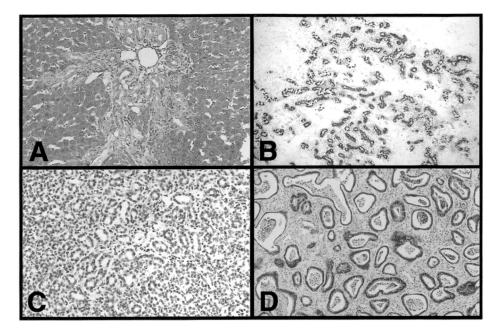

Fig. 4. (A) Light photomicrograph of typical bile ductular hyperplasia in rat liver at 7 wk after bile duct ligation and prior to perfusion of the liver *in situ* with collagenase-type 1 (hematoxylin and eosin, ×66). (B) Light photomicrograph of freshly isolated hyperplastic biliary tissue from rat liver at several weeks after bile duct ligation. In this tissue preparation, the hyperplastic biliary epithelial cells are selectively charac terized by their prominent histochemical red staining for γ-glutamyl transpeptidase activity (×13). (C) Representative histological section from the right liver lobe of a 7-wk bile duct-ligated/6-wk furan-treated rat, in which the entire hepatic parenchyma has become replaced with well differentiated hyperplastic biliary tissue (hematoxylin, ×33). (D) Representative histopathology of a transplantable rat cholangiocarcinoma derived from a furan-induced intrahepatic biliary cancer (hematoxylin, ×33).

has been demonstrated to be an important and useful experimental model for amplifying biliary epithelium in liver through stimulation of a well differentiated bile ductal/ductular hyperplasia, which is largely localized to the area of the portal tracts *(35)*. This type of biliary cell hyperplasia, which has been termed "typical ductular proliferation" *(23,34,35)*, is exemplified by the photomicrograph shown in **Fig. 4A**. It results principally from the multiplication of preexisting portal bile ducts/ductules, thereby leading to an elongation of the intrahepatic biliary tree. Moreover, proliferated bile ductal/ductular epithelial cells obtained from the liver of bile duct-ligated rats have been found to retain, in large part, their phenotypic and functional properties *(5,34)*, to also maintain their commitment to differentiate along the biliary lineage *(1,27,36,37)*, to exhibit a diploid karyotype in cell culture *(1)*, to be nontransformed and to exhibit a finite life span in culture (*see* **Note 1**) *(27)*, and not to undergo neoplastic change following their cell transplantation in vivo *(1,37)*.

Fig. 5 schematically depicts our modified protocol *(27)* used to establish primary cultures of a nontransformed well differentiated biliary epithelial cell population isolated in high yield, viability, and purity from the liver of the bile duct-ligated adult rat (*see* **Note 2**). The specific steps of this protocol are as follows:

1. Perfuse the adult rat liver at 6–15 wk following bile duct ligation *in situ* via the portal vein with perfusion medium.
2. Maintain the temperature of the perfusion medium at 37°C using a temperature-controlled water bath.
3. Regulate the perfusion rate using a peristaltic pump to give a flow rate of 12 mL/min.
4. Bubble 95% oxygen/5% CO_2 mixture constantly into the medium during the entire time of *in situ* perfusion.
5. After 15 min, add 220,000 U/L of collagenase to the medium.
6. Remove the liver carefully and place in a 150-mm diameter glass or plastic culture dish containing ice-cold perfusion medium.
7. Gently comb the liver with a fine-tooth comb, examples of which are shown in **Fig. 1**, to separate intact hyperplastic biliary tissue from enzyme-dissociated hepatic parenchymal and sinusoidal components.
8. To obtain an essentially pure isolate of hyperplastic biliary tissue, shake the combed out tissue fragments for 10 min at 37°C in a flask containing 100 mL perfusion medium to which 30,000 U collagenase and 13,000 U DNase I have been added.
9. This treatment serves to remove residual hepatic parenchymal cells from the biliary tissue fragments. As shown in **Fig. 4B**, the freshly isolated hyperplastic biliary tissue obtained in this manner is composed of biliary ductal structures selectively stained by histochemistry for γ-glutamyl transpeptidase (*see* **Note 3**) and supported only by a loose fibrotic stroma.
10. Mince the isolated biliary tissue fragments in 50 mL enzyme solution.
11. Shake the mixture moderately in a temperature-regulated shaking water bath for 50 min at 37°C.
12. Cool the resulting crude biliary cell suspension on ice to 4°C.
13. Filter through consecutive Nitex Swiss nylon monofilament screens with mesh pore diameters ranging from 253–20 μm, respectively.
14. Centrifuge the cell filtrate at 850*g* for 10 min at 4°C to obtain a crude nonparenchymal cell pellet.
15. Resuspend the pelleted cells in 32% isotonic Percoll and layer on a cushion of 90% isotonic Percoll in 12-mL centrifuge tubes.
16. Centrifuge at 1250*g* for 6 min at 4°C.
17. The viable hyperplastic biliary epithelial cells band at a density of between 1.065 and 1.075 g/cm^3 as determined by the use of commercially available density

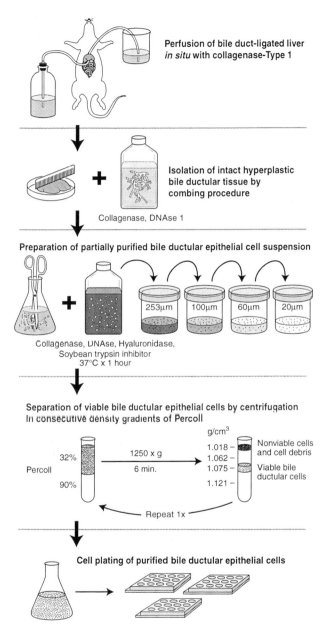

Perfusion of bile duct-ligated liver *in situ* with collagenase-Type 1

Isolation of intact hyperplastic bile ductular tissue by combing procedure

Collagenase, DNAse 1

Preparation of partially purified bile ductular epithelial cell suspension

253µm 100µm 60µm 20µm

Collagenase, DNAse, Hyaluronidase, Soybean trypsin inhibitor 37°C x 1 hour

Separation of viable bile ductular epithelial cells by centrifugation In consecutive density gradients of Percoll

g/cm³

Percoll 32% 90%

1250 x g 6 min.

1.018 — Nonviable cells and cell debris
1.062 —
1.075 — Viable bile ductular cells
1.121 —

Repeat 1x

Cell plating of purified bile ductular epithelial cells

Fig. 5. Schematic diagram of procedure developed to isolate and culture nontransformed well differentiated hyperplastic biliary epithelium from rat liver at 6–15 wk after bile duct ligation. This figure represents a modification of **Fig. 1**, originally published in **ref. 27**, and is reproduced with permission from *Cancer Research*. (American Association for Cancer Research, Inc.).

marker beads. Parallel Percoll gradients are run, one of which contains the cells, and the other which contain the color-coded density marker beads. After centifugation, the density beads band at their designated densities. Cell densities are then determined by matching the band in the cell gradient to the color banding patterns formed in the parallel gradient containing the color-coded density marker beads.

18. Collect the banded cells and wash in L-15 medium. This can either be unsupplemented or supplemented with 100 U/mL penicillin and 100 µg/mL streptomycin.
19. Repeat the Percoll gradient step.
20. Recover the final hyperplastic biliary epithelial cell isolate from the same density region of the Percoll gradient.
21. Wash in L-15 medium.
22. Determine viability of the cells using Trypan blue dye exclusion.
23. Carry out cell counts using a hemocytometer.
24. Plate the isolated biliary epithelial cells out to form a primary monolayer culture at densities ranging between 4 and 6×10^6 cells/cm^2 in plastic tissue culture wells coated with type I rat tail tendon collagen.
25. The isolated biliary epithelial cells could also be readily established as primary gel cultures, in which case the cells are plated onto either type I collagen gels *(27,28)* or onto basement membrane Matrigel *(27)*. Although the cells culture well on Matrigel, we do not use this substratum for our studies. These rat biliary cells can be effectively cultured on a number of different extracellular matrix substitutes.
26. Maintain rat hyperplastic biliary epithelial cells in growth medium. Typically, these cells are cultured on type I collagen-coated wells or on type I collagen gels, with daily medium changes in a standard water-jacketed CO_2 incubator. They are difficult to subculture, but this is possible for a finite number of passages (i.e., 4 to 6) employing gentle enzymatic treatments with either trypsin for cells cultured on collagen-coated plates, type I collagenase for cells cultured on collagen gels, or a mixture of Dispase and type I collagenase for cells cultured on Matrigel.

3.2. Isolation and Culturing of Nontransformed Well-Differentiated Biliary Epithelium from the Liver of Bile Duct-Ligated/Furan-Treated Rats

As already cited, in 1994, we developed a unique rat model of massive intrahepatic biliary hyperplasia, in which liver becomes almost totally replaced with nontransformed well differentiated hyperplastic bile ductules *(30)*. We have taken advantage of this model to develop a simplified cell isolation procedure to obtain and culture viable hyperplastic diploid biliary epithelial cells in high numbers and with a high degree of purity from mainly right lateral lobe and a portion of median lobe resected from livers of 7-wk bile duct-ligated/6-wk furan-treated rats (*see* **Note 4**). A schematic of this procedure is shown in **Fig. 6A**. Because much if not all of the resected liver tissue was composed of hyperplas-

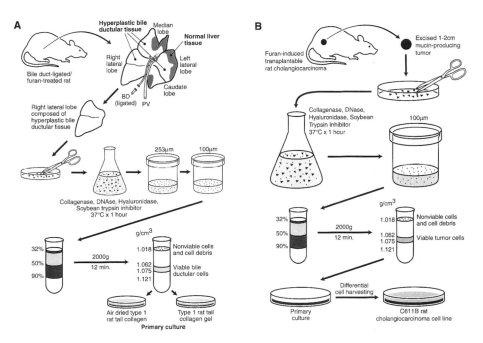

Fig. 6. (**A**) Schematic diagram of procedure developed to isolate and culture a highly enriched nontransformed hyperplastic biliary epithelial cell fraction derived mostly from right liver lobe of 7-wk bile duct-ligated/6-wk furan-treated rats. Modified from **Fig. 1**, originally published in **ref. 28**, and reproduced with permission from *Hepatology* (W.B. Saunders). (**B**) Schematic diagram of procedure for isolating and culturing malignant biliary epithelial cells from a furan-induced transplanted rat cholangiocarcinoma. Reproduced from **ref. 29** with permission from *Carcinogenesis* (Oxford University Press).

tic biliary tissue, this abrogated the need for the enzyme perfusion and combing steps in **Subheading 3.1.**

1. Carry out a bile duct ligation on the rats, by double-ligating the common bile duct and then resecting the intervening segment.
2. One week later, administer furan in corn oil by gavage at 45 mg/kg body weight to these animals.
3. Continue to administer the furan once daily, 5 times/wk, for a period of 6 wk.
4. **Fig. 4C** is a light photomicrograph of a section of right liver lobe of a 7-wk bile duct-ligated/6-wk furan-treated rat, in which the entire normal liver parenchyma has been replaced with proliferated well differentiated bile ductules supported by a fine fibrotic stroma.
5. Resect the right lateral lobe and a portion of median lobe from the livers of the rats.
6. As depicted in **Fig. 6A**, finely mince the resected liver in a dissociation medium.

7. Transfer this mixture to a flask and shake for 1 h at 37°C.
8. Cool on ice to 4°C.
9. Follow **Subheading 3.1., steps 13–26**.
10. It is possible to induce the biliary epithelial cells to form into branching 3-dimensional ductal structures whose morphological and phenotypic features closely resemble those of polarized hyperplastic bile ducts/ductules in vivo *(28,38)* (*see* **Figs. 2A**, **C**, and **3A–D**).
11. To do this, culture the biliary epithelial cells on rat tail tendon type I collagen gels in growth medium 2.

3.3. Establishment of a Novel Rat Biliary Cancer Cell Line from a Furan-Induced Transplantable Cholangiocarcinoma

Recently, we adopted the procedure described in **Subheading 3.2.** to establish a unique rat cholangiocarcinoma cell culture model *(29)*. The procedure for isolating and culturing rat cholangiocarcinoma cells derived from a transplantable cholangiocarcinoma (**Fig. 4D**) originally induced in the liver of a rat subjected to long-term furan treatment is shown schematically in **Fig. 6B**. As depicted, this procedure closely follows the steps outlined in **Subheading 3.2.** for the isolation and culturing of hyperplastic biliary epithelium induced in the liver of 7-wk bile duct-ligated/6-wk furan-treated rats, except that transplantable biliary tumor tissue is used as the source of the malignant cells. Primary cholangiocarcinoma cell cultures are readily established with these isolated cells (**Figs. 2B**, **D**). In contrast to rat hyperplastic biliary epithelium, rat cholangiocarcinoma cells cultured on type I collagen gels in the presence of 25 ng/mL epidermal growth factor and 10% FBS do not typically become organized into 3-dimensional bile duct-like structures. Rather, they exhibit evidence of the loss of contact inhibition, tending to pile up at the medium surface (**Figs. 2D** and **3E**). However, occasional adenocarcinomatous glandular structures can be observed within the gel cultures of these malignant transformed cells (**Figs. 3E**, **G**). Like rat hyperplastic biliary epithelium in gel culture, the cultured rat cholangiocarcinoma cells exhibit strong cytoplasmic immunoreactivity for cytokeratin 19 (**Figs. 3F**, **G**), but unlike hyperplastic biliary epithelium, the cultured cholangiocarcinoma cells, similar to neoplastic glandular epithelium of the parent tumor, give a positive histochemical reaction for mucin *(29)* (**Fig. 3H**).

Utilizing differential cell harvesting, involving selective trypsinzation and serial passaging of cultured rat cholangiocarcinoma cells, we established a novel rat cholangiocarcinoma epithelial cell line designated C611B *(29)*. Under basal medium conditions without the addition of exogenous growth factors like epidermal growth factor, the C611B cell line exhibited a cell doubling time of approx 24 h, was aneuploid with 72% of the analyzed chromosome spreads having chromosome counts ranging from 43–46 (diploid number = 42), exhibited up-regulation of the proto-oncogene-encoded receptor tyrosine kinases c-Met and c-Neu when compared with cultured nontransformed rat hyperplastic biliary epithelial cells *(29)*, aberrantly expressed cyclooxygenase-2 *(31)*, and spontaneously produced hepatocyte growth factor/scatter factor *(31)*, the ligand for c-Met. Moreover, when transplanted in the inguinal fat pad or liver of Fischer 344 syngeneic rats, C611B cholangiocarcinoma cells gave rise to a 100% incidence of mucin-producing cytokeratin19-positive adenocarcinomas, whose histopathological features were essentially identical to those of the parent tumor from which this tumorigenic cell line was derived *(29)*.

4. Notes

1. Under our standard culture conditions *(1,27,28)*, we have maintained rat hyperplastic biliary epithelium in culture for between 100 and 140 d before they became senescent. However, for the majority of our studies related to biliary cell growth regulation, morphogenesis, and functional properties, we utilize primary cultures that are typically between 1 and 14 d old *(27,28,39,40)*. To date, we have not been successful in obtaining in vitro neoplastic transformation of cultured rat hyperplastic biliary epithelium using protocols involving the use of either direct-acting chemical carcinogens, such as N-methyl-N'-nitro-N-nitrosoguanidine or transforming oncogenes, such as activated neu oncogene.

2. At 6–12 wk after bile duct ligation, between 10^7 and $3–5 \times 10^8$ biliary epithelial cells at approximately 95% purity, and with viabilities ranging between 90 and 98% as judged by trypan blue dye exclusion can routinely be obtained from a single liver using the procedure described in **Subheading 3.1.** The freshly isolated hyperplastic biliary epithelial cells were determined to have a mean peak density of 1.07 g/mL in Percoll and to range between 10 and 15 μm in diameter *(5,36)*.

3. Histochemically, γ-glutamyl transpeptidase has been shown to be specifically localized to the intrahepatic biliary epithelium of normal and bile duct-ligated rat liver. Together with cytokeratin 19, histochemically-detectable γ-glutamyl transpeptidase is a very reliable and selective phenotypic marker of isolated normal and hyperplastic rat biliary epithelial cells *(5,23,34)*.

4. In **Subheading 3.2.**, we have obtained a mean biliary cell yield of 19.4×10^7 per 3 to 3.5 wet weight of liver tissue, having a mean cell viability of 87.1 ± 3.9%. More than 90% of the cells in the freshly isolated hyperplastic biliary cell fraction obtained with this protocol exhibited strongly positive staining reactions for both cytokeratin 19 and γ-glutamyl transpeptidase *(28)*.

Acknowledgments

This work was supported by Grant Nos. R01 CA39225 and R01 CA 83650 to A.E.S. from the National Cancer Institute, National Institutes of Health. The author wishes to express his thanks to Ms. Paula Morris for typing the final draft of the manuscript for this chapter.

References

1. Sirica, A. E., Sattler, C. A., and Cihla, H. P. (1985) Characterization of a primary bile ductular cell culture from the livers of rats during extrahepatic cholestasis. *Am. J. Pathol.* **120,** 67–78.
2. Yang, L., Faris, R. A., and Hixson, D. C. (1993) Long-term culture and characteristics of normal rat liver bile duct epithelial cells. *Gastroenterology* **104,** 840–852.
3. Okamoto, H., Ishii, M., Mano, Y., Igarashi, T., Ueno, Y., Kobayashi, K., and Toyota, T. (1995) Confluent monolayers of bile duct epithelial cells with tight junctions. *Hepatology* **22,** 153–159.
4. Vroman, B. and LaRusso, N. F. (1996) Development and characterization of polarized primary cultures of rat intrahepatic bile duct epithelial cells. *Lab. Invest.* **74,** 303–313.
5. Sirica, A. E. (1992) Biology of biliary epithelial cells, p. 63–87. In *Progress in liver diseases* (Boyer J. L. and Ockner, R. K., eds.). W. B. Saunders, Philadelphia.
6. Strazzabosco, M., Mennone, A., and Boyer, J. L. (1991) Intracellular pH regulation in isolated rat bile duct epithelial cells. *J. Clin. Invest.* **87,** 1503–1512.
7. McGill, J. M., Basavappa, S., and Fitz, J. G. (1992) Characterization of high-conductance anion channels in rat bile duct epithelial cells. *Am. J. Physiol.* **262,** G703–G710.
8. Katayanagi, K., Kono, N., and Nakanuma, Y. (1998) Isolation, culture and characterization of biliary epithelial cells from different anatomical levels of the intrahepatic and extrahepatic biliary tree from a mouse. *Liver* **18,** 90–98.
9. Yahagi, K., Ishii, M., Kobayashi, K., et al. (1998) Primary culture of cholangiocytes from normal mouse liver. *In Vitro Cell. Dev. Biol. Anim.* **34,** 512–514.
10. Paradis, K. and Sharp, H. L. (1989) *In vitro* duct-like structure formation after isolation of bile ductular cells from a murine model. *J. Lab. Clin. Med.* **113,** 689–694.
11. Hu, W., Blazar, B. R., Carlos Manivel, J., Paradis, K., and Sharp, H. L. (1996) Phenotypic and functional characterization of intrahepatic bile duct cells from common duct ligated mice. *J. Lab. Clin. Med.* **128,** 536–544.
12. Asakawa, T., Tomioka, T., and Kanematsu, T. (2000) A method for culturing and transplanting biliary epithelial cell from syrian golden hamster. *Virchows Arch.* **436,** 140–146.
13. Sakisaka, S., Gondo, K., Yoshitake, M., Harada, M., Sata, M., Kobayashi, K., and Tanikawa, K. (1996) Functional differences between hepatocytes and biliary epithelial cells in handling polymeric immunoglobulin A2 in humans, rats, and guinea pigs. *Hepatology* **24,** 398–406.
14. Talbot, N. C. and Caperna, T. J. (1998) Selective and organotypic culture of intrahepatic bile duct cells from adult pig liver. *In Vitro Cell. Dev. Biol. Anim.* **34,** 785–798.
15. Blair, J. B., Ostrander, G. K., Miller, M. R., and Hinton, D. E. (1995) Isolation and characterization of biliary epithelial cells from rainbow trout liver. *In Vitro Cell. Dev. Biol. Anim.* **31,** 780–789.
16. Joplin, R., Strain, A. J., and Neuberger, J. M. (1989) Immuno-isolation and culture of biliary epithelial cells from normal human liver. *In Vitro Cell. Dev. Biol. Anim.* **25,** 1189–1192.

17. Matsumoto, K., Fujii, H., Michalopoulos, G. K., Fung, J. J., and Demetris, A. J. (1994) Human biliary epithelial cells secrete and respond to cytokines and hepatocyte growth factors *in vitro*: interleukin-6, hepatocyte growth factor and epidermal growth factor promote DNA synthesis *in vitro. Hepatology* **20,** 376–382.
18. Joplin, R., Strain, A. J., and Neuberger, J. M. (1990) Biliary epithelial cells from the liver of patients with primary biliary cirrhosis: isolation, characterization, and short-term culture. *J. Pathol.* **162,** 255–260.
19. Nakanuma, Y., Katayanagi, K., Kawamura, Y., and Yoshida, K. (1997) Monolayer and three-dimensional cell culture and living tissue culture of gallbladder epithelium. *Micros. Res. Tech.* **39,** 71–84.
20. Kuver, R., Savard, C., Nguyen, T. D., Osborne, W. R., and Lee, S. P. (1997) Isolation and long-term culture of gallbladder epithelial cells from wild-type and CF mice. *In Vitro Cell. Dev. Biol. Anim.* **33,** 104–109.
21. Hreha, G., Jefferson, D. M., Yu, C.-H., Grubman, S. A., Alsabeh, R., Geller, S. A., and Vierling, J. M. (1999) Immortalized intrahepatic mouse biliary epithelial cells: immunologic characterization and immunogenicity. *Hepatology* **30,** 358–371.
22. Grubman, S. A., Perrone, R. D., Lee, D. W., et al. (1994) Regulation of intracellular pH by immortalized human intrahepatic biliary epithelial cell lines. *Am. J. Physiol.* **266,** G1060–G1070.
23. Sirica, A. E., Gainey, T. W., Harrell, M. B., and Caran, N. (1997) Cholangiocarcinogenesis and biliary adaptation responses in hepatic injury. p229–290. In: *Biliary and pancreatic ductal epithelia-pathobiology and pathophysiology.* (Sirica A. E. and Longnecker, D. S., eds.). Marcel Dekker, New York.
24. Sirica A. E. and Longnecker, D. S. eds.) (1997) *Biliary and pancreatic ductal epithelia-pathobiology and pathophysiology,* p. 1–575. Marcel Dekker, Inc., New York, Basel and Hong Kong.
25. Baiocchi, L. LeSage, G., Glaser, S., and Alpini, G. (1999) Regulation of cholangiocyte bile secretion. *J. Hepatol.* **31,** 179–191.
26. Strazzabosco, M., Spirli, C., and Okolicsanyi, L. (2000) Pathophysiology of the intrahepatic biliary epithelium. *J. Gastroenterol. Hepatol.* **15,** 244–253.
27. Mathis, G. A., Walls, S. A., and Sirica, A. E. (1988) Biochemical characteristics of hyperplastic rat bile ductular epithelial cells cultured "on top" and "inside" different extracellular matrix substitutes. *Cancer Res.* **48,** 6145–6152.
28. Sirica, A. E. and Gainey, T. W. (1997) A new rat bile ductular epithelial cell culture model characterized by the appearance of polarized bile ducts *in vitro. Hepatology* **26,**537–549.
29. Lai G.-H. and Sirica, A. E. (1999) Establishment of a novel rat cholangiocarcinoma cell culture model. *Carcinogenesis* **20,** 2335–2339.
30. Sirica, A. E., Cole, S. L., and Williams, T. (1994) A unique rat model of bile ductular hyperplasia in which liver is almost totally replaced with well-differentiated bile ductules. *Am. J. Pathol.* **144,** 1257–1268.
31. Sirica, A. E., Lai, G.-.H., and Zhang, Z. (2001) Biliary cancer growth factor pathways, cyclo-oxygenase-2 and potential therapeutic strategies. *J. Gastroenterol. Hepatol.* **16,** 363–372.

32. Michalopoulos, G. and Pitot, H. C. (1975) Primary culture of parenchymal liver cells on collagen membranes. *Exp. Cell Res.* **94,** 70–78.

33. Sirica, A. E., Richards, W., Tsukada, Y., Sattler, C. A., and Pitot, H. C. (1979) Fetal phenotypic expression by adult hepatocytes on collagen gel/nylon meshes. *Proc. Natl. Acad. Sci. U.S.A.* **76,** 283–287.

34. Sirica, A. E., Mathis, G. A., Sano, N., and Elmore, L. W. (1990) Isolation, culture, and transplantation of intrahepatic biliary epithelial cells and oval cells. *Pathobiology* **58,** 44–64.

35. Sirica, A. E. (1995) Ductular hepatocytes. *Histol. Histopathol.* **10,** 433–456.

36. Sirica, A. E., Elmore, L. W., and Sano, N. (1991) Characterization of rat hyperplastic bile ductular epithelial cells in culture and *in vivo. Dig. Dis. Sci.* **36,** 494–501

37. Sirica, A. E. (1996) Biliary proliferation and adaptation in furan-induced rat liver injury and carcinogenesis. *Toxicol. Pathol.* **24,** 90–99.

38. Sirica, A. E., Radaeva, S., and Lai, G.-H. (1999) Proliferation and Ductal morphogenesis of bile duct epithelial cells, p. 3–20. In *Diseases of the liver and the bile ducts-new aspects and clinical implications* (_pi_ák, J., Boyer, J., et al.). Kluwer Academic Publishers, Dordrecht.

39. Mathis, G. A., Walls, S. A., D'Amico, P., Gengo, T., and Sirica, A. E. (1989) Enzyme profile of rat bile ductular epithelial cells in reference to the resistance phenotype in hepatocarcinogenesis. *Hepatology* **9,** 477–485.

40. Mathis, G. A. and Sirica, A. E. (1990) Effects of medium and substratum conditions on the rates of DNA synthesis in primary cultures of bile ductular epithelial cells. *In Vitro Cell. Dev. Biol.* 26, 113–118.

6

Liver Epithelial Cell Culture

Rolf Gebhardt

1. Introduction

The establishment of liver epithelial cell lines or strains from newborn or adult rat liver has been reported by many investigators *(1–6)*. The cells of these lines are smaller in size and morphologically more simple than hepatocytes, have a considerable growth potential, and are easy to passage. These features are different from normal rat hepatocytes, which usually do not proliferate without addition of growth factors *(7)*, as well as from biliary epithelial cells that quickly proliferate in culture, but cannot simply be subcultured in the absence of factors such as hybridoma growth factor (HGF) *(8,9)*. The behavior is also different from that of isolated oval cells, which are much more reluctant to proliferate in culture *(10)*. Despite this fact, a relationship with oval cells has been claimed *(11)*, but is still not proven. Since other nonparenchymal cells do not show an epithelial morphology, it is rather unlikely that such cells could be the origin of these epithelial cells. Thus, the ultimate precursors of these cell lines are still not known, despite many efforts to characterize them using enzyme patterns and other antigens *(5,6,12–15)*.

One particular reason considerably hampering in tracing back the clonogenic origin of these cells is the fact that they rapidly undergo changes in the number and composition of chromosomes as revealed by karyotyping. This, of course, results in many alterations of their phenotype and potentially explains why so many different cell lines or strains have been established over the decades. Nonetheless, there remains a good chance that these cells are related to rare liver stem cells as has occasionally been hypothesized *(12)*. Indeed, there have been reports claiming the transition of these epithelial cells into hepatocytes as well as bile duct cells *(16–18)*. Whether this is true remains to be carefully

From: *Methods in Molecular Biology, vol. 188: Epithelial Cell Culture Protocols*
Edited by: C. Wise © Humana Press Inc., Totowa, NJ

investigated. Also, the design of culture conditions that favor the karyotypic stability of these cells without affecting their potent clonogenicity seems to be a valuable challenge. On the other hand, the study of these epithelial cells may considerably aid in the understanding of hepatocarcinogenesis *(16,19)*. Moreover, the above mentioned genetic instability, demonstrated usually in culture, may reflect basic mechanisms that might occur also in vivo either sporadically or initiated by carcinogens. Thus, these cells may enable us to study the development and the consequences of genetic instability on liver epithelial cell growth and apoptosis, as they may likewise happen in liver carcinomas. Because of these perspectives and advantages, the following protocols for establishing liver epithelial cell lines may provide more than an isolation technique for as yet undefined but remarkable cell populations.

General protocols have been described for the isolation of liver epithelial cells from newborn *(3,4,15,20)* and from adult rat liver *(12,21)*. Usually, newborn rat liver is superior over adult liver, if high numbers of cells are wanted, but qualitative differences between cells from these tissues cannot be neglected *(6)*. Based on the various modifications of the isolation techniques published, we have developed a protocol that combines high yields with excellent clonogenic properties irrespective of the starting material *(6)*.

2. Materials

1. Hank's solution (enriched with HEPES): 8 g/L sodium chloride, 0.4 g/L potassium chloride, 0.1 g/L magnesium sulfate (7 H_2O), 0.1 g/L magnesium chloride (6 H_2O), 0.06 g/L disodium hydrogen phosphate (2 H_2O), 0.06 g/L potassium dihydrogenphosphate, 0.01 g/L calcium chloride, 0.48 g/L HEPES in double-distilled water, adjusted to pH 7.4. Sterilize the buffer by passing through a 0.22-μm filter and store at 4°C for up to 6 mo.
2. Calcium-free Hank's solution (without HEPES): omit calcium chloride and HEPES from the formulation given above.
3. 0.2% (w/v) Trypsin in Hank's solution.
4. Williams' medium E: the formulation without glutamine can be stored at 4°C for several months. Add 2 mM L-glutamine before use.
5. Isolation medium: 135 mM sodium chloride, 5.4 mM potassium chloride, 1.2 mM magnesium sulfate (7 H_2O), 0.79 mM disodium hydrogenphosphate (2 H_2O), 0.15 mM potassium dihydrogenphosphate, 1 mM calcium chloride, 10 mM HEPES, 0.1% glucose in double-distilled water, adjusted to pH 7.4. Sterilize the buffer by passing through a 0.22-μm filter and store at 4°C for up to 6 mo.
6. Dispase: neutral protease from *Bacillus polymyxa*. Dilute to 100 pronase U/mL in Williams medium E supplemented with 10 mM HEPES, pH 7.4.
7. Accutase: 3 mL/75-cm^2 flask (PAA Laboratories).
8. Culture medium: Williams' medium E supplemented with 10% newborn calf serum, 2 mM L-glutamine, 50 U/mL penicillin, 50 μg/mL streptomycin.

9. Freezing medium: Williams' medium E supplemented with 2 mM L-glutamine, 15% (v/v) fetal calf serum, 10% (v/v) dimethyl sulfoxide (DMSO), 50 U/mL penicillin, 50 µg/mL streptomycin.
10. 70% (v/v) Ethanol.
11. CO_2 incubator.
12. Centrifuge.
13. Shaking water bath.
14. Inverted light microscope.
15. Sterile scalpels.
16. Nylon mesh (250 and 100 µM pore size).
17. Hemocytometer.
18. Cloning ring (inner diameter 5 mm, outer diameter 13 mm, height 8 mm).
19. Silicon grease.
20. Tissue culture plastic: sterile pipets, culture flasks, Petri dishes.

3. Methods

3.1. Isolation from Newborn Rat Liver

1. Remove liver from 10-d-old rats (*see* **Note 1**) and transfer to a 35-mm Petri dish.
2. Add 2 mL of Hank's solution.
3. Mince the liver with scalpels to pieces not larger than 1 mm^3 (*see* **Note 2**).
4. Transfer the contents of the Petri dish to an Erlenmeyer flask containing 8 mL of serum-free Williams medium E and 10 mL of 0.2% trypsin solution.
5. Incubate at 37°C in a shaking water bath.
6. After 10 min, allow the tissue debris to sediment for 1 to 2 min.
7. Aspirate 15 mL of the supernatant by means of a pipet and centrifuge at 200g for 3 min.
8. After the centrifugation, retransfer the trypsin-containing supernatant to the Erlenmeyer flask, which is then incubated for further 10 min (repetition of steps 6–9, *see* **Note 3**).
9. Resuspend the pellet from the centrifugation in 5 mL of culture medium (*see* **Note 4**) and transfer the resulting cell suspension to culture flasks (e.g., 2.5 mL/50-mL culture flask).
10. Gently shake the culture flask to ensure equal distribution of the cells and cultivate in a humidified incubator at 37°C in an atmosphere containing 5% CO_2.
11. After 2 d, change the culture medium (*see* **Note 5**).
12. Check the outgrowth of epithelial cell colonies by phase contrast microscopy each day. Do not allow the cells to form confluent cell layers in the flask (*see* **Note 6**).
13. Select those flasks that contain the highest number of colonies of epithelial cells and aspirate the medium.
14. Add 2 mL of 0.2% trypsin solution and leave the flasks at room temperature for 2 min. Then discard most of the solution, such that only a thin film of trypsin solution remains on the cells.

15. View the cultured cells under the phase contrast microscope. If the epithelial cells start to contract and round up, add 5 mL of culture medium containing 10% newborn calf serum (*see* **Note 7**).
16. Gently shake the flasks to remove all epithelial cells from the substratum (*see* **Note 8**).
17. Seed the cells liberated from one flask into two new culture flasks and ensure homogeneous distribution of the cells by gently shaking the flasks.
18. Incubate the cells in a humidified incubator at 37°C under an atmosphere containing 5% CO_2.
19. Change culture medium every second day (*see* **Note 5**).
20. Before the cells reach confluency, steps 4–6 should be repeated. Thereafter, cloning of the epithelial cells should be performed (*see* **Subheading 3.3.**).

3.2. Isolation from Adult Rat Liver

1. Perform the common 2-step dissociation technique for the preparation of hepatocytes including perfusion of the liver with a calcium-free preperfusion medium and a high-calcium collagenase containing perfusion medium.
2. After perfusion with collagenase for 15–20 min, switch to the perfusion of the liver at 20 mL/min for 4 min with dispase (*see* **Note 9**).
3. Stop the perfusion and transfer the liver to a beaker containing 50 mL of isolation medium.
4. Perforate the liver capsule with a pair of scissors several times without cutting off the different lobes.
5. Hold the liver with forceps at the remainder of the hepatic vein and gently shake the tissue in the isolation medium to liberate the hepatocytes (*see* **Note 10**).
6. Filter the resulting cell suspension through double layers of gauze to remove undissociated tissue and large aggregates of cells.
7. Repeat filtration first through nylon mesh of 250 μm pore size and then through nylon mesh of 100 μm pore size.
8. After filtration of the cell suspension and centrifuging at 50g for 5 min, the pellet containing primarily hepatocytes should be discarded (*see* **Note 11**).
9. The supernatant should be recentrifuged at 100g for 5 min, and the supernatant discarded.
10. Resuspend the cells in the pellet in isolation medium and steps 9–10 should be repeated 3 times.
11. Finally resuspend the cells in the pellet in culture medium and count.
12. Plate the cells in 50-mL culture flasks at a seeding density of approx 0.6×10^6 cells per flask (*see* **Note 12**).
13. Change the culture medium every second day (*see* **Note 5**).
14. Check the outgrowth of epithelial cell colonies by phase contrast microscopy each day. Do not allow the cells to form confluent cell layers in the flask (*see* **Note 13**).
15. Select those flasks that contain the highest number of colonies of epithelial cells and aspirate the medium.

16. Add 2 mL of Hank's solution containing 0.2% trypsin and leave the flasks at room temperature for 2 min. Then discard most of the solution, such that only a thin film of trypsin solution remains on the cells.
17. View the cultured cells under the phase contrast microscope (*see* **Note 14**). When the epithelial cells start to contract and round up, add 5 mL of culture medium containing 10% newborn calf serum (*see* **Note 15**).
18. Gently shake the flasks to remove all epithelial cells from the substratum (*see* **Note 8**).
19. Seed the cells liberated from one flask into two new culture flasks and ensure homogeneous distribution of the cells by gently shaking the flasks.
20. Incubate the cells in a humidified CO_2 incubator at 37°C. Change culture medium every second day (*see* **Note 5**).
21. Before the cells reach confluency, steps 16–18 should be repeated. Thereafter, cloning of the epithelial cells should be performed.

3.3. Cloning of Liver Epithelial Cells

1. To clone the cells with the ring technique (*see* **Note 16**), cells are first detached from the substratum by trypsin treatment, as before.
2. Dilute the resulting cell suspension with culture medium to concentrations of 5, 10, and 20 cells/mL.
3. Seed 90-mm Petri dishes with cell densities of 0.5, 1, and 2 cells/cm² (*see* **Note 17**).
4. Incubate in a CO_2 incubator at 37°C for several days until small colonies have formed.
5. Using sterile forceps, take one cloning ring and dip its base on sterile silicon grease. Then press the ring on a sterile Petri dish to ensure that the whole base of the ring is covered with a thin film of silicon grease.
6. Examine the Petri dishes for suitable cell colonies. These should be sufficiently isolated from neighboring colonies (>1 cm) and should have a diameter of 1–3 mm.
7. Mark appropriate colonies that you wish to isolate with a felt tip marker on the underside of the dish. Up to 3 colonies per dish can be marked and picked.
8. Remove medium from the dish.
9. Place ring around the desired cell colony (*see* **Note 18**). Make sure that ring tightens safely.
10. Add 0.2% trypsin in culture medium (0.4 mL), leave for 30 s, and remove.
11. Cover the dish and place in incubator for 5 to 10 min. Carefully check when cells lift off.
12. Add 0.5 mL of culture medium to each ring.
13. To pick the clones, pipet medium up and down to disperse the cells. Transfer to a 25-cm² flask (*see* **Note 19**). Make sure to use a separate pipet for each clone.
14. Rinse the ring once with 0.5 mL culture medium and transfer to the same flask.
15. Add another 1 mL of culture medium to each flask and incubate in CO_2 incubator at 37°C.
16. When cells have grown to near confluency, they should be detached with trypsin and subcultured (*see* **Note 20**).

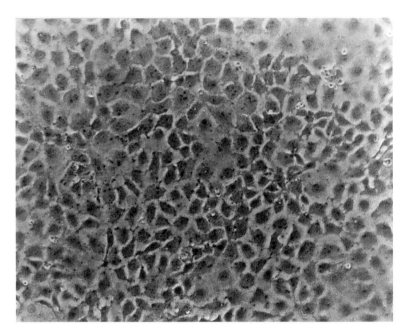

Fig. 1. Appearance of rat liver epithelial cells (line RL-ET-14, *[6]*) at the time when confluency was reached. Phase contrast micrograph (magnification, 40×).

3.4. Cultivation

1. Pure epithelial cells are maintained in culture medium with changes of the culture medium every third day (*see* **Note 5**) until they reach confluency (**Fig. 1**).
2. Nearly confluent or confluent cultures have to be passaged (*see* **Note 21**).
3. Remove culture medium and add 2 mL (per 50-mL culture flask) calcium-free Hank's solution (*see* **Note 22**).
4. After 3 min, replace the calcium-free Hank's solution with 2 mL 0.2% trypsin solution (*see* **Note 23**).
5. View the cultured cells under the phase contrast microscope. If the cells start to contract, round up and disunite the cell layer, add culture medium containing 10% newborn calf serum.
6. Gently shake the flasks to remove all cells from the substratum (*see* **Note 8**).
7. Transfer the cell suspension to a centrifuge tube and centrifuge at 150g for 5 min.
8. Discard the supernatant and gently resuspend the cells in normal culture medium at a concentration of $1–3 \times 10^5$ cells/mL.
9. Seed the cells into new culture flasks at a density of $13–40 \times 10^3$ cells/cm^2 (10 mL/75-cm^2 flask) (*see* **Note 24**) and ensure homogeneous distribution of the cells by gently shaking the flask.
10. Allow incubation without disturbance in a humidified CO_2 incubator at 37°C.

3.5. Storage of Liver Epithelial Cells

3.5.1. Freezing and Storage

1. Use cultures that are nonconfluent and in exponential growth phase (*see* **Note 25**).
2. Detach cells with 0.2% trypsin.
3. Add culture medium and centrifuge at 100*g* for 5 min.
4. Resuspend the cells in freezing medium at a concentration of 10^6 cells/mL (*see* **Note 26**).
5. Place cell suspension (1 mL) into small freezing vials or ampules and seal tightly.
6. Allow to stand at room temperature for 20 min.
7. Place vials into a polystyrene foam box containing cotton wool for insulation, transfer to the freezer (–80°C) and allow to cool down slowly (at approx –1°C/min) (*see* **Note 27**).
8. After 12 h, transfer vials to liquid nitrogen (*see* **Note 28**).

3.5.2. Thawing

1. Retrieve vial from the liquid nitrogen.
2. Rapidly place into a bucket with at least 1 L of water at 37°C (*see* **Note 29**).
3. Try to thaw the cells as quickly as possible by gently rotating the vial.
4. When thawed, swab the vial with 70% EtOH and open in a sterile hood.
5. Transfer the contents to a 25-cm^2 culture flask (*see* **Note 30**).
6. Add 1 mL of culture medium and incubate in a CO_2 incubator at 37°C.
7. Subculture when the cells are in exponential growth phase.

4. Notes

1. Rats (adults or pubs) should be maintained and treated according to ethical standards and the specific national regulations for animal care. For removal of the liver, animals should be anesthesized with diethylether or should be killed directly by cervical dislocation, whatever is appropriate and meets the required ethical rules. It is of utmost importance that the animals are cleaned with a disinfectant and that sterile equipment is used for removal of the liver.
2. Alternatively, slices of liver tissue (50–100 μm) can be prepared with the aid of a tissue chopper.
3. Each round of incubation will lead to 2 culture flasks. It is advisable to go through 8–10 rounds and to mark the flasks carefully, since the fraction of epithelial cells liberated from liver tissue varies from round to round. Usually, the highest proportion is found in the flasks from rounds 2 to 4, but sometimes many epithelial cells may also be found in cultures established from subsequent rounds. The optimal flasks are selected after visual examination.
4. The culture medium can be supplemented with antibiotics. For this purpose, a combination of penicillin (50 U/mL) and streptomycin (50 μg/mL) is added. This is recommended in laboratories with less experience in aseptic cell culture techniques, at least for the initial steps, until stable cell lines have been established.

However, it should be taken into account that the addition of antibiotics does not substitute for careful aseptic manipulation of the cells and, thus, can often be omitted without enhanced risk of loosing the lines.

5. Regularly changing the culture medium every second or third day is sufficient for freshly established and cloned epithelial cells, respectively. However, if the color of the culture medium changes to orange or yellow, the medium should be changed immediately.

6. Since these initial cultures have a very heterogeneous cellular composition, a confluent stage may lead to the lift-off of the cells of interest or to other drawbacks, particularly the impeded liberation of the cells from the monolayer. Therefore, it is recommended to redisperse the cells already in a subconfluent state.

7. The behavior of the epithelial cell should be carefully observed. It may be that other cell types detach earlier or later than the epithelial cells. These features may be used to further enhance the fraction of the epithelial cells, if appropriate times for detachment are selected.

8. Sometimes the epithelial cells do not readily detach by simply shaking the flask. In such cases, it may be useful to rinse them away by a steady stream of medium using a pipet.

9. Dispase (neutral protease) is preferred over pronase.

10. Alternatively, cells can be liberated by combing as described *(21)*.

11. Although the hepatocytes usually have a high viability, it is not recommended to use them for cultivation, because their properties differ from those isolated by collagenase only.

12. Seeding density may vary because of the presence of different amounts of hepatocytes and other cell types. Preferentially, they should cover between one-third and half of the culture area.

13. In confluent cultures, the epithelial cells may be hard to detach, because of the stabilizing influence of adjacent hepatocytes.

14. Eventually, the flasks should be incubated at 37°C in between, since epithelial cells from adult rat liver do not as readily detach as cells from newborn liver.

15. Usually, hepatocytes are detached and destroyed sooner than epithelial cells. If there are many remaining hepatocytes, wash first with serum-free Williams' medium E to remove the hepatocytes and then continue incubation after the re-addition of trypsin.

16. Alternatively, dilution cloning techniques can be applied as described in **ref. 22**.

17. Use at least 3 different cell densities (one above and one below the optimal density of 1 cell/cm^2) to ensure that the optimal sparse cultures can be obtained. Note that sparse cultures grow less efficiently and more slowly.

18. Make sure that the colony is right in the center of the ring. If a colony is already too large, the ring may exceptionally be placed over some of the cells. However, take into account that large colonies often derive from more than one cell and thus are not monoclonal.

19. Sometimes it is preferable to culture the cells in 24-well plates and to enhance growth by diluting them less. Make sure that cells are transferred before reaching confluency.

20. Usually, at least two rounds of this cloning procedure are required before the monoclonal origin of the cells can be assumed with high probability.
21. Confluency usually leads to phenotypic alteration of the cells characterized by enhanced production of extracellular matrix, decreased ability to grow, and possibly further features of senescence. Therefore, it is highly recommended to passage the cells before confluency is reached and to split the cultures each time at a similar state of development.
22. The use of calcium-free Hank's solution is not necessarily required, as preincubation with normal Hank's solution is sufficient for many cell lines. For other cells, addition of EDTA (0.37 g/L) may be necessary to shorten the incubation with trypsin. Thus, the conditions for this preincubation step have to be optimized for each individual cell line.
23. For established clones, trypsin could be successfully replaced by Accutase for detaching the cells. In fact, Accutase may produce less cell damage than trypsin (unpublished observation).
24. If the cells have a stable phenotype, splitting could be performed without prior counting of the cells. In that case, the cells from one flask are seeded into 3–8 flasks.
25. Only cells in exponential growth phase have a high survival and proliferation state after freezing.
26. DMSO is a powerful solvent and has hazardous potential. Handle with special care.
27. Controlled cooling rates can be obtained by use of a programmable cooler (expensive).
28. Storage for several years is possible, but large variations in storage temperature may result in considerable loss of viability over the years. Therefore, check viability and proliferation status at least every 2 yr, in order not to lose your clones.
29. If samples were kept in the liquid phase, the bucket should be covered by a lid, since there is danger that vials may explode.
30. Some cell lines do not tolerate the presence of DMSO. In this case, cell suspensions should be centrifuged at 100*g*, and the cell pellet resuspended in 1 mL of culture medium.

References

1. Gerschenson, L. E., Anderson, M., Molson, J., and Okigaki, T. (1970) Tyrosine transaminase induction by dexamethasone in a new rat liver cell line. *Science* **170,** 859–861.
2. Borek, E. (1972) Neoplastic transformation *in vitro* of a clone of adult liver epithelial cells into differentiated hepatoma-like cells under conditions of nutritional stress. *Proc. Natl. Acad. Sci. U.S.A.* **69,** 956–959.
3. Williams, G. M., Weissburger, E. L., and Weissburger, J. H. (1971) Isolation and long-term culture of epithelial-like cells from rat liver. *Exp. Cell Res.* **69,** 106–112.
4. Grisham, J. W. (1983) Cell types in rat liver: their identification and isolation. *Mol. Cell. Biochem.* **53,** 23–33.
5. Marceau, N., Germain, L., Goyette, R., Noel, M., and Gourdeau, H. (1986) Cell of origin of distinct cultured rat liver epithelial cells, as typed by cytokeratin and surface component selective expression. *Biochem. Cell Biol.* **64,** 788–802.

6. Gebhardt, R., Schrode, W., and Eisenmann-Tappe, I. (1998) Cellular characteristics of epithelial cell lines from juvenile rat liver: selective induction of glutamine synthetase by dexamethasone. *Cell Biol. Toxicol.* **14,** 55–67.

7. Gebhardt, R. and Jonitza, D. (1991) Different proliferative response of periportal and perivenous hepatocytes to EGF. *Biochem. Biophys. Res. Commun.* **181,** 1201–1207.

8. Eisenmann-Tappe, I., Wizigmann, S., and Gebhardt, R. (1991) Glutamate uptake in primary cultures of biliary epithelial cells from normal rat liver. *Cell Biol. Toxicol.* **7,** 315–325.

9. Joplin, R., Hishida, T., Tsubouchi, H., Daikuhara, Y., Ayres, R., Neuberger, J. M., and Strain, A. J. (1992) Human intrahepatic biliary epithelial cells proliferate *in vitro* in response to human hepatocyte growth factor. *J. Clin. Invest.* **90,** 1284–1289.

10. Sirica, A. E., Mathis, G. A., Sano, N., and Elmore, L. W. (1990) Isolation, culture, and transplantation of intrahepatic biliary epithelial cells and oval cells. *Pathobiology* 58, 44–64.

11. Tsao, M.-S., Smith, J. D., Nelson, K. G., and Grisham, J. W. (1984) A diploid epithelial cell line from normal adult rat liver with phenotypic properties of oval cells. *Exp. Cell Res.* **154,** 38–52.

12. Grisham, J. W., Thal, S. B., and Nagel, A. (1975) Cellular derivation of continuously cultured epithelial cells from normal rat liver, p. 1–23. In, *Gene expression and carcinogenesis in cultured liver* (Gerschenson, L. E. and Thompson, E. B., eds.). Academic Press, New York.

13. Gebhardt, R. and Williams, G. M. (1986) Amino acid transport in established adult rat liver epithelial cell lines. *Cell Biol. Toxicol.* **2,** 9–20.

14. Kässner, G., Neupert, G., Scheibe, R., and Wenzel, K.-W. (1991) Isoenzymes of pyruvate kinase, lactate dehydrogenase and alkaline phosphatase in epithelial cell lines of rat liver. *Exp. Pathol.* **43,** 51–56.

15. Neupert, G., Langbein, L., and Karsten, U. (1987) Characterization of established epitheloid cell lines derived from rat liver: expression of cytokeratin filaments. *Exp. Pathol.* **31,** 161–167.

16. Tsao, M. S. and Grisham, J. W. (1987) Hepatocarcinomas, cholangiocarcinomas, and hepatoblastomas produced by chemically transformed cultured rat liver epithelial cells. *Am. J. Pathol.* **127,** 168–181.

17. Mayer, D. and Schäfer, B. (1982) Biochemical and morphological characterization of glycogen-storing epithelial liver cell lines. *Exp. Cell Res.* **138,** 1–14.

18. Lazaro, C. A., Rhim, J. A., Yamada, Y., and Fausto, N. (1998) Generation of hepatocytes from oval cell precursors in culture. *Cancer Res.* **58,** 5514–5522.

19. Braun, L., Mikumo, R., and Fausto, N. (1989) Production of hepatocellular carcinoma by oval cells: cell cycle expression of c-myc and p53 at different stages of oval cell transformation. *Cancer Res.* **49,** 1554–1561.

20. Williams, G. M. (1976) Primary and long-term culture of adult rat liver epithelial cells. *Methods Cell Biol.* **14,** 357–364.

21. Furukawa, K., Shimada, T., England, P., Mochizuki, Y., and Williams, G. M. (1987) Enrichment and characterization of clonogenic epithelial cells from adult rat liver and initiation of epithelial cell strains. *In Vitro Cell. Develop. Biol.* **23,** 339–348.
22. Freshney, I. (1987) *Culture of animal cells. A manual of basic technique.* 2nd ed. Alan R. Liss, New York.

7

Pulmonary Epithelial Cell Culture

Ben Forbes

1. Introduction
1.1. Background

The respiratory epithelium changes dramatically in cellular composition as the conducting airways give way to the alveolar regions of the lung. This chapter will concentrate on the culture of cells that make up the epithelial monolayer of the peripheral gas exchange (pulmonary) region of the lung. The pulmonary epithelium is composed of alveolar type I and type II epithelial cells, which are present in a 1:2 ratio. Alveolar type II cells differentiate into type I cells as part of the normal physiological replacement or repair mechanism, but the two cell types (also known as pneumocytes) are functionally and morphologically distinct (*see* **Table 1**). Despite their greater numbers compared to type I cells, alveolar type II cells comprise less than 10% of the epithelial surface area, even when their apical microvilli are taken into account. The type II cells are cuboidal in shape and can be distinguished by their lamellar bodies, which are unique to these cells *(1)*. Alveolar type I cells are squamous, contain few mitochondria or cellular inclusions, and make up over 90% of the epithelial surface *(2)*.

While immortalized cell lines are emerging, which represent the different cells of the bronchial epithelium *(3)*, there are no cell lines that possess satisfactorily the properties of alveolar epithelial cells. Primary culture is, therefore, used to supply cells for most research applications that require alveolar epithelial cells. The primary culture of alveolar epithelial cells involves the isolation, purification, and culture of cells from the lungs of laboratory animals. Similar methods have been used to isolate and culture human alveolar epithelial cells *(4)*, but lack of availability of human tissue prevents the routine use of human cells.

From: *Methods in Molecular Biology, vol. 188: Epithelial Cell Culture Protocols*
Edited by: C. Wise © Humana Press Inc., Totowa, NJ

Table 1
Properties of Human Alveolar Type II and Type I Cells

	Type II cells	Type I cells
Description	Cuboidal cells containing distinctive lamellar bodies and numerous cytoplasmic inclusions.	Squamous cells with an extended cytoplasm and few cytoplasmic inclusions.
Approximate dimensions[a]	Volume: 900 μm^3 Surface area: 200 μm^2 Perimeter: 50 μm Thickness: 1 μm	Volume: 1800 μm^3 Surface area: 5100 μm^2 Perimeter: 250 μm Thickness: 0.1 μm
Functions	Active ion and water transport. Processing alveolar surfactant. Type I cell progenitor.	Provides the thin blood–air interface of the gas exchange region.

[a]Rat type I and type II cells are smaller than their human counterparts *(1,2)*.

Isolation of type I cells has been attempted *(2)*, but the methods are poorly developed, and the results have not been well characterized. In contrast, methods for the isolation and culture of type II cells have been progressively refined over the last 25 yr *(5–13)*. Following isolation, type II cells should be used within 48 h for applications that require their metabolic, functional, and toxicological responses to be maintained. Alternatively, using the methods first reported by Kim and coworkers *(5,6)*, type II cells can be cultured to produce alveolar type I cell-like monolayers, which represent the permeability barrier of the alveolar epithelium. The methods described here aim to produce tight alveolar type I cell-like monolayers with high transepithelial electrical resistances, which are suitable to study alveolar permeability and drug transport *(7)*.

The isolation of alveolar type II cells from the laboratory rat, the commonest source of these cells, is described. Since the method for the isolation of type II cells was first published in 1974 *(8)*, a variety of methods for dissociating the epithelial cells from the lung and purifying alveolar type II epithelial cells from the resultant crude cell suspension have been developed *(9,10)*. The method described is based on well-established techniques, but notable alternative methods have been identified in the notes. The surgical isolation of the intact lung and enzymatic dissociation of the cells requires some practice to achieve the quick efficient technique that is important to the quality of the final cell preparation. Once alveolar type II cells have been obtained, little proliferation occurs, but cell culture conditions can be modified to maintain type II cell phenotype or to promote the formation of a confluent type I cell-like monolayer.

1.1.1. Isolation of Alveolar Type II Cells

The objective of the isolation procedure is to achieve a high yield of viable cells while minimizing the amount of non-type II cells. The first step is the surgical isolation of the lung and perfusion of the pulmonary circulation to remove blood cells. Lavage is used to remove nonepithelial cells from the pulmonary airspaces; these cells will be mainly macrophages in healthy animals. After removal of mobile cells from the vasculature and airspaces of the peripheral lung, a proteolytic enzyme solution is introduced into the lung to dissociate the pulmonary epithelial cells from their basement membrane. The composition of the enzyme solution used is critical to the quality of the cell suspension obtained (*see* **Note 1**). The use of elastase is less damaging to the cells than trypsin and has become accepted as the proteolytic enzyme of choice for most investigators.

1.1.2. Purification of Alveolar Type II Cells

The method described for separating type II cells from the crude cell suspension uses centrifugation on a discontinuous Percoll gradient followed by differential adherence to a Petri dish (*see* **Fig. 1**). This method selects type II cells on the basis of their size and density then uses a short incubation in a Petri dish to remove further contaminating cells, predominately macrophages, which adhere to the dish more readily than type II cells. The major alternative method for purification of the crude cell suspension is based on the removal of macrophages and leukocytes using IgG-coated plates (*see* **Note 2**).

The isolation and purification processes should be routinely monitored for the number of cells obtained (yield), the proportion of type II cells obtained (purity), and the health of the cells (viability). A simple method for the identification of the type II cells is to stain for their distinctive surfactant phospholipid-containing lamellar bodies using the Papanicoulou method *(9)*. Other methods for determining type II phenotype include lectin-binding, ectoenzyme expression or activity, and electron microscopy. The relative merits of different methods of type II cell dissociation, purification and characterization have been reviewed *(9,10)*.

1.1.3. Culture to Alveolar Type I Cell-Like Phenotype

The tendency of alveolar type II cells to dedifferentiate in culture must be combated if type II cell properties are to be retained for longer than 48 h. Expression of the type II cell phenotype can be prolonged and the cuboidal morphology of these cells retained by adjustment of the composition of the substratum and culture conditions *(9)*. Otherwise, the transformation to type I-like cells begins almost immediately in culture, and over 4–6 d, the cells come to

**CLEAR
THE LUNGS**

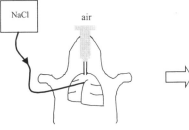

Flush the pulmonary circulation in situ

Excise the lungs and
lavage the airspaces

**OBTAIN A CELL
SUSPENSION**

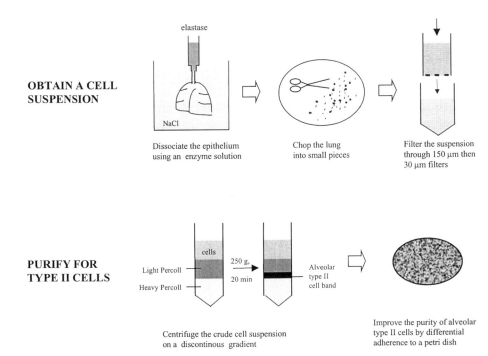

Dissociate the epithelium
using an enzyme solution

Chop the lung
into small pieces

Filter the suspension
through 150 μm then
30 μm filters

**PURIFY FOR
TYPE II CELLS**

Light Percoll

cells

250 g,

20 min

Alveolar
type II
cell band

Heavy Percoll

Centrifuge the crude cell suspension
on a discontinous gradient

Improve the purity of alveolar
type II cells by differential
adherence to a petri dish

Fig. 1. Schematic showing the major stages in the isolation procedure to obtain alveolar type II cells.

resemble type I cells. When cultured on permeable cell culture inserts (*see* **Fig. 2**), the cells assume the morphology and many biochemical features of type I cells. Despite accumulating evidence to suggest that these cells are acquiring the type I cell phenotype, most investigators still cautiously refer to such cultures as type I cell-like. The formation of tight monolayers (monolayers with high transepithelial electrical resistances) is critically dependent on the reagents used

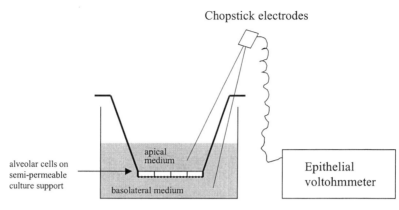

Transwell cell culture system

Fig. 2. Schematic showing the culture of type I-like alveolar epithelial cells in a Transwell cell culture system and the measurement of transepithelial electrical resistance using a voltohmmeter with chopstick electrodes.

to isolate the cells, cell seeding density, cell culture medium, and time in culture *(6,7)*.

2. Materials

2.1. Isolation of Alveolar Type II Cells

1. Infection free rats, 150–250 g bodyweight (*see* **Note 3**).
2. Pentobarbitone.
3. Dissection kit, including curved scissors for chopping the lung into small pieces.
4. Syringes for lavage and administration of digestion medium.
5. Luer lock blunt teflon cannulas and suture thread.
6. 0.15 *M* NaCl (sterile) for use as pulmonary circulation perfusion solution (*see* **Note 4**) and lavage solution (*see* **Note 5**).
7. 0.15 *M* NaCl (sterile).
8. Buffer solution A: 133 m*M* NaCl, 5.2 m*M* KCl, 1.89 m*M* CaCl$_2$, 1.29 m*M* MgSO$_4$, 1 m*M* NaH$_2$PO$_4$, 6 m*M* Na$_2$HPO$_4$, 10.3 m*M* HEPES, 5.6 m*M* glucose, pH 7.4.
9. Buffer solution B (Mg^{2+} and Ca^{2+}-free): 133 m*M* NaCl, 5.2 m*M* KCl, 1 m*M* NaH$_2$PO$_4$, 6 m*M* Na$_2$HPO$_4$, 10.3 m*M* HEPES, 5.6 m*M* glucose, pH 7.4.
10. Enzyme solution (*see* **Note 6**): elastase 2 U/mL (Worthington Biochemical) in buffer solution A.
11. Fetal bovine serum (FBS).
12. Deoxyribonuclease I (DNase I) type IV.

2.2. Purification of Alveolar Type II Cells

1. Heavy Percoll solution: 6.5 mL Percoll, 0.05 mL FBS, 2.5 mL distilled water, 0.95 mL buffer solution A (*see* **Subheading 2.1.**).

2. Light Percoll solution: 2.7 mL Percoll, 0.05 mL FBS, 6.3 mL distilled water, 0.95 mL buffer solution A (*see* **Subheading 2.1.**), one drop of phenol red.
3. Sterile centrifuge tubes, bacteriological Petri dishes.
4. Refrigerated centrifuge with swingout rotor.
5. Cell culture medium: Dulbecco's modified Eagle's medium (DMEM) supplemented with 10% FBS, 8 m*M* glutamine, 100 U/mL penicillin, 50 µg/mL gentamicin, 0.1 µ*M* dexamethasone.
6. 0.4% Trypan blue (w/v).
7. Harris's Hemotoxylin.
8. Lithium carbonate solution (*see* **Note 7**).
9. Phase contrast microscope, hemocytometer, microscope slides.
10. Xylene, ethanol, distilled water.

2.3. Culture to Alveolar Type I Cell-Like Phenotype

1. Cell culture-treated polycarbonate cell culture inserts, 0.4 µm pore size (Transwell® system [Costar] or equivalent). Other cell culture plasticware may be used according to experimental requirements.
2. Cell culture medium: *see* **Subheading 2.2.**
3. Cell culture CO_2 incubator.
4. Evom epithelial voltohmmeter.

3. Methods

3.1. Isolation of Alveolar Type II Cells

1. Anesthetize the rat by lethal peritoneal injection of pentobarbital.
2. Lay the rat on its back, expose the trachea and cut carefully half way through its diameter (*see* **Note 8**).
3. Insert the tracheal cannula approximately 1.5 cm into the trachea to rest above the bifurcation into the major bronchi.
4. Tie the cannula in place using suture thread and use a syringe to partially inflate the lungs with air (1 cm^3).
5. Open the abdomen by midline incision and exsanguinate the rat by cutting the major abdominal arteries.
6. Expose the thoracic cavity by trimming away the diaphragm, cut along the sternum, and maximize access to the lungs by carefully fracturing the ribs and cutting away the thymus (*see* **Note 9**).
7. Make an incision at the base of the right ventricle and insert a cannula (slowly leaking perfusion solution, 0.15 *M* NaCl) into the pulmonary artery.
8. Push the cannula up the artery to where it emerges at the top of the heart.
9. The right atrium will immediately swell. It should be cut promptly to allow the unrestricted efflux of fluid from the pulmonary circulation.
10. Perfuse sterile 0.15 *M* NaCl through the pulmonary circulation using a gravity feed (positioned 30–50 cm above the rat). Simultaneously, inflate the lungs 10 times with 1 cm^3 of air. The lungs should immediately and uniformly blanch to appear completely white.

11. Lift the lungs by the tracheal cannula and trim them free of the thorax, then suspend them from the tracheal cannula.
12. Attach the barrel of a 20-mL syringe to the opening of the tracheal cannula and pour 8 mL 0.15 M NaCl into the lung, detach the syringe from the tracheal cannula and pour the lavage fluid from the lung. Repeat this procedure at least 6 times to remove as many macrophages as possible.
13. Fill the lungs with 10 mL of filter-sterilized enzyme solution and suspend them in a beaker of 0.15 M NaCl at 37°C. Top up the enzyme solution over 20 min using a total of 40 mL of enzyme solution containing 80 U elastase (*see* **Note 10**).
14. Transfer the lungs to a Petri dish. Trim away the trachea and major bronchi, then use curved scissors to chop the lung parenchyma into small 1 to 2 cm^2 pieces.
15. Add 5 mL FBS to stop the digestion, then 15 mL of buffer solution B supplemented with 0.025% (w/v) DNase to prevent cell aggregation. Transfer the suspension to a 50-mL centrifuge tube and shake it in a waterbath at 37°C for 4 min.
16. Filter the suspension through progressively smaller diameter filters: (*i*) gauze, (*ii*) 150-µm nylon filter, and (*iii*) 30-µm nylon filter. This cell suspension is a crude alveolar cell isolate.

3.2. Purification of Alveolar Type II Cells (see Note 11)

1. Layer the crude cell suspension on top of a sterile discontinuous Percoll gradient (*see* **Note 12**). The Percoll gradient should be prepared in a sterile 50-mL centrifuge tube by layering 10 mL light Percoll solution (1.040 g/mL) on top of 10 mL heavy Percoll solution (1.089 g/mL) (*see* **Note 13**).
2. The preparation is centrifuged at 250g for 20 min at 4°C using a swingout rotor to produce an alveolar type II cell rich layer at the interface between the percoll gradients (*see* **Note 14**).
3. Using a Pasteur pipet, transfer the alveolar type II cell rich layer to a fresh centrifuge tube. Wash the cells by mixing with 40 mL of ice-cold buffer solution B supplemented by 0.005% (w/v) DNase and pellet the type II cells by centrifugation (250g for 20 min at 4°C).
4. Resuspend the type II cell pellet in 10 mL cell culture medium and transfer to a Petri dish for 90 min (37°C, 95% air, 5% CO_2). Rock the cells gently back and forth to collect the type II cells, but leave behind the adherent cells.
5. The cell suspension should be sampled for counting (*see* **Note 15**), viability testing, and Papanicolaou staining. The cell suspension should then be pelleted by centrifugation (250g for 20 min) before resuspension in cell culture medium (**Subheading 3.3.**).
6. The viability of the cells can be tested by addition of 100 µL Trypan blue to 400 µL of cell suspension for 5–15 min. Exclusion of dye by healthy cells and uptake of dye by damaged cells allows a differential count to be performed with viability expressed as the proportion of cells (%), which exclude the dye (*see* **Note 16**).
7. Type II cells are readily identified by the modified Papanicolaou staining method described by Dobbs (*9*). To monitor the purification method, it is recommended

that the proportion of type II cells in the cell suspension is assessed before and after each purification step. The staining procedure is performed as follows.

8. First, prepare microscope slides of isolated cells at 2×10^5 cells/cm^2 and air-dry overnight.
9. Incubate the slides in Harris's hemotoxylin for 3 to 4 min.
10. Rinse 2 to 3 times with distilled water, then incubate with lithium carbonate solution for 2 min.
11. Rinse with distilled water, then incubate sequentially in (v/v) 50, 80, 95, and 100% ethanol for 90, 15, 15, and 30 s, respectively.
12. Finally, incubate in xylene:ethanol (1:1) mixture for 30 s, then pure xylene for 60 s. Inspect the cells at ×1000 magnification (*see* **Note 17**).

3.3. Culture to Alveolar Type I Cell-Like Phenotype

1. Resuspend the type II cells in cell culture medium at a concentration that will allow seeding on microporous cell culture inserts (or other cell culture plasticware) at 1×10^6 cells/cm^2 (*see* **Note 18**).
2. Incubate the cells at 37°C, 95% air, 5% CO_2 with cell culture medium in the apical and basolateral chamber of the Transwell (*see* **Notes 19** and **20**). The cell purity is further improved when nonattached cells are discarded at the first medium change (48 h). By d 2, the purity of the culture should be >90% type II cells.
3. The cells are cultured for 4–7 d with the medium changed every 48 h. The cells will spread to form a confluent monolayer and assume type I cell morphology (*see* **Table 1**).
4. A concomitant increase in transepithelial electrical resistance can be measured using an Evom epithelial voltohmmeter. By d 6 in culture, the cells should be have a transepithelial electrical resistance of >1500 Ohm cm^2.

4. Notes

1. Trypsin and elastase are the proteolytic enzymes upon which most methods for the isolation of alveolar type II cells are based *(9)*. The merits of using elastase *(11)* or trypsin *(10)* have been reviewed, and the effect of the enzyme on the isolated cells is an important consideration. Elastase is more selective in dissociating alveolar cells while leaving the basement membrane intact *(11)* and must be used if tight type I cell-like monolayers are to be cultured.
2. The major alternative method for purification of type II cells is based on the expression of Fc receptors by the contaminating cells. Plates can be coated with IgG that binds Fc receptors, resulting in the retention and removal of contaminating cells. Advantages in cell yield and purity are claimed for the adapted IgG panning technique *(9,12)*, although purification on a discontinuous gradient remains a commonly used method. Because of the damage to Fc receptors during isolation by trypsin, IgG panning cannot be used to purify cells obtained using this enzyme.
3. The size and condition of the rat affects the yield and purity of cells. The use of smaller (<250 g) specific pathogen-free rats gives better cell yields. If specific pathogen-free rats are not used, the use of non-sawdust bedding is a sensible precaution.

4. Some investigators have heparinized rats before commencing surgery to assist clearance of the lungs. However, if dissection is performed quickly this is not necessary to improve the purity or yield of the final cell suspension.

5. The inclusion of EDTA in the lavage solution has been suggested to improve the removal of macrophages, and the use of NaCl (or other Mg^{2+}- and Ca^{2+}-free buffer) probably has an equivalent effect. However, it is important that Mg^{2+} and Ca^{2+} are present in the enzyme solution for optimal proteolytic enzyme activity.

6. Commercial supplies of enzymes are subject to inter-batch variation in quality. The source of elastase also needs to be carefully selected, and the activity of the batch must be carefully checked *(9)*. Elastase is also susceptible to autolysis, and it may be worth confirming the activity by assay *(10)*. It is important to note that different units of activity are used to measure the activity of elastase. One unit of activity, measured by the succinyl-(L-analine)$_3$-p-nitroanilide method, is equivalent to seven units measured by the orcein–elastase method *(9)*. Elastase (approx 4 U/mg, succinyl-(L-analine)$_3$-p-nitroanilide method) supplied by Worthington Biochemical (Lorne diagnostics, Reading, UK) is a preferred source of elastase for many investigators.

7. Lithium carbonate solution is prepared by addition of 2 mL of saturated lithium carbonate solution (1 g in 100 mL water) to 158 mL distilled water.

8. The lungs will deflate when the trachea is cut. Be careful not to cut through the entire diameter or the trachea will retract into the unexposed thorax.

9. It is important not to damage the lungs at any point. If the lungs are punctured the enzyme solution will leak from the lungs excessively. If the lungs are bruised, cells will not be obtained from edematous areas.

10. The lungs will become progressively leaky, requiring the solution to be topped up, but care is needed to avoid the introduction of air bubbles, which may block the airways.

11. Sterile technique and materials should be used from this point onwards.

12. The cell suspension should be well mixed to disperse any cell aggregates.

13. The light Percoll solution is carefully layered on top of the heavy gradient. The discontinuous gradient should be cooled on ice before adding the cell suspension. Other solutions, particularly metrizamide (which is more expensive), have been used to form the discontinuous gradient. These have been suggested to offer theoretical advantages over Percoll (less toxic, not metabolized), although all effectively select type II cells according to their size and density.

14. Phenol red is added to the light Percoll solution to aid the identification of the light/heavy Percoll interface, from which the type II cells are harvested. The use of a swingout centrifuge rotor head improves the banding pattern of the cells at the interface.

15. Although the yield of alveolar type II cells will vary between preparations, $>10^7$ cells should be obtained after purification. This represents about 10% of the total number alveolar type II cells in the adult rat lung.

16. Uptake of the Trypan blue dye is time-dependant. If the culture is left too long, viable cells may also begin to take up the dye.

17. The lamellar bodies of type II cells are stained blue. Contaminating cells are not stained by the Papanicolaou procedure and may include macrophages or fibroblasts (which are distinctive elongated cells in culture).
18. Cell seeding density is important. If the seeding density is too low, the cells may not achieve a confluent monolayer, whereas higher seeding densities allow less cell spreading and can result in monolayers with lower transepithelial electrical resistances.
19. Cell culture on microporous cell culture inserts allows access to the apical and basolateral sides of the epithelial monolayer and allows permeability to be studied. It is also possible to culture type I cell-like monolayers on cell culture-treated plastic, in flasks or cluster wells, in which case cell culture medium bathes the apical surface of the cells only.
20. The development of tight type I cell-like monolayers depends on the cell culture medium, particularly the serum component *(7)*. A defined medium has been reported and which may allow more control over the influence of serum factors on alveolar cells in culture *(13)*.

References

1. Mason, R. J., Shannon, J. M. (1997) Alveolar type II cells, p. 543–556. In *The lung: scientific foundations. vol. 1* (Chrystal, R. G., West, J. B., and Barnes, P. J., eds.). Lippincott-Raven, Philadelphia.
2. Schneeberger, E. E. (1997) Alveolar type I cells, p. 535–542. In *The lung: scientific foundations. vol. 1* (Chrystal, R. G., West, J. B., and Barnes, P. J., eds.). Lippincott-Raven, Philadelphia.
3. Forbes, B. (2000) Human airway epithelial cell lines for *in vitro* drug transport and metabolism studies. *Pharm. Sci. Tech. Today* **3,** 18–27.
4. Elbert, K. J., Schafer, U. F., Schafers, H-J., Kim, K-J., Lee, V. H. L., and Lehr, C-M. (1999) Monolayers of human alveolar epithelial cells in primary culture for pulmonary absorption and transport studies. *Pharm. Res.* **16,** 601–608.
5. Kim, K-J., Suh, D-J., Lubman, R. L., Danto, S. I., Borok, Z., and Crandall, E. D. (1992) Studies on the mechanism of active ion fluxes across alveolar epithelial cell monolayers. *J. Tiss. Cult. Methods* **14,** 187–193.
6. Cheek, J. M., Kim, K-J., and Crandall, E. D. (1989) Tight monolayers of rat alveolar epithelial cells: bioelectric properties and active sodium transport. *Am. J. Physiol.* **256,** C688–C693.
7. Dickinson, P. A., Evans, J. P., Farr, S. J., Kellaway, I. W., Appelqvist, T. P., Hann, A. C., and Richards, R. J. (1996) Putrescine uptake by alveolar epithelial cell monolayers exhibiting differing transepithelial electrical resistances. *J. Pharm. Sci.* **85,** 1112–1116.
8. Kikkawa, Y. and Yoneda, K. (1974) The type II epithelial cell of the lung. I. Method of isolation. *Lab. Invest.* **30,** 76–84.
9. Dobbs, L. G. (1990) Isolation and culture of alveolar type II cells. *Am. J. Physiol.* **258,** L134–147.

10. Richards, R. J., Davies, N., Atkins, J., and Oreffo, V. I. C. (1987) Isolation, biochemical characterisation, and culture of lung type II cells of the rat. *Lung* **165,** 143–158.
11. Dobbs, L. G., Geppert, E. F., Williams, M. C., Greenleaf, R. D., and Mason, R. J. (1980) Metabolic properties and ultrastructure of alveolar type II cells isolated with elastase. *Biochim. Biochem. Acta* **618,** 510–523.
12. Dobbs, L. G., Gonzalez, R., and Williams M. C. (1986) An improved method for isolating type II cells in high yield and purity. *Am. Rev. Respir. Dis.* **134,** 141–145.
13. Borok, Z., Danto, S. I., Zabski, S. I., and Crandell, E. D. (1994) Refined medium for primary culture de novo of adult rat alveolar epithelial cells. *In Vitro Cell. Dev. Biol.* **30A,** 99–104.

8

Prostate Epithelial Cell Isolation and Culture

David L. Hudson

1. Introduction

The prostate constitutes part of the male reproductive system and is a small gland located at the base of the bladder surrounding the urethra. Although the functions of the prostate are unclear, prostatic secretions comprise around 30% of the components of seminal fluid *(1)* and may provide nutrients for sperm. One component, prostate specific antigen (PSA), a form of chymotrypsin, functions as an anticoagulant maintaining the fluidity of semen. Unfortunately, it is a gland with a high tendency to develop diseases later in life. One of these is benign prostatic hyperplasia (BPH), a proliferative disorder of the transition region of the prostate that surrounds the urethra. Growth of both epithelial and mesenchymal cells in this region causes constriction of the urethra, leading to obstruction of the bladder outflow, and serious urinary problems. BPH affects many men from middle age onwards and is one of the most frequent reasons for surgery in elderly men *(2)*. Another major disease is prostatic carcinoma, which originates in the epithelial cells and is currently the most frequently diagnosed cancer in men in the USA *(3)*.

Increasing interest in research into the causes of prostatic diseases over recent years has led to a burst of activity in the development of culture systems for prostate cells. Human and rodent prostates differ significantly from each other in many anatomical aspects. Although the use of transgenic animals has led to some useful murine models of prostate cancer *(4)*, rodent cells are not ideal for the study of human disease. Two experimental animals, the dog and the chimpanzee *(5)*, have been shown to suffer from BPH-like symptoms. However, the hyperproliferation found in the dog is not comparable to that found in the human condition, and neither are available to the majority of researchers.

From: *Methods in Molecular Biology, vol. 188: Epithelial Cell Culture Protocols*
Edited by: C. Wise © Humana Press Inc., Totowa, NJ

As a better alternative to the rodent models, it therefore became essential to develop ways of culturing human prostatic epithelial and mesenchymal cells.

Following the pioneering work of Ham *(6)*, several serum-free culture media for prostate have been developed. Until recently, there were two main media in use. One, based on WAJC-404 basal medium, was originally developed for rat cell culture *(7)* and has since been adapted for human cell growth from epithelial organoids *(8)*. A second was developed by Donna Peehl et al. *(9)* using optimization of PFMR-4 medium *(10)*. Both of these media use additives that include cholera toxin, epidermal growth factor, insulin, and bovine pituitary extract. The latter was found to be vital for the maintenance of good clonal growth at low seeding densities *(9)*. Although these media perform well in some laboratories, they are based on complex basal media, which are difficult to make up from the many ingredients. Recently, a medium called PrEGM, one of the Clonetics™ optimized media from a range manufactured by BioWhittaker was introduced for prostate epithelial cell culture. This is provided as a base medium with frozen aliquots of 9 separate additives, including bovine pituitary extract. PrEGM compares favorably with WAJC-404 *(11)* and produces similar colony forming efficiencies, for primary cells, to that reported by Peehl et al. *(9)* with PFMR-4A *(12)*.

Since we obtained good results using PrEGM, we believe that this is a good option for anyone venturing into prostate cell culture. Therefore, the procedures outlined below will be based on this medium. One limitation for PrEGM, however, results from the manufacturer's reluctance to disclose the full recipe of the medium and the concentrations of the additives. This may be important for some studies. The techniques described for isolating epithelial organoids and single-cell suspensions are common to all methods of culture, however, and should be suitable for other media.

Suitable tissue for nonmalignant prostate cell growth can be obtained from surgical procedures such as radical prostatectomy, needle biopsies, autopsies, cystectomies, and transurethral resections of the prostate (TURP). Normal prostate tissue, lacking either cancer or BPH, will generally only be obtained from younger glands removed during kidney harvest from organ donors. BPH tissue, a good source of nonmalignant epithelial cells, is readily obtained from needle biopsies or TURP specimens, and the latter are the main source we use. All experimental use of human tissue will require ethical approval from local hospital committees, and this will require advance planning prior to commencement of any projects. This may be most difficult to obtain for the use of fresh cadaver material. It will also be necessary to coordinate with local histopathology departments, who will require tissue from any exploratory procedures for diagnostic purposes. This will also assist in determining the disease status of the tissue taken for cell culture.

This chapter will describe the separation of the epithelial ductal tissue from the fibroblast containing stroma and explore ways of growing these cells either from duct segments, or organoids, or as a single-cell suspension on a feeder layer. Histocytochemical methods to determine the characteristics and origin of the cells are covered elsewhere in this book.

2. Materials

1. Transport medium: RPMI 1640 with 20 mM HEPES. Weigh out 0.48 g of tissue culture grade HEPES (Sigma) per 100 mL of RPMI-1640 (Life Technologies) into a universal tube. Add 10 mL of RPMI to the tube and agitate until dissolved (this may take several min). Filter-sterilize the HEPES solution through a 0.2-μm syringe filter and add to the remainder of the RPMI. Supplement this with 5% fetal calf serum (FCS) (heat-inactivated) (Sigma), 1% penicillin–streptomycin (Life Technologies), and 1% fungizone (Life Technologies).
2. Collagenase solution: RPMI 1640 supplemented with 5% FCS (heat inactivated), and 200 U/mL collagenase type 1 (Sigma). Weigh out the required amount of enzyme into a universal container. Add RPMI with 5% serum to a concentration of 200 U/mL and agitate to dissolve the powder. Filter-sterilize through a 0.2-μm syringe filter into a clean sterile tube.
3. Sterile calcium and magnesium-free phosphate-buffered saline (PBS) (Life Technologies).
4. 0.25% Trypsin and 0.02% EDTA solution in isotonically buffered saline (Life Technologies).
5. PrEGM growth medium with BulletKit® additives (Clonetics). PrEGM is purchased with the epidermal growth factor, hydrocortisone, epinephrine, transferrin, insulin, retinoic acid, triiodothyronine, antibiotics, and bovine pituitary extract provided separately in frozen aliquots. Aliquots should be stored frozen and thawed at room temperature just before use. Complete medium should be stored at 4°C in the dark, and only the required volume should be prewarmed to 37°C.
6. Vitrogen 100 (Nutacon, Postbus 94, 2450 AB Leimuiden, Netherlands) purified bovine dermal collagen diluted to 10 μg/mL in sterile PBS.
7. Mouse embryo Swiss-3T3 cells (ATCC), confluent T75 flasks (*see* **Note 1**).
8. Mitomycin C solution. Prepare by dissolving mitomycin C powder (Sigma) in PBS to a concentration of 0.4 mg/mL and filter-sterilize. Store as frozen aliquots at –20°C.
9. Instruments, pre-sterilized:
    a. Two scalpels with size 11 blades.
    b. Fine forceps.
    c. Sharp scissors.
10. Sterile 30-mL universal containers
11. Disposable 1- and 10-mL pipets.
12. 10-cm tissue culture dishes

13. 25-cm^2 tissue culture plastic flasks.
14. Orbital platform shaker.

3. Methods

3.1. Tissue Acquisition

1. Tissues must be collected as soon as possible after removal from the patient or donor. Operating theater staff should be provided with a universal container containing chilled transport medium in which to place the tissue.
2. After collection, this should be carried back to the laboratory on ice and kept cool until processed. Although it is preferable to process immediately, physiological responses and cell viability are maintained for at least 24 h after removal.
3. To allow for histological examination of the tissue, a small section of each sample should be cut under sterile conditions and placed in formaldehyde for histological analysis (*see* **Note 2**). If the tissue is from patients undergoing TURP procedures, a longitudinal section should be taken from each chip to ensure the absence of cancer.
4. As is always the case when handling human tissue, it is important to refer to local biological hazard regulations for recommendations on the safe handling and disposal of all waste from these procedures. This will involve the wearing of gloves at all stages and bleach treatment of any instruments and containers before cleaning or disposal. Excess pieces of tissue should be fixed overnight in 4% formaldehyde and disposed of as hazardous waste.

3.2. Tissue Preparation and Digestion

1. Remove the transport medium.
2. Wash the tissue pieces by filling the universal container with fresh transport medium, inverting to suspend the tissue, and then allowing the tissue to settle before aspirating the medium.
3. Repeat twice.
4. Tip the tissue into a sterile 10-cm Petri dish and trim away clotted blood and charred areas (in the case of TURP chips), using scissors and scalpels. At this stage the tissue can be weighed for future reference.
5. Mince the tissue as finely as possible (approx 1-mm^3 pieces) initially using sharp scissors, then with crossed scalpels (such as size 11 blade) (*see* **Note 3**).
6. To wash the minced tissue free of blood, transfer it to a fresh universal container.
7. Add 20 mL of PBS, mix by inverting the tube and allow the tissue to settle to the bottom.
8. After 5 min, remove the PBS using a 5-mL pipet, taking care not to pick up any tissue pieces.
9. Repeat 2 or 3 times until the PBS is clear after the tissue has settled.
10. Add 7.5 mL of collagenase solution per gram of tissue and digest by gentle agitation on an orbital platform shaker at 37°C for 18–20 h. Very small samples such as needle biopsies require significantly less time and may be digested in 2–4 h.
11. After the appropriate incubation time, the tissue is reduced to a cloudy broth with no large pieces visible.

12. Break up any remaining clumps by repeated pipetting up and down in a 10-mL pipet, then in a 5-mL pipet to produce a broth-like mixture (*see* **Note 4**).
13. To sediment the epithelial acini from the digested stroma, centrifuge for 20 s at 170g in a centrifuge such as a Denley.
14. Remove and discard the supernatant carefully, using a wide-bore pipet, such as a transfer pipet or 5-mL pipet, taking care not to dislodge the loose cell pellet.
15. Resuspend the pellet in 10 mL of PBS and repeat the procedure twice. The pellet now contains a fairly pure population of epithelial cell organoids, which can either be plated directly or further digested to produce a single-cell suspension (*see* below).

3.3. Organoid Culture Plating

1. The organoid suspension should be suspended in 12 mL of PrEGM medium per gram of original tissue and pipetted up and down vigorously to break up any large aggregates.
2. Add 4-mL aliquots to collagen-coated T25 flasks (*see* **Note 5**).
3. Place the flasks at 37°C, ensuring that the incubator shelf is level, and leave undisturbed for 6 d.
4. After 6 d, replace the medium with fresh PrEGM, taking care not to disturb the cell organoids. Outgrowth from the organoids can be monitored under the microscope from this point on, and cells should reach confluence over the following 10 d (*see* **Note 6**). **Fig. 1A** shows the appearance of cells 6 d after plating.
5. Any visible contaminating mesenchymal cells from the stroma can be removed by differential trypsinization. Smooth muscle or fibroblasts may be seen growing out from the edge of epithelial colonies or explants (*see* **Fig. 1B**).
6. Mark areas containing contamination on the base of the flask with a marker pen to allow their identification.
7. Wash the culture with 5 mL sterile PBS and add 1 mL of trypsin-versene solution.
8. Incubate for 2 min, then aspirate the trypsin over the marked area gently 2 or 3 times.
9. Examine the flask under the microscope to check that all contaminating cells have been removed, then remove the trypsin and replace the growth medium (*see* **Note 6**).

3.4. Plating of Single Cell Suspension

1. Prepare a feeder layer by splitting mitomycin C-treated 3T3 cells (*see* **Note 7**) at one-third confluence into fresh T25 flasks. This should be done between 2 and 24 h prior to use.
2. To the preparation of epithelial cell organoids (*see* **Subheading 3.2.**), add 5 mL of trypsin-versene and mix vigorously by pipetting up and down several times.
3. Incubate with gentle shaking at 37°C for 20 min to separate the cells.
4. Rinse twice by adding 10 mL of PBS and sediment by centrifugation at 170g.
5. After 2 washes, resuspend the cell pellet in 5 mL PrEGM and count the cells.
6. Seed between 10^3 and 10^4 cells per T25 onto feeders and return to the incubator. Small colonies should become visible within 6 d, and cultures will reach confluence in 10 to 14 d. **Fig. 1** shows the appearance of colonies seeded at low (**Fig. 1C**) or high (**Fig. 1D**) density after 6 d.

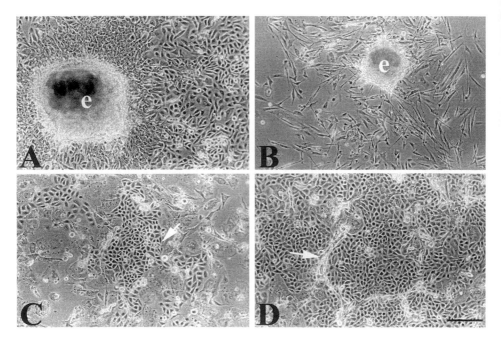

Fig 1. Appearance of primary prostate cells grown in PrEGM for 6 d. (**A,B**) Explants (e) on collagen-coated plastic showing outgrowth of epithelial cells (**A**) or stromal cells (**B**). (**C,D**) Single-cell suspension of epithelial cells plated at 10^3 (**C**) or 5×10^3 (**D**) cells per 6-cm dish, on a 3T3 feeder layer. Arrow in panel **C** indicates edge of epithelial colony, and the arrow in panel **D** indicates detaching 3T3 cells at junction between 2 coalescing epithelial colonies. All photographed at ×100 magnification. Bar = 200 μm.

4. Notes

1. Mouse 3T3 cells can be maintained in culture until required. The cells are grown routinely in Dulbecco's modified Eagle's medium (DMEM) medium with 10% FCS at 37°C with 5% CO_2. The cells should be passaged at preconfluence by washing the monolayer once with PBS, then detaching the cells by adding 2 mL of trypsin-versene for 3–5 min. Make the cell suspension up to 10 mL with serum containing DMEM, and pellet the cells by centrifugation at 170*g* for 5 min. Seed the 3T3s into fresh flasks at a split of 1:3 to 1:10. Splitting the cells 1:3 will give confluent cultures in 3 d, or 5–7 d for a 1:10 split.
2. Tissue removed from the patient will be sent for pathological examination, and, while this may be sufficient to confirm the clinical diagnosis, it will not determine the histology of individual TUR chips.
3. It is worth spending as much time as possible at this stage to produce finely minced tissue. This will maximize the efficiency of the collagenase digestion.
4. At this point, the mixture contains a suspension of released stromal cells and digested connective tissue (mostly collagen), together with epithelial acini and ducts.

5. To coat flasks with collagen, dilute sterile Vitrogen 100 (a solution consisting mainly of bovine type I collagen) to 10 µg/mL in sterile PBS. Add 3 mL per T25 or 5 mL per T75 flask to be coated. Incubate at 37°C for 1 h or, if more convenient, at 4°C overnight. After this time, remove the coating solution and wash the flasks twice with sterile PBS. Add culture medium and place the flasks at 37°C, ready for use.

6. It is possible, if required, to establish stromal cell cultures from the cells removed from the epithelial cultures. The trypsin solution containing the stromal cells can be inhibited with DMEM containing 10% serum and then centrifuged for 5 min at 170g. Resuspend the cells in 5 mL of RPMI containing 10% FCS and add to a T25 flask. The cells will grow over the following 7 d.

7. Swiss 3T3 cells have been used for many years as feeder layers for various epithelial cells types and provide a supply of growth factors and extracellular matrix support, allowing clonal growth of epithelial cells from lower seeding densities than would otherwise be needed *(6)*. To use 3T3 cells as a feeder layer, the cells are pretreated with mitomycin C. This inhibits cell division. The main advantage of mitomycin C is that it requires no specialist equipment (unlike irradiated feeder layers) and can be performed easily when cells are required. However, it is necessary to have cells growing at all times to ensure availability when clinical tissue is obtained. Prepare cells as a feeder layer by adding mitomycin C to the growth medium in a flask of confluent 3T3 cells at a final concentration of 4 µg/mL (1:100 dilution of stock solution). Incubate at 37°C for 2 h, then remove medium, wash twice with sterile PBS before trypsinizing the cells, as described in **Note 1**, and plating in collagen-coated flasks (*see* **Note 5**) at a 1:3 split (approximately 1.5×10^4 cell/cm^2).

References

1. Cunha, G. R., Donjacour, A. A., Cooke, P. S., Mee, S., Bigsby, R. M., Higgins, S. J., and Sugimura, Y. (1987) The endocrinology and developmental biology of the prostate. *Endocr. Rev.* **8,** 338–362.
2. Oesterling, J. E. (1995) Benign prostatic hyperplasia. Medical and minimally invasive treatment options [see comments]. *N. Engl. J. Med.* **332,** 99–109.
3. Landis, S. H., Murray, T., Bolden, S., and Wingo, P. A. (1999) Cancer statistics, 1999 [see comments]. *CA Cancer J. Clin.* **49,** 8–31, 1.
4. Sharma, P. and Schreiber-Agus, N. (1999) Mouse models of prostate cancer. *Oncogene* **18,** 5349–5355.
5. Steiner, M. S., Couch, R. C., Raghow, S., and Stauffer, D. (1999) The chimpanzee as a model of human benign prostatic hyperplasia [see comments]. *J. Urol.* **162,** 1454–1461.
6. Ham, R. G. (1974) Nutritional requirements of primary cultures: a neglected problem of modern biology. *In Vitro.* **10,** 119–129.
7. McKeehan, W. L., Adams, P. S., and Rosser, M. P. (1984) Direct mitogenic effects of insulin, epidermal growth factor, glucocorticoid, cholera toxin, unknown pituitary factors and possibly prolactin, but not androgen, on normal rat prostate epithelial cells in serum-free, primary cell culture. *Cancer Res.* **44,** 1998–2010.

8. Collins, A. T., Robinson, E. J., and Neal, D. E. (1996) Benign prostatic stromal cells are regulated by basic fibroblast growth factor and transforming growth factor-beta 1. *J. Endocrinol.* **151,** 315–322.
9. Peehl, D. M., Wong, S. T., and Stamey, T. A. (1988) Clonal growth characteristics of adult human prostatic epithelial cells. *In Vitro Cell. Dev. Biol.* **24,** 530–536.
10. Lechner, J. F., Babcock, M. S., Marnell, M., Narayan, K. S., and Kaighn, M. E. (1980) Normal human prostate epithelial cell cultures. *Methods Cell Biol.* 195–225.
11. Fry, P. M., Hudson, D. L., O'Hare, M. J., and Masters, J. R. W. (2000) Comparison of marker protein expression in benign prostatic hyperplasia *in vivo* and *in vitro*. *Br. J. Urol.* **85,** 504–513.
12. Hudson, D. L., O'Hare, M. J., Watt, F. M., and Masters, J. R. W. (2000) Proliferative heterogeneity in the human prostate: evidence for epithelial stem cells. *Lab. Invest.* **80,** 1243–1250.

9

A Bovine Mammary Endothelial/Epithelial Cell Culture Model of the Blood/Milk Barrier

Albert Guidry and Celia O'Brien

1. Introduction

The circulatory system is the body's inter-organ highway for transporting nutrients to the various organs and removing waste products. It also delivers cellular and soluble defense mechanisms to protect the body against invading pathogens. The circulatory system is complex but well defined and relatively easy to study. However, the movement of nutrients and humoral and cellular defense mechanisms from blood to the various organs of the body is much more complex and difficult to study. Each organ has specific requirements that must be satisfied by the blood. Study of the mechanism(s) for satisfying these requirements from blood requires a close look at the cells lining the blood vessels (endothelium) and the specific organ tissues. In studies of the mucosal organs, epithelial cells transport or synthesize and secrete organ-specific products, i.e., mammary gland, milk and colostrum; lungs, absorb O_2 and expel CO_2; gut, digestive enzymes, mucous, and antibodies. Epithelial cells also serve as the first line of defense against the onslaught of bacteria, viruses, parasites, chemicals, and other biological hazards.

The study of host–pathogen interactions during bacterial infection of the mammary gland has been hampered by the complex nature of the gland. This chapter describes an in vitro model of the blood/milk barrier in the bovine mammary gland consisting of mammary endothelial and epithelial cells separated by an extracellular matrix. This model allows for the direct observation of the function of each cell type as a result of bacteria or parasite challenge, variation in nutrition, and antibiotic therapy, etc. This model also enables the study of antibiotic diffusion from the blood to the lumen of the gland or from the lumen of the gland to the blood, transport of nutrients from blood to secretory

From: *Methods in Molecular Biology, vol. 188: Epithelial Cell Culture Protocols*
Edited by: C. Wise © Humana Press Inc., Totowa, NJ

cells, synthesis and secretion of lacteal secretions, secretion of cytokines by the various cells of the mammary gland, and the transport of cellular defense mechanisms from blood to the alveoli. A similar model could be constructed for other organs of other species.

In this chapter, we describe in detail the protocols used to prepare a model of the blood/milk barrier in the bovine mammary gland. This includes procedures for the isolation of bovine mammary gland endothelial cells *(1)*, epithelial cells of the teat sinus and milk ducts *(2)*, secretory epithelial cells *(3)*, fibroblast *(3)*, cryopreservation of cells *(3)*, immunocytochemistry *(1,3)*, and preparation of the endothelial/epithelial cell culture model *(4)*.

2. Materials

2.1. Endothelial Cell Isolation and Culture

2.1.1. Reagents and Media

1. Betadine® (The Purdue Frederick Company).
2. HBSSs: 494 mL Hank's balanced salt solution (HBSS) (Sigma), 1 mL 1 mol/L HEPES buffer (Sigma), and 5 mL of antibiotic-antimycotic solution (Life Technologies).
3. Sterile dissection kit.
4. Endothelial cell culture medium: 439 mL Dulbecco's modified Eagle's medium (DMEM) F12 K medium (Life Technologies), 50 mL fetal bovine serum (FBS) (Hyclone), 5 mL antibiotic-antimycotic solution, 5 mL 200 m*M* L-glutamine (Life Technologies), and 1.0 mL 50 mg/mL heparin (Sigma).
5. Kreb's Ringer bicarbonate solution: 0.1 g MgCl$_2$ · 6 H$_2$O, 7.0 g NaCl, 0.1 g anhydrous sodium phosphate (dibasic), 0.18 g anhydrous sodium phosphate (monobasic), 1.26 g sodium bicarbonate, and 0.54 g D-glucose. Bring volume up to 1 L with double-distilled (dd)H$_2$O. Filter through a 0.22-μm filter.
6. Collagenase solution I: 100 mg collagenase (Sigma), 48 mL Kreb's Ringer bicarbonate solution, and 2 mL bovine serum albumin (BSA) (Hyclone).
7. Dil-Ac-LDL: dilute stock Dil-Ac-LDL (Biomedical Technologies, cat. no. BT-902) (5 μg/mL) 1:40 in culture medium.
8. Dulbecco's phosphate-buffered saline (PBS) (Sigma).
9. Trypsin-EDTA, undiluted (Sigma).
10. Rabbit anti-von Willebrand factor antiserum (Dako Corporation): diluted 1:40 in PBS.
11. 0.5% Triton-X 100 (Sigma) in PBS.
12. Fluorescein isothiocyanate (FITC) goat anti-rabbit IgG (Kirkegaard & Perry, cat. no. 02-15-06): diluted 1:20 in PBS.
13. Normal rabbit serum (Sigma): diluted 1:40 in PBS.
14. Mounting fluid: 1:1 Glycerol:PBS.
15. 0.1% Calf-skin collagen in 0.1 *M* acetic acid (Sigma).
16. 3.7% Formaldehyde in PBS.

2.1.2. Cultureware and Equipment

1. 15-mL Sterile screw-capped conical centrifuge tubes.
2. 50-mL Sterile screw-capped conical centrifuge tubes.
3. 25-cm^2 Tissue culture flask (Corning Costar).
4. Flow cytometer equipped with two argon lasers, a 514-nm laser blocking filter, a 550 nm pass filter and cell sorting capabilities.
5. Fluorescence microscope with rhodamine filter.
6. Inverted microscope.

2.2. Epithelial Cell Isolation

2.2.1. Reagents and Media

1. Betadine.
2. HBSSs: (*see* **Subheading 2.1.1., step 2.**).
3. Epithelial cell culture medium: 462 mL RPMI 1640 (JRH Biosciences, cat. no. 51502-78), 462 mL DMEM, 100 mL FBS, 10 mL antibiotic-antimycotic solution, 10 mL sodium pyruvate (1 mM) (Sigma), 10 mL L-glutamine (2 mM), 40 mL HEPES buffer (40 mM) (Sigma), 0.5 mL bovine insulin (5 µg/mL) (Sigma), 1.0 mL hydrocortisone (1 µg/mL) (Sigma), and 2 mL bovine prolactin (1 µg/mL) (National Hormone and Pituitary Program, Los Angeles County Harbor—UCLA Medical Center, 1000 W. Carson Street, Torrance, CA 90502, USA).
4. Collagenase solution II: 100 mL HBSSs, 40 mg collagenase.
5. Trypsin-EDTA.
6. 0.1% Calf-skin collagen in 0.1 M acetic acid (Sigma).
7. Trypan blue: 1% in 0.01 M PBS pH 7.4 (Sigma).
8. 70% Ethanol.

2.2.2. Cultureware and Equipment

1. 15-mL Sterile screw-conical centrifuge tubes.
2. 50-mL Sterile screw-capped conical centrifuge tubes.
3. 60-mm Culture dishes precoated with rat tail collagen (Becton Dickinson).
4. 25-cm^2 Tissue culture flask.
5. 2-Chambered tissue culture slides (Fisher Scientific).
6. 200-µm Nylon mesh (Spectrum Laboratories, cat. no. 146487).
7. Laminar flow hood.
8. Fluorescence microscope.
9. Inverted microscope.

2.3. Cryopreservation and Thawing of Cells

2.3.1. Reagents and Media

1. Dimethyl sulfoxide (DMSO) (Sigma).
2. Trypan blue.
3. Freezing medium: 70% RPMI or DMEM, 10% DMSO, 20% FBS.

2.4. Culture of Epithelial Cells

2.4.1. Reagents and Media

1. Trypsin-EDTA.
2. Trypan blue.
3. Culture medium II: as before.
4. HBSS.

2.4.2. Cultureware and Equipment

1. Fluorescence microscope.
2. Inverted microscope.
3. 15-mL Sterile screw-conical centrifuge tubes.
4. 60-mm Culture dishes coated with rat-tail collagen.
5. 25-cm^2 Tissue culture flask.
6. 2-Chambered tissue culture slides.
7. 22×30 mm Cover glass.

2.5. Immunocytochemistry

2.5.1. Reagents and Media

1. Calf-skin collagen (type 1).
2. HBSS.
3. FBS.
4. PBS.
5. Bouin's solution (Sigma).
6. Aqueous mounting medium (Biogenex, cat. no. HK099-5K).
7. Gamma globulin-free horse serum diluted to 5% in 0.01 M PBS, pH 7.4, with 0.05% Tween 20 (Life Technologies).
8. Rabbit anti-von Willebrand factor antiserum 1:40 in PBS.
9. Mouse monoclonal anti-α-smooth muscle actin 1:200 in PBS (Sigma).
10. Rabbit anti-cytokeratin, undiluted (Biogenex, cat. no. PA071-5P).
11. Mouse monoclonal anti-vimentin, undiluted (Biogenex, cat. no. MA074-5C).
12. Fluorescein-labeled goat anti-rabbit IgG diluted 1:20 in PBS.
13. Fluorescein-labeled goat anti-mouse IgG diluted 1:20 in PBS (Kirkegaard & Perry, cat. no. 02-18-07).

2.5.2. Cultureware and Equipment

1. CO$_2$ incubator.
2. Platform rocker.
3. Fluorescence microscope.
4. 2-Chambered tissue culture slides.

2.6. Preparation of Cell Culture Model

2.6.1. Reagents and Medium

1. Trypsin-EDTA.
2. Calf-skin collagen (type 1).
3. Culture medium II: as before.

2.6.2. Cultureware and Equipment

1. CO_2 incubator.
2. UV light.
3. Millicell-ERS resistance system (ohm meter).
4. Microtiter plate reader.
5. 15-mL Sterile conical centrifuge tubes.
6. Tissue culture inserts, 12 mm diameter, 12.0 µm pore size (Millipore, cat. no. PIXP01250).
7. 24-Well tissue culture plates (Corning Costar).
8. 6-Well tissue culture plates (Corning Costar).
9. 96-Well microtiter plate (Corning Costar).

3. Methods

3.1. Endothelial Cell Isolation

1. At necropsy, remove mammary gland (*see* **Note 1**).
2. Wash the udder with Betadine, rinse with water, then with 70% ethanol.
3. Remove as much of the mammary artery as possible.
4. Place the artery in a 1-L beaker containing cold sterile HBSSs and transport to the laboratory on ice.
5. In sterile hood, place the artery in a dish deep enough to submerse the artery in HBSSs.
6. Remove extraneous tissue with scissors.
7. Rinse the interior of the artery with HBSSs.
8. Clamp off one end with forceps, fill the artery with 37°C collagenase solution I, and clamp off the other end and all branches of the artery to prevent leakage of the collagenase.
9. Wrap the vessel and forceps in aluminum foil and place in 37°C, 5% CO_2 for 15 min.
10. Remove the forceps from one end of the artery and decant the contents into a 50-mL centrifuge tubes (*see* **Note 2**).
11. Rinse the interior of artery 3× with endothelial cell culture medium and collect rinse in 50-mL centrifuge tubes.
12. Fill the artery with endothelial cell culture medium, clamp with forceps, and massage the artery with forceps to release cells from the interior surface.
13. Remove the forceps and collect the culture medium with suspended cells into 50-mL centrifuge tubes. Repeat steps 12 to 13 twice.
14. Centrifuge tubes at 850g, at 15°C for 10 min.
15. Resuspend the pellets in 5 mL endothelial cell culture medium and transfer to a 25-cm² culture flask.
16. Incubate at 37°C, 5% CO_2, overnight.
17. Endothelial cells will adhere to flask (*see* **Note 3**).
18. Remove the medium, rinse the flask with 37°C medium, and add 5 mL fresh 37°C endothelial cell culture medium.

19. Continue to incubate at 37°C, 5% CO_2, changing the culture medium every 2 d until confluent.
20. Check for confluence using the inverted microscope. When endothelial cells are 90–95% confluent (10 to 11 d), aspirate off medium.
21. Add 1 mL 37°C trypsin-EDTA/25-cm^2 culture flask, rock the flask to make sure all cells come into contact with the trypsin, and incubate for 5 min at 37°C, 5% CO_2 (see **Note 4**).
22. View cells with inverted microscope (see **Note 5**).
23. Add a volume of 37°C endothelial cell culture medium equal to or greater than the volume of trypsin (see **Note 6**).
24. Aspirate suspended cells and place in 75-cm^2 culture flask along with 15 mL of 37°C endothelial cell culture medium and incubate at 37°C, 5% CO_2, until confluent.
25. Label cells with Dil-Ac-LDL by aspirating off the medium and adding 3 mL Dil-Ac-LDL/75cm^2 culture flask.
26. Incubate for 2 h at 37°C, 5% CO_2.
27. After incubation, remove Dil-Ac-LDL, and rinse confluent monolayer with 10 mL HBSS.
28. Remove HBSS and add 3 mL 37°C trypsin-EDTA/75-cm^2 culture flask, rock the flask to make sure all cells come into contact with the trypsin, and incubate for 5 min at 37°C, 5% CO_2.
29. View cells with inverted microscope.
30. Tap the flask to loosen adhered cells.
31. Aspirate suspended cells and place in 15 mL centrifuge tube with 50% FBS to neutralize the trypsin, and centrifuge at 850g, at 15°C, for 10 min.
32. Resuspend pellet in a 0.5-mL endothelial cell culture medium and transfer to small round bottom 2.0-mL cryotube.
33. Transport cells (at room temperature) to cell sorter.
34. Tune laser to 514 nm at 100 mW with voltage set at 900 V.
35. Gate cells according to peak fluorescence and debris and collect highly fluorescing cells into 15-mL centrifuge tubes containing 10 mL endothelial cell culture medium.
36. Place in 75-cm^2 culture flask and incubate at 37°C, 5% CO_2, until confluent.
37. Repeat steps 25 through 35 (see **Note 7**).
38. To check for purity, place 1×10^5 cells in each chamber of 2-chambered tissue culture slides coated with 0.1% calf-skin collagen and incubate at 37°C, 5% CO_2, until confluent, changing culture medium every 2 d (see **Note 8**).
39. When cells on slides are confluent, remove culture medium.
40. Fix cells by placing slides in a coplin jar containing 3.7% formaldehyde in PBS and incubate for 20 min at room temperature.
41. Remove excess formaldehyde by blotting.
42. Permeabilize cells by immersing slides in 0.5% Triton X-100 in PBS for 15 min at room temperature.
43. Remove excess Triton X-100 by blotting and add a 1:40 dilution of antiserum to von Willebrand factor in PBS to one chamber of the slide and a 1:40 dilution of normal rabbit serum as a serum control to the other chamber (see **Note 9**).

44. Incubate the slides in the humidity chamber at 37°C for 30 min.
45. Rinse slides in PBS 3× for 3 min each rinse.
46. Incubate slides with FITC-labeled goat anti-rabbit antibody diluted 1:20 in PBS and incubate 37°C for 30 min (*see* **Note 9**)
47. Wash slides in PBS 3× for 10 min each.
48. Blot excess PBS and mount with mounting fluid (1:1 glycerol:PBS).
49. Examine using the fluorescent microscope equipped with a rhodamine filter (*see* **Note 10**).
50. Once a pure culture has been verified by morphology and staining, expand the culture in a 75-cm^2 culture flask.
51. After trypsinization, determine cell count and number of viable cells by mixing equal volumes (50 µL) of the cell suspension and trypan blue on a microscope slide and transferring a small amount to a hemocytometer (*see* **Note 11**).
52. Calculate the number of live cells.
53. Centrifuge and resuspend cells to a concentration of 5×10^6 cells/mL in culture medium for preparation of the model or in freezing medium for cryopreservation as described below.

3.2. Epithelial Cell Isolation

3.2.1. Teat Sinus Epithelial Cell Isolation

1. Immediately after slaughter, remove the udder, wash with Betadine, and rinse with water, and then with 70% ethanol.
2. Clamp teats at the base with forceps to occlude the teat sinus and aseptically remove from the udder using a scalpel.
3. Submerge in a beaker of HBSSs and cover with aluminum foil for transport to the laboratory.
4. Flush the teat twice with 5 mL HBSSs via cannula through the streak canal and milk out the HBSSs.
5. Infuse 5 mL collagenase solution II into the teat sinus and place the entire teat in HBSSs.
6. Incubate at 37°C, 5% CO_2, for 30 min.
7. Remove the teat from the HBSSs, gently dislodge the epithelial cells lining the teat sinus by flushing the collagenase solution back and forth with a cannula and syringe before aspirating the suspended cells and placing them in a 15-mL centrifuge tube.
8. Rinse the teat sinus twice with HBSSs to obtain residual dislodged cells.
9. Infuse fresh collagenase solution II and incubate in HBSSs at 37°C for 30 min.
10. Repeat enzymatic digestion every 30 min for 5 h, keeping the 30-min samples in separate aliquots.
11. Filter each aliquot through a 200-µm nylon mesh into 50-mL centrifuge tubes, using HBSSs to facilitate filtration.
12. Centrifuge at 100g for 5 min and wash twice with 10 mL HBSSs to eliminate enzyme residue.

13. Suspend in 10 mL HBSSs.
14. Determine cell count and number of viable cells by mixing equal volumes (50 μL) of the cell suspension and trypan blue on a microscope slide and transfer a small amount to a hemocytometer (*see* **Note 11**).
15. Calculate the number of live cells.
16. Centrifuge and resuspend cells to a concentration of 5×10^6 cells/mL in epithelial cell culture medium and overlay 1 mL on 60-mm culture dishes containing 4 mL warm epithelial cell culture medium for immediate culturing or suspend in freezing medium for cryopreservation as described in **Subheading 3.3.**

3.2.2. Ductal Epithelial Cell Isolation

1. Immediately after slaughter, remove the udder, wash with Betadine, and rinse with water, and then with 70% ethanol.
2. Aseptically remove a section of the large duct network immediately anterior to the gland cistern.
2. Expose the lining of the duct using forceps and scalpel.
3. Rinse the epithelium with HBSSs.
4. Gently scrape the epithelium with a scalpel and suspend the scrapings in HBSSs.
5. Filter the cells through a 200-μm nylon mesh into 50-mL centrifuge tubes using HBSSs to facilitate filtration.
6. Centrifuge at 100*g* for 5 min and wash twice with 10 mL HBSSs.
7. Suspend in 10 mL HBSSs.
8. Determine cell count and number of viable cells by mixing equal volumes (50 μL) of the cell suspension and trypan blue on a microscope slide and transferring a small amount to a hemocytometer (*see* **Note 11**).
9. Calculate the number of live cells.
10. Centrifuge and resuspend cells to a concentration of 5×10^6 cells/mL in epithelial cell culture medium and overlay 1 mL on 60-mm culture dishes containing 4 mL warm epithelial cell culture medium dishes for immediate culturing or suspend in freezing medium for cryopreservation as described in **Subheading 3.3.**

3.2.3. Secretory Epithelial Cell Isolation

1. Immediately after slaughter, remove the udder, wash with Betadine, and rinse with water, and then with 70% ethanol.
2. Excise several 50-g sections of secretory tissue dorsal to the large duct network, avoiding large blood vessels and milk ducts.
3. Immerse in HBSSs at room temperature for transport to the laboratory.
4. Wash twice with HBSSs to eliminate residual milk and place in a sterile 100-mm Petri dish.
5. Moisten with HBSSs and slice into 5-g sections.
6. Wash sections twice with HBSSs.
7. Finely mince tissue with forceps and scissors.
8. Transfer minced tissue to a flask containing 50 mL HBSSs and rock for 5 min at room temperature.

9. Allow large pieces of tissue to settle and decant supernatant.
10. Repeat until the supernatant appears clear.
11. Replace the HBSSs with 5 mL of collagenase solution II per gram of tissue and rock at 37°C for 30 min.
12. Filter through a 200-μm nylon mesh to collect dispersed cells, using additional 37°C HBSSs to facilitate filtration.
13. Return undigested tissue to the digestion flask and repeat the digestion procedure every 30 min for 5 h.
14. Centrifuge the filtrates at 100g for 5 min and wash twice with 10 mL HBSSs.
15. Suspend in 10 mL HBSSs.
16. Determine cell count and number of viable cells by mixing equal volumes (50 μL) of the cell suspension and trypan blue on a microscope slide and transferring a small amount to a hemocytometer (*see* **Note 11**).
17. Calculate the number of live cells.
18. Centrifuge and resuspend cells to a concentration of 5×10^6 cells/mL in epithelial cell culture medium and overlay 1 mL on 60-mm culture dishes containing 4 mL warm epithelial cell culture medium for immediate culturing or suspend in freezing medium for cryopreservation as described in **Subheading 3.3.**

3.2.4. Fibroblast Isolation

Cells obtained from enzymatic digestion of teat and secretory tissue from 3 to 5 h yields approximately 50% fibroblasts. Fibroblasts appear as single stellate and spindle-shaped cells between the epithelial islands. Because fibroblasts grow more rapidly on collagen than epithelial cells, they can be purified by repeated subculturing with mild trypsin elution of each subculture early in the culturing of the cells.

3.3. Cryopreservation and Thawing of Cells

1. Centrifuge and resuspend endothelial and epithelial cells and fibroblasts to a concentration of 5×10^6 cells/mL in freezing medium as described in **Subheadings 3.1.** and **3.2.**
2. Aliquot 1 mL in 2-mL cryotubes.
3. Freeze at –20°C for 15 min, then transfer to –80°C (*see* **Note 12**).
4. Thaw by placing in a 37°C water bath until only a few ice crystals are present. Cells are ready for cell culturing.

3.4. Epithelial Cell Culture

1. Suspend freshly isolated cells or cryopreserved cells in epithelial cell culture medium at 5×10^5 cells/mL (*see* **Note 13**).
2. Overlay 5 mL of the cell suspension on 60-mm culture dishes and gently shake to evenly distribute the cells.
3. Incubate cultures at 37°C, 5% CO_2, changing culture medium every 48 h (*see* **Note 14**).

4. When epithelial cells become 80% confluent, approximately 10 to 14 d, remove culture medium and wash twice with HBSS.
5. Replace HBSS with 5 mL trypsin-EDTA and incubate at 37°C, 5% CO_2, observing periodically with the inverted microscope to determine when most of the cells have become dislodged (*see* **Note 4**).
6. Transfer the suspended cells to a 15-mL centrifuge tube with an equal volume of HBSS enriched with 50% FBS to stop further trypsinization.
7. Wash the cells twice with HBSS and resuspend the cells in culture medium at 5 × 10^6 cells/mL for further culturing on 60-mm culture dishes or 25-cm^2 culture flask for expanding the cell population and for culturing on chambered slides for immunocytochemistry.

3.5. Immunocytochemistry

1. To coat culture slides with collagen place 0.5 mL calf-skin collagen solution in each well of 2-well culture slides and allow to dry overnight at 4°C.
2. Wash with HBSS.
3. Overlay 10^5 cells/chamber in epithelial cell culture medium and incubate at 37°C, 5% CO_2, changing culture medium every 48 h until cells appear confluent.
4. When cells are confluent remove medium and wash the cultures twice with HBSS at 37°C for 5 min.
5. Fix the cells by adding 1 mL Bouin's solution and incubating for 15 min with rocking.
6. Rinse with PBS until the PBS is clear.
7. Add 1 mL diluted gamma globulin-free horse serum to each chamber to block nonspecific binding of primary antibodies.
8. Incubate for 30 min at room temperature with rocking.
9. Remove blocking agent and add 1 mL diluted primary antibody specific for either epithelial cells (rabbit anti-cytokeratin), endothelial cells (rabbit anti-von Willebrand factor), smooth muscle cells (mouse monoclonal anti-α-smooth muscle actin), or fibroblast (mouse monoclonal anti-vimentin) to respective chambers (*see* **Notes 9** and **15**).
10. Incubate for 1 h at room temperature with rocking.
11. Remove primary antibodies and wash 3× with PBS for 5 min each.
12. Add 1 mL diluted fluorescein-labeled goat anti-rabbit IgG or fluorescein-labeled goat anti-mouse and incubate in the dark for 45 min at room temperature with rocking.
13. Remove fluorescein-labeled antibodies and wash 3× with PBS.
14. Remove chamber walls from the slide and mount the slide with aqueous mounting medium.
15. Examine slides for specific staining for each cell type, using the fluorescence microscope (*see* **Note 16** and **17**).

3.6. Preparation of Cell Culture Model (see Note 18)

1. Coat the bottom of the Millipore inserts (epithelial cell side of the insert) with calf-skin collagen by inverting the insert and layering the collagen on the epithelial side of the membrane (*see* **Note 19**).

2. Dry overnight at room temperature.
3. Turn insert over and coat the endothelial side of the insert in a like manner.
4. Place inserts in 6-well plates and fill plates with epithelial culture medium (*see* **Note 20**).
5. Remove excess medium and layer 75 µL of fibroblasts (3×10^5 cells/75 µL) on the collagen.
6. Incubate for 8 h at 37°C in 5% CO_2.
7. Attenuate fibroblast by exposing the inserts to UV light for 15 min at room temperature (*see* **Note 21**).
8. Turn plate 180° and expose fibroblast to UV light for an additional 15 min.
9. Place 75 µL of calf-skin collagen on top of the fibroblasts and incubate at 37°C, 5% CO_2, overnight.
10. Place 75 µL of epithelial cells (1×10^5 cells/75 µL) on top of the collagen and incubate at 37°C, 5% CO_2, for 8 h.
11. Invert inserts and add 10^5 endothelial cells in 100 µL endothelial culture medium to the chamber side of the inserts.
12. Incubate for 6 d or until the cell layers become confluent, changing the culture medium, both epithelial and endothelial every 2 d.
13. Determine confluence daily by measuring resistance across the cell layers using the ohm meter. Place the short pole of the ohm meter inside the insert and the long pole in the well of a 24-well plate (*see* **Note 22**).
14. To determine the reliability of the ohm meter to measure confluence, wash one of the inserts 2 times with HBSS and add 200 µL Trypan blue to the insert well.
15. At 30-min intervals for 6 h, transfer 50 µL of medium from the well of the 24-well plate to 96 well microtiter plate wells and measure the absorbance at 570 nm using the microtiter plate reader. Use membranes coated with collagen as positive controls. The absorbance readings from these wells should rise rapidly, whereas the absorbance of the wells with the monolayers should remain close to 0 absorbance when the monolayer is confluent (*see* **Note 23**).
16. Once confluence is established, the model can be used for further studies, i.e., diapedesis of neutrophils, transport of substances across the membranes, etc. (*see* **Fig. 1**).

4. Notes

1. All work, except initial removal of arteries, is performed under sterile conditions.
2. The end of the artery may become sealed and may need to be cut off.
3. Small aggregates will be apparent, cell debris and nonadherent cells will appear in the medium.
4. Trypsin incubation should be kept to a minimum (approx 5 min) to avoid cell damage.
5. The cells should be rounded.
6. Serum in the culture medium will neutralize the trypsin.
7. Repeat culturing and sorting until a pure culture of endothelial cells is obtained.
8. Continue the remaining cells in culture.
9. Dilution may vary with lots of antisera.

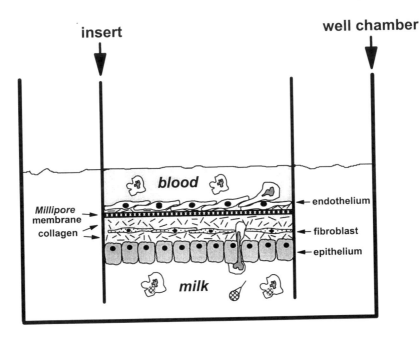

Fig. 1. Depicts the model of the blood/milk barrier during polymorphonuclear leu-kocyte diapedesis and phagocytosis of opsonized bacteria.

10. Dil-Ac-LDL and von Willebrand factor are classical endothelial markers. Smooth muscle and fibroblast do not stain for these markers.
11. Dead cells will stain with Trypan blue.
12. If cells are to be stored for longer than 6 mo, they should stored at –150°C.
13. Freshly isolated cells will contain small (2–6 cells) and large clumps (20–100 cells) of cells.
14. Observing the cells after a 2- to 4-h incubation, using the inverted microscope, should reveal adhered cells, clumps of cells, and numerous nonadhered cells float-ing in the medium. Adhered cells may be singular or in clumps. Cell clumps proliferate into islands with a dense core of cells from which cell projections radiate. By 7 d, cells surrounding the dense core increase, and the core will atro-phy. The cells will begin to form islands of cells with large cells around the periphery of the islands *(3,5)*. The islands will eventually merge into a confluent monolayer. In addition to specific immunostaining, mammary cells display dis-crete morphological characteristics. Epithelial cells are cuboidal and form a cobblestone-like monolayer. Pure epithelial cell cultures can best be obtained from teat and ductal tissue by culturing the earlier collagenase digestion times for the teat and using the scrapings from the ductal tissue *(2,3,5–7)*. Fibroblasts appear as single stellate and spindle-shaped cells between the epithelial islands *(3)*. Unlike myoepithelial, they are broad in the middle and have multiple spike-

like projections. Fibroblast may condense into bundles surrounding the epithelial islands *(2)*. Pure cultures of fibroblasts form loose cell layers with cells oriented in parallel. Fibroblast are difficult to control when culturing secretory epithelial cells, but can be kept to a minimum by frequent trypsinization as described below. Mammary endothelial cells tend to be more elongated with fewer spindle-like projections than fibroblast. Unlike fibroblasts, endothelial cells will form a monolayer in pure culture. However, there is considerable heterogeneity in the structure, function, antigenic composition, metabolic properties, and response to growth factors among endothelial cells of different organs *(1)*. Therefore, von Willebrand and Dil-Ac-LDL staining should be the major identifying criteria. Myoepithelial cells cultured on collagen at low density appear spindle like projections. When confluent, they do not show the cobblestone morphology of epithelial cells nor the fusiform morphology of fibroblasts *(5–8)*. Should these criteria prove inadequate for the differentiation of fibroblast and myoepithelial cell, contraction of the cells following exposure to oxytocin could be used to confirm the presence of myoepithelial cells. Myoepithelial cell contamination was not a problem when mammary epithelial cells were isolated and cultured as described above.

15. Add PBS to one chamber as the negative control.
16. Care must be taken to avoid drying of slides during the staining process.
17. Epithelial cells: cytokeratin filaments appear as interconnected bundles in the cytoplasm. The cytokeratin network is more dense around the nucleus, cytoplasmic vesicles, and in the periphery of the cell where cytokeratin filaments run parallel to the cell surface *(3)*. Some of the peripheral filaments may extend into neighboring cells via desmosomes. After several subcultures, cells may show a reduced cytokeratin network restricted to the area surrounding the nucleus. Epithelial cells will not stain for vimentin, but will stain to a small extent for actin. Fibroblasts: appear as single stellate and spindle-shaped cells between growing islands of epithelial islands *(3)*. After confluence, fibroblasts condense into bundles surrounding the epithelial islands. Pure cultures of fibroblasts form loose cell layers with cells oriented in the same parallel direction. They stain specifically for vimentin. Endothelial cells: endothelial stained with fluorescein-tagged anti-von Willebrand display intense granular perinuclear immunofluorescence *(1)*. When examined with an epifluorescence microscope equipped with a rhodamine excitation-emission filter, cells stained with Dil-Ac-LDL display a granular pattern of fluorescence in their cytoplasm. This staining is due to the accumulation of acetylated lipoprotein in secondary lysosomes. Myoepithelial cells: contain many densely packed myofilaments, very few cytoplasmic organelles elongated surface projections, and dense irregularly shaped nuclei *(9)*. They contain an extensive network of cytoskeletal proteins, including á-smooth muscle actin, á-actinin, and vimentin. Myoepithelial cells also contain vimentin, but the vimentin fibers terminate at the nuclei. Myoepithelial cell ultrastructure resembles smooth muscle in the content of filamentous tracts, which fill most of the cytoplasmic volume in differentiated cells. Myoepithelial cells were not used in this model, but

detailed description is presented to determine purity of the fibroblast *(9–12)*.
18. Have plates of confluent fibroblasts and epithelial and endothelial cells available.
19. Care should be taken so that the collagen does not flow through the membrane.
20. Turn inserts over so that there are no bubbles on the epithelial side of the insert.
21. Timing will depend on the strength of the UV lamp and the distance from insert to lamp.
22. Depending on the adjustment of the ohm meter, the reading should be 1000 ohms or greater when the cells are confluent.
23. Trypan blue is toxic to cells. Therefore, the trypan blue insert serves only as a test for confluence and cannot be use for further studies.

References

1. Aherne, K. M., Davis, M. R., and Sordillo, L. M. (1995) Isolation and characterization of bovine mammary endothelial cells. *Methods Cell Sci.* **17,** 41–46.
2. Cifrian, E., Guidry, A. J., O'Brien, C. N., and Keys, J. E. (1994) Bovine mammary teat and ductal epithelial cell cultures. *Am. J. Vet. Res.* **55,** 239–246.
3. Cifrian, E., Guidry, A. J., O'Brien, C. N., Nickerson, S. C., and Marquardt, W. W. (1994) Adherence of *Staphylococcus aureus* to cultured mammary epithelial cells. *J. Dairy Sci.* **77,** 970–983.
4. Guidry, A. J. and O'Brien, C. N. (1998) A bovine mammary endothelial/epithelial cell culture model of the blood/milk barrier. *Can. J. Vet. Res.* **62,** 117–121.
5. Smits, E., Burvenich, C., and Guidry, A. J. (2000) Adhesion receptor CD11b/ CD18 contribution to neutrophil diapedesis across the blood/milk barrier. *Vet. Immunol. Immunopathol.* **15,** 255–650.
6. Smits , E., Burvenich, C., Guidry, A. J., Hayneman, R., and Massart-Leen, A. (1999) Diapedesis across mammary epithelium reduces phagocytic and oxidative burst of bovine neutrophils. *Immunol. Immunopathol.* **68,** 169–176.
7. Smits , E., Burvenich, C., Guidry, A. J., and Roets, E. (1998) *In vitro* expression of adhesion receptors and diapedesis by polymorphonuclear neutrophils during experimentally induced *Streptococcus uberis* mastitis. *Infect. Immun.* **66,** 2529–2534.
8. Smits, E., Cifrian, E., Guidry, A. J., Rainard, Pl, Burvenich, C., and Paape, M. J. (1996) Cell culture system for studying bovine neutrophil diapedesis. *J. Dairy Sci.* **79,** 1353–1360.
9. Zavizion, B. Politis, I., and Gorewit, R. C. (1992) Bovine mammary myoepithelial cells. 1. Isolation, culture, and characterization. *J. Dairy Sci.* **75,** 3367–3380.
10. Zavizion, B. Politis, I., and Gorewit, R. C. (1992) Bovine mammary myoepithelial cells. 2. Interactions with epithelial cells *in vitro. J. Dairy Sci.* **75,** 3381–3393.
11. Zavizion, B., van Duffelen, M., Schaeffer, W., and Politis, I. (1995) Use of microinjection to generate an immortalized bovine mammary cell line with both epithelial and myoepithelial characteristics. *Methods Cell Sci.* **17,** 271–282.
12. Zavizion, B., van Duffelen, M., Schaeffer, W., and Politis, I. (1996) Establishment and characterization of a bovine mammary myoepithelial cell line. *In Vitro Cell. Dev. Biol. Anim.* **32,** 149–158.

10

The Blood–CSF Barrier in Culture

Development of a Primary Culture and Transepithelial
Transport Model from Choroidal Epithelial Cells

Wei Zheng and Qiuqu Zhao

1. Introduction

The chemical stability of the central nervous system (CNS) is safeguarded by two major barrier systems that separate the systemic circulation from the cerebral compartment. Within the cerebral compartment, the interstitial fluid (ISF) flows between neurons and the cerebrospinal fluid (CSF) circulates among major brain structures and ventricles. The direct continuity of ISF and CSF allows for the free exchange of substances within the extracellular space of the cerebral compartment. Thus, the barrier that separates the systemic compartment from ISF is defined as the blood-brain barrier, while the one that discontinues the circulation between systemic and CSF compartments is named the blood-CSF barrier. The choroid plexus, located within brain ventricles, is the tissue where the blood-CSF barrier is formed *(1)*.

Under the microscope, the choroid plexus consists of three cellular layers: (*i*) the apical epithelial cells; (*ii*) the underlying supporting connective tissue; and (*iii*) the inner layer of endothelial cells. These choroidal epithelial cells have the tight junctions near their apical surface, which seal one to another. The tight junctions constitute a structural basis for the blood-CSF barrier. The barrier impedes the diffusion of water soluble small molecules, proteins, other macromolecules, and ions from the blood to the CSF. The barrier also secretes CSF, which comprises approximately 80–90% of the total CSF. Furthermore, the barrier actively participates in the regulation of the homeostasis of the cere-

From: *Methods in Molecular Biology, vol. 188: Epithelial Cell Culture Protocols*
Edited by: C. Wise © Humana Press Inc., Totowa, NJ

bral compartment. For example, the choroid plexus transports, bidirectionally between blood and CSF, a variety of amino acids (e.g., glycine, L-alanine), hormones (e.g., thyroid hormones, melatonin, growth hormone), peptides (e.g., atriopeptin, vasopressin), proteins (e.g., transthyretin), and drug molecules (e.g., β-lactam antibiotics, cimetidine, benzylpenicillin) *(1,2)*.

Keeping pace with the rapid growth in blood-CSF barrier research, we have developed a primary choroidal epithelial cell culture derived from rat choroid plexus. The plexus tissues are collected from Sprague-Dawley rats, digested, and then mechanically dissociated. The cells are then cultured. Usually the yield is around $2–5 \times 10^5$ cells from pooled plexuses of 3 to 4 rats, and they have a viability of 77–85%. Two days after initial seeding, the culture medium is replaced with medium containing cis-hydroxyproline (cis-HP) for 3–5 d to control the growth of fibroblastic cells. The cells are then cultured in the normal medium without cis-HP. The cultures display a dominant polygonal type of epithelial cells, with a population doubling time of 2 to 3 d. Immunocytochemical studies using rabbit anti-rat TTR polyclonal antibody reveal a strong positive stain of transthyretin (TTR), a protein exclusively produced by the choroidal epithelia in the brain. In addition, reverse transcription polymerase chain reaction (RT-PCR) confirms the presence of specific TTR mRNA in the cultures.

We have further adapted this primary culture of choroidal epithelial cells on a freely permeable membrane sandwiched between two culture chambers. The formation of an impermeable confluent monolayer occurs within 5 d after seeding and can be verified by the presence of a steady electrical resistance across the membrane (100–180 ohm × cm^2).

This primary cell culture system and the pertinent in vitro model of the blood-CSF barrier have proven useful in studies of thyroxine transport at the blood-CSF barrier and the mechanisms of lead toxicity on CSF transthyretin *(3,4,5)* (for comments on species other than rat, see **Note 1**).

2. Materials

2.1. Coating of Culture Dishes

1. 1.0 mg/mL Mouse laminin (Sigma).
2. Hank's balanced salt solution (HBSS) (Life Technologies).
3. Transwell culture chambers, 12 mm in diameter, 0.4 μm pore size (Corning Costar).
4. 35-mm Tissue culture grade Petri dishes (Falcon).
5. Coverslips.
6. 0.1% Collagen, type I from rat tail (Sigma), diluted in distilled, deionized water.

2.2. Tissue Separation

1. Sprague-Dawley rats, both sexes, 4–6 wk old, 80–90 g (Hilltop Inc.).
2. Pentobarbital.

3. Dissection kit.
4. 75% Ethanol.
5. Phosphate-buffered saline (PBS): to 800 mL of distilled-deionized water add 8.0 g NaCl, 0.2 g KCl, 1.44 g Na_2HPO_4, and 0.24 g KH_2PO_4. Adjust the pH to 7.4 with HCl, and bring the volume up to 1000 mL. Autoclave and store at 4°C.

2.3. Primary Cell Culture

1. Digestion solution: 4mg/mL pronase (Calbiochem-Novobiochem). Dissolve 6 mg in 1.5 mL HBSS. The solution should then be transferred to a syringe and passed through an attached 0.22-μm low-protein-binding filter unit. The final stock solution (4 mg/mL or 0.4%) should be kept on ice in the culture hood until use. This digestion solution must be made fresh on the day of experiment.
2. Low-protein-binding filter units (Millex-GV4, 0.22 μm) (Millipore).
3. 0.4% Trypan blue.
4. cis-HP (CalBiochem-Novabiochem).
5. 0.25% Trypsin, 1 mol/L EDTA (Life Technologies).

2.3.1. Growth Medium

The normal growth medium consists of three major components in Dulbecco's modified Eagle's medium (DMEM): (*i*) antibiotics to prevent infection; (*ii*) FBS to provide nutrients; and (*iii*) epidermal growth factor (EGF) to stimulate the growth of epithelia. The growth medium is normally made on the day of use.

1. DMEM (Life Technologies).
2. Antibiotic-antimycin (100×) solution (Life Technologies), which contains 10,000 U/mL penicillin, 10,000 μg/mL streptomycin, and 25 μg/mL amphotericin. Keep frozen at –20°C and thaw on the day of use.
3. FBS (Life Technologies). The solution of FBS arrives in a frozen state. To thaw FBS, the frozen solution should be placed in a refrigerator (4°C) overnight, prior to the experiment. Warm the FBS solution in a 37°C water bath, and then inactivate by incubating at 56°C for 30 min on the day of medium preparation. Inactivated FBS is now commercially available from Life Technologies.
4. 0.1 mg/mL Mouse EGF (Life Technologies). This solution is delivered in a package of 0.1 mg EGF/mL in a vial. Upon arrival, the stock solution should be dispensed into 100-μL aliquots and stored at –20°C until use. The solution is stable for at least 3 mo.

To 450 mL of DMEM, add stock individual solutions in sequence to yield a total volume of 500 mL.

Volume of Stock Solution	Final Concentration
5 mL of antibiotic-antimycin (100×)	100 U/mL penicillin
	100 μg/mL streptomycin
	0.25 μg/mL amphotericin
50 μL of EGF (0.1 mg/mL)	10 ng/mL EGF
50 mL of inactivated FBS	10% FBS

FBS is usually added into the medium immediately before use. The unused medium can be stored at 4°C for the next medium change.

2.3.2. Serum-Free Culture Medium

Some experiments require the use of serum-free culture medium.

1. Insulin-transferrin-sodium selenite medium supplement (25 mg/mL, 25 mg/mL, 25 µg/mL stock) (Sigma).
2. Fibroblast growth factor (FGF), from bovine pituitary glands (10 µg/vial) (Sigma).

To prepare total 500 mL medium, the following stock solutions should be added in sequence to 494 mL of DMEM:

Volume of Stock Solution	Final Concentration
5 mL of antibiotic-antimycin (100×)	100 U/mL penicillin
	100 µg/mL streptomycin
	0.25 µg/mL amphotericin
50 µL of EGF (0.1 mg/mL)	10 ng/mL EGF
1 mL of 2.5 mg/mL insulin,	5 µg/mL insulin
2.5 mg/mL transferrin, and	5 µg/mL transferrin
2.5 µg/mL sodium selenite	5 ng/mL sodium selenite
25 µL of FGF (10 µg/mL)	5 ng/mL FGF

Store the serum-free medium at 4°C.

2.4. Two-Chamber Transepithelial Model

1. Epithelial voltohmmeter (model EVOM) (World Precision Instruments, Sarasota, FL).

2.5. Immunocytochemical Studies

Purified rat plasma TTR and specific rabbit anti-rat TTR polyclonal antibody were the gifts of Dr. W. Blaner at the Institute of Human Nutrition, Columbia University.

1. 4% Paraformaldehyde in PBS.
2. 0.05% Tween-20 in PBS.
3. 1:1250 Rabbit anti-rat TTR antibody, diluted in PBS.
4. 1:200 Biotinylated goat anti-rabbit antibody (Vector Laboratories), diluted in PBS.
5. ABC Reagent (Vectastain®) (Vector Laboratories).
6. Fluorescein-conjugated goat anti-rabbit antibody (Amersham).
7. Microscope with fluorscein isothiocyanate (FITC) and phase contrast optics.

2.6. RT-PCR

1. RNAzol B RNA isolation solvent (Tel-Test, Newark, NJ).
2. RNA PCR core kit, including murine leukemia virus (MuLv) reverse transcriptase *Taq* DNA polymerase, and random hexamers (Perkin-Elmer).

3. DNase I (Rnase-free) from bovine pancreas (Sigma).
4. Isopropanol (Sigma).
5. Diethylpyrocarbonate (DEPC) (Sigma).
6. Chloroform.
7. Ethanol.
8. Primers specifically selected for rat TTR (synthesized by Keystone).
9. RT buffer: 10 mM Tris-HCl (pH 8.3), 50 mM KCl, 5 mM MgCl$_2$, 1 mM each dATP, dTTP, dCTP, and dGTP, and 20 U of RNase inhibitor (GeneAmp).
10. 0.15 µM specific oligonucleotide pairs
11. PCR buffer: 10 mM Tris-HCl (pH 8.3), 50 mM KCl, and 2 mM MgCl$_2$.
12. DEPC-treated Rnase-free solution: 10 mM Tris (pH 8.0), 1 mM EDTA, and 20 mM NaCl in DEPC-treated water, which is prepared by adding 1 mL of DEPC to 1000 mL of distilled, deionized water, standing overnight, and autoclaving prior to use.

3. Method
3.1. Coating of Culture Dishes.

Laminin is the major glycoprotein component of basement membranes and functions to facilitate cell attachment, spreading, and growth *(6)*. Collagen is much less expensive than laminin, but still as effective for cell attachment.

1. To coat dishes or membranes of Transwell inner chambers with laminin, dilute the stock laminin solution (1 mg/mL) 1:10 with HBSS.
2. Add an aliquot (100 µL) of diluted laminin solution to 35-mm dishes or Transwell inserts. Swirl the dishes or inserts to ensure an even distribution of the coating solution.
3. Incubate at room temperature in a culture hood for 10 min.
4. Remove the excess fluid and allow to air-dry in the hood for at least 1 h prior to cell seeding.
5. To coat dishes with collagen, dilute collagen with distilled-deionized water to obtain the working concentration of 0.01%.
6. Apply 0.8 mL of this solution to a 35-mm dish. This is approx 6–10 µg/cm^2, since the dish is about 9.6 cm^2.
7. Place the dish in the culture hood at room temperature for 4 to 5 h.
8. Remove excess fluid and allow the coated dishes air-dry in the hood overnight.
9. Be careful to avoid contamination during the coating process.

3.2. Tissue Separation

Fig. 1 illustrates the flowchart of the procedures pertaining to primary culture of choroidal epithelial cells.

1. Anesthetize the rats with an i.p. injection of 30 mg/kg pentobarbital.
2. To minimize the amount of blood present in choroid plexus tissues, draw as much blood as possible from the inferior vena cava using a syringe.

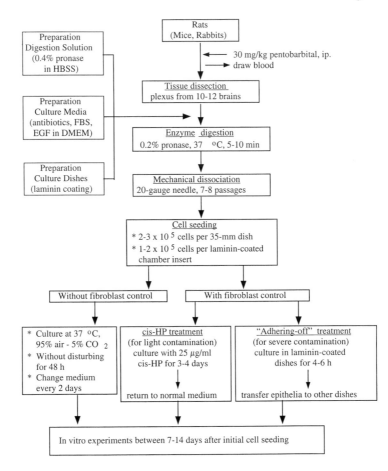

Fig. 1. Flowchart of the procedures in establishing primary culture of choroidal epithelial cells.

3. Remove the hair on the back of the head with a pair of scissors.
4. Sterilize the exposed skin using cotton wool saturated with 75% ethanol.
5. Remove the brain from the skull and place in a beaker containing PBS on ice, to chill the tissues, and wash off excess blood.
6. When you have a pool of 5–8 brains, place into the culture hood for dissection of the choroid plexus.
7. Dissect the choroid plexuses from both the lateral and third ventricles and immerse in 2 mL of HBSS.
8. After tissues have been collected from 10–15 brains, rinse the pool of choroid plexuses in HBSS, and transfer to another beaker containing 0.5 mL of HBSS.
9. Mince the plexus tissues with fine ophthalmologic scissors, so that they are about 1-mm cubes.

10. Bring the total volume up to 1 mL.

3.3. Primary Cell Culture

3.3.1. Tissue Digestion

1. Add 1 mL of digestion solution to the beaker, to give a final pronase concentration of 0.2%.
2. Shake the beaker lightly by hand to allow a complete mixing of the digestion solution with tissues.
3. Incubate at 37°C for 5–10 min.
4. Stop the digestion reaction by adding 4 mL of HBSS solution to the digestion mixture (*see* **Note 2**).
5. Centrifuge at 800g for 5 min, and then decant the supernatant, which contains primarily nonepithelial cells.
6. Wash the pellet, which consists of cell clumps of primary epithelial cells (probably joined by tight junctions), in 4 mL of HBSS.
7. Resuspend in 4 mL of growth medium.
8. Mechanically dissociate the cells by 7 to 8 forced passages through a 20-gauge needle (*see* **Note 2**).
9. Remove an aliquot (0.1 mL) of cell suspension and mix with 0.1 mL of 0.4% Trypan blue to count cell numbers and to assess the viability.
10. The procedure for cell isolation described here yields around $0.8–1 \times 10^5$ epithelial cells per rat.

3.3.2. Culture of Epithelial Cells

1. Prior to cell seeding, dilute the cell preparations with growth medium to approx $1–2 \times 10^5$ cells/mL (*see* **Note 3**).
2. Plate the cells onto 35-mm coated Petri dishes (2 to 3×10^5 cells per dish) and culture in a humidified incubator with 95% air/5% CO_2 at 37°C.
3. Leave the cultures undisturbed for at least 48 h following initial seeding, to ensure a good cell attachment.
4. Change the medium every 2 d thereafter for the duration of the culture.
5. Two days after initial seeding, remove the culture medium, and replace with fresh medium containing 25 µg/mL of cis-HP to control fibroblast contamination (*see* **Note 4**).
6. Usually the treatment with cis-HP suffices for the purpose of inhibition of the growth of fibroblasts. Typical microphotographs of cultured choroidal epithelia under phase contrast microscope are presented in **Fig. 2**.
7. After 3–5 d culture with cis-HP, return the cells to normal growth medium without cis-HP, providing that there are no visible fibroblasts under the microscope.
8. From our own experience, if the digestion procedure works well, the epithelia usually attaches and grows rapidly. Therefore, the treatment with cis-HP may not be necessary.

A

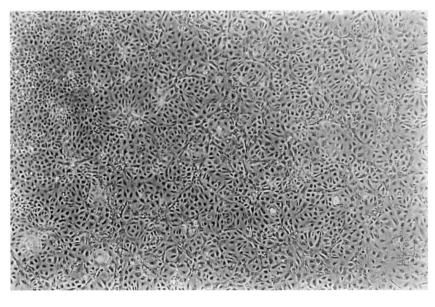

B

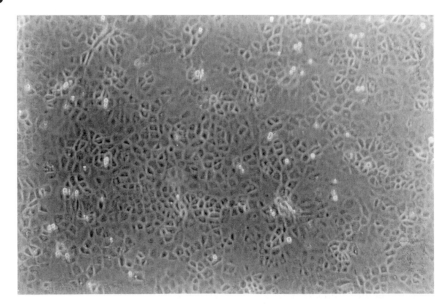

Fig. 2. Primary culture of choroidal epithelial cells after 7 d in culture: (**A**) ×40, (**B**) ×100. Note the confluent layer of the cells with predominant polygonal cell type. The choroid plexuses were obtained from 5-wk-old Sprague-Dawley rats.

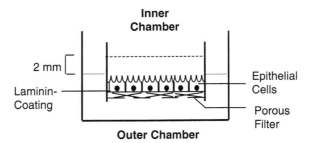

Fig. 3. Transepithelial model of blood-CSF barrier used to study transepithelial transport. Epithelial cells are connected by tight junctions and form a barrier between fluids in the inner and outer chambers. Fluid in the inner chamber is in contact with the apical surface of the cells, while the fluid in the outer chamber has access to the basal surface of the cells.

9. If the choroid plexus tissues are harvested from older animals, e.g., >4–6 mo old, the contamination of the culture with fibroblasts can sometimes become a serious problem. A method of "fibroblast adhering-off" should be used to deal with this problem.
10. Initially, seed the cell preparation onto laminin-coated dishes.
11. Six hours after seeding, transfer the culture medium containing the majority of unattached epithelial cells to another dish, to continue epithelial culture.
12. This treatment effectively leaves fibroblasts behind in the laminin-coated dishes, because fibroblasts usually attach to the laminin-coated surface much faster (4- to 6-h incubation) than the epithelial cells (16–24 h).
13. To detach the cells for bioassays, incubate the culture with trypsin-EDTA in PBS at 37°C for 10 min.
14. Harvest the cells, centrifuge, and wash. They can then be used for further studies.

3.4. Two-Chamber Transepithelial Model

1. The procedure for preparation of epithelial suspension is the same as described in **Subheading 3.3.**
2. Prior to seeding the cells in Transwell inner chambers (inserts), coat the permeable membranes attached to the inserts with laminin as described in **Subheading 3.1.** (*see* **Note 5**).
3. Plate aliquots (0.5 mL) of cell suspension onto 12-mm laminin-coated culture wells (2×10^5 cells/well).
4. Insert the inner chambers into the outer (basal) chambers, which should already contain 1 mL of growth medium (**Fig. 3**).
5. Allow cells to grow for 48 h.
6. Change the medium every 2 d thereafter.
7. The formation of confluent impermeable cell monolayers is judged by two criteria: (*i*) the height of the culture medium in the inner chamber has to be at least 2 mm higher than that in the outer chamber for at least 24 h; and (*ii*) the electrical resistance across the cell layer has to fall into the range of 100–180 ohm $\times$ cm^2.

8. Transepithelial electrical resistance can be measured using an epithelial voltohmmeter after cells have been cultured in the chambers for at least 4 d.
9. The net value of electrical resistance is calculated by subtracting the background (which is measured on laminin-coated cell-free chambers) from values of epithelial cell-seeded chambers.

3.5. Immunocytochemical Studies

A reliable method for identification of choroidal epithelial cells is visualization of TTR (*see* **Note 6**), a unique marker for choroidal epithelial cells. TTR is a 55,000-Da protein consisting of 4 identical subunits in tetrahedral symmetry. Per unit of weight, rat choroid plexus contains 10 times more TTR mRNA than liver, and per gram of tissue, synthesizes TTR 13 times faster than the liver, which is the major organ producing serum TTR *(7,8)*.

1. Culture cells that are to be stained on a laminin-coated glass coverslip for 5–7 d.
2. Fix the cells in 4% paraformaldehyde in PBS.
3. Wash 3 times with PBS.
4. Permeabilize cell monolayers by washing with 0.05% Tween-20 in PBS 3 times.
5. Incubate the cells with rabbit anti-rat TTR antiserum at room temperature for 30 min.
6. Rinse with 0.05% Tween-20 in PBS one more time to reduce the background.
7. Incubate the cultures for 30 min with biotinylated goat anti-rabbit secondary antibody.
8. Stain the cultures with ABC reagent (Vectastain®) to form avidin-biotin-horseradish peroxidase complex.
9. For immunofluorescent staining, treat the cells in the same way as described above, except that the secondary antibody should be fluorescein-conjugated goat anti-rabbit antibody.
10. Examine the cells under FITC fluorescence and phase contrast optics (**Fig. 4**).

3.6. RT-PCR Analysis

While immunohistochemical staining of TTR proteins is regarded as the best approach to identify choroidal epithelial cells, there is no anti-rat TTR antibody commercially available in the current market. Thus, one may use an alternative approach to examine the mRNA encoding TTR by using a reverse PCR technique.

1. Extract total RNA from the cultured cells or rat liver (as a positive control) according to the procedure described by Sambrook et al. *(9)* or using an RNA isolation kit (RNAzol B).
2. Homogenize cells or tissues in RNAzol B solution, followed by a chloroform extraction to remove DNA and proteins.
3. Precipitate RNA in isopropanol and wash with 75% ethanol.
4. Resuspend in DEPC-treated RNase-free solution.
5. Prior to transcription, digest RNA extracts with DNase to eliminate contaminated DNA.

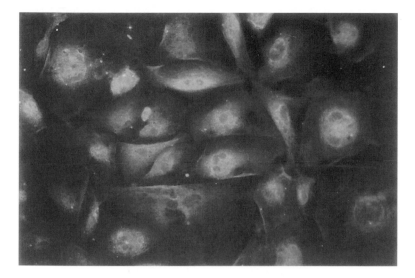

Fig. 4. Cultured choroidal epithelial cells possess cytosolic TTR by immunofluorescent staining. Cells were treated with anti-TTR primary antibody followed by secondary antibody conjugated with fluorescein. Note the positive staining in cytosol (×300).

6. Carry out the RT on 1 μg of total RNA, using MuLv reverse transcriptase with random hexamers (2.5 μmol/L) or selected antisense primer (0.75 μmol/L) in 20 μL RT buffer.
7. Carry out the reaction at 42°C for 45 min.
8. For PCR amplification, one set of specific oligonucleotide pairs should be incubated with the above reaction mixture.
9. Add 80 μL PCR buffer, containing 2.5 U *Taq* DNA polymerase, giving rise the total volume of 100 μL.
10. The cycle parameters are: 5 min at 94°C for initial denaturation, 1 min at 55°C for annealing, and 0.5 min at 72°C for extension. The subsequent cycle: 1 min at 94°C, 1 min at 55°C, and 0.5 min at 72°C for 35 cycles. Follow this with a final 5-min incubation at 72°C.
11. An aliquot (10 μL) of each reaction mixture should be analyzed by electrophoresis on 1.5% agarose gels containing 0.5 μg/mL ethidium bromide (**Fig. 5**).
12. The primers (custom-synthesized) designed by us specifically for rat TTR consist of:
    Primer sense: 5'-CCTGGGGGGTGCTGGAGAAT-3'
    Primer anti-sense: 5'-ATGGTGTAGTGGCGATGAC-3'
    This amplifies a product of 317 bp covering most of the TTR mature peptide region from rats *(7)*.

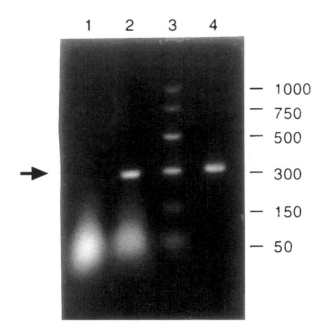

Fig. 5. Cultured choroidal epithelial cells express TTR mRNA by RT-PCR analysis. All samples underwent DNase digestion and RT-PCR unless otherwise stated. Arrow indicates bands corresponding to TTR mRNA. Lane ID: 1, cultured plexus cells, total RNA for PCR without RT; lane 2, cultured plexus cells, mRNA with selected primer; lane 3, base pair markers; and lane 4, liver, mRNA with selected primer.

4. Notes

1. Adaptability of the current protocol to plexus tissues obtained from other species. We have tried to adapt this protocol to establish the primary culture of choroidal epithelial cells derived from mice, rabbits, and dogs. The morphology, as well as the growth property, of cells from mice and rabbits shared many similarities with those from rats; however, cultures from dogs were problematic. Canine plexus cells appear to be very sensitive to pronase treatment, as few attached epithelial clusters could be seen after digestion. From the economic point of view, culturing one dish of rat plexus cells (usually requiring three rats) costs the dollar equivalent to that of rabbit (one per dish). Thus, the option as to which species is chosen is solely dependent upon the purpose of the study.

2. Isolation of epithelial cells from the choroid plexus. To ensure a high yield of epithelial cells, the digestion procedure is critical. We have tried collagenase (2 mg/mL) and pronase (2 mg/mL) to digest tissues, and found that collagenase treatment results in low cell viability and poor cell attachment. Digestion with pronase, on the other hand, effectively releases epithelial cells. However, the

duration and the concentration of pronase must be well controlled. The time for an ideal digestion varies depending upon the tissue mass. The rule of the thumb is to watch carefully the color change of the culture medium. With a complete digestion, the medium usually turns from light red to yellowish orange and from relatively transparent to cloudy. A thin layer of cell clumps will visibly smear the bottom of the beaker. Digestion with pronase should not last for over 10 min, since prolonged digestion reduces cell attachment in the later stage. It should also be noted that the activity of pronase often varies among different batches of shipment. Thus, an ideal digestion condition needs to be tested out for each shipment. The other seemingly trivial, yet absolutely important procedure, is the mechanical dissociation of the cells. The epithelial clumps after enzyme digestion normally attach to the surface of the dish; but tend to form less colonies if they are not further disintegrated. Forcing the cell preparation to pass through the needle effectively triturates the cell clumps and produces the maximal yield of epithelia, thus increasing the cell colonies and plate efficiency.

3. Density of cells for initial seeding. The healthy growth of choroidal epithelia requires a sufficient number of cells at the stage of cell seeding. When the cells are initially plated at total numbers that are less than 10^4/mL, the cell proliferation can become very slow. We recommend seeding the cells at a density of 2 to 3×10^5 cells/35-mm dish, which is about 2 mL of 1 to 2×10^5 cells/mL after digestion. The other technical detail worthy of mention pertains to the transfer of the cells from centrifuge tubes to culture dishes. The tips of glass pipets must be moistened with culture medium prior to the transfer of cells. This procedure minimizes the loss of dissociated cells, which are prone to sticking to the dry tip of a glass pipet.

4. Control of fibroblasts. One clear challenge for successful culture of choroidal epithelial cells is the control of contamination by fibroblasts. Under the light microscope, fibroblasts are typically elongated in the direction of cell stretch, and their nuclei are condensed. Fibroblasts usually spread in the space between epithelial clusters. We have tried several methods to block fibroblast growth. Initially, we attempted to exclude or reduce serum, which contains FGF, from the culture medium. By reducing the FBS to 5% of the culture medium, however, the overall growth of the culture was significantly weakened as evidenced by slow growth of epithelial cells and decreased viable cell numbers. We then experimented with a specific fibroblast inhibitor cis-HP *(10,11)*. The presence of cis-HP did inhibit the growth of fibroblasts, but it also affected the normal growth of epithelia. Our experience suggests that both the concentration of cis-HP and the time of its addition to the medium are critical. Higher concentration and earlier treatment, while most effectively inhibiting fibroblastic contamination, killed the epithelia as well. We found that the optimal condition for cis-HP treatment is to add 25 μM cis-HP to the culture medium at 48 h after initial seeding. This procedure achieves a good result with the plexus culture derived from young animals, since the young plexus tissues contain fewer fibroblasts, and their epithelia tend to tolerate cis-HP treatment. During the second week of culture, cis-HP can be withdrawn from the medium, if fibroblastic cells do not become visible under

phase contrast microscope. For the choroid plexus obtained from the older animals (4–6 mo old) or from other larger species such as dog, the fibroblast adhering-off approach proves practical in eliminating fibroblasts. This approach takes advantage of a higher affinity of fibroblasts than epithelia to collagen or laminin-coated surfaces in the early cell selection stage. A relatively complete fibroblast adhering would occur 12 h after incubation of digested cells in coated dishes. However, appreciable numbers of epithelial clusters could also attach to the coated wall during this period and, therefore, suffer loss in subsequent cell transfer procedure. Thus, the adhering treatment for 4–6 h is a reasonable approach.

5. Culture on Transwells. The procedure for culture of choroidal epithelia on Transwell membrane is the same as that used in the routine cultures, except that the cells must be seeded on a laminin-coated membrane. Cells grown on the membrane of the inner chambers display similar morphology to those observed in the culture dishes and survived for at least 2 wk. Since the epithelial cells are connected by tight junctions when they grow to a confluent monolayer, the cells actually form an impermeable barrier between the media in the inner and outer chambers. The net electrical resistance across this barrier in our study (100–180 ohm × cm^2) is comparable to those reported by others, e.g., 99 ± 15 ohm · cm^2 *(3)* and 170 ohm × cm^2 *(12)*. It is worth noting that many factors can interfere with the determination of electrical resistance, such as the difference in preparations (tissue vs cultured cells), temperature, pH (physiological solutions vs culture media), age of tissues or cultures, and the freshness of culture medium. In our own experiments, a higher pH, colder culture medium, or fresher preparation usually resulted in a higher resistance reading. We have used an 8-d culture to study thyroxine transport in this in vitro model of blood-CSF barrier and demonstrate that lead (Pb) exposure hinders the transepithelial transport of thyroxine *(4,5)*. This appears to be due to the inhibitory effect of Pb on the production and secretion of TTR by the choroid plexus *(13,14)*. Recently, we have also applied this model to study iron transport at the blood-CSF barrier (data not shown). From these studies, we observe that transepithelial transport of metal ions appears to be a rather slow process; sometimes it takes more than 24 h to reach equilibrium. A short time course of the study would probably fail to reveal the steady state transport of substances across the blood-CSF barrier. Thus, caution must be taken to allow for sufficient time for the substances to reach steady-state equilibrium.

6. Characterization of choroidal epithelial cells. Immunohistochemical staining with anti-TTR antibody is the most reliable method to distinguish choroidal epithelia from the cells of other origins, since TTR has been repeatedly demonstrated to present exclusively in the choroidal epithelia in the brain *(15,16)*. Because of the lack of commercial TTR antibody, the reverse PCR to examine TTR mRNA seems to be an indispensable checkmark for the choroidal epithelia. The sequence of TTR mRNA was originally reported by Dickson et al. *(7)*. We have designed the primer set for the purpose of RT-PCR of TTR mRNA from rat. The method presented in this article exhibits a good consistency in our cultured cells, freshly isolated choroid plexus tissues, and liver cytosolic preparations. In summary, the

establishment of choroidal epithelial cell culture has been described in the literature for cells from various sources, including mouse *(17,18)*, rat *(18–20)*, rabbit *(6)*, sheep *(21)*, and cow *(10,22)*. Some have the advantages over others. We describe here a simple and reproducible method to culture epithelial cells derived from rat, mouse, and rabbit. The cultures possess relatively uniform epithelial cell type with minor contamination from fibroblasts. The epithelial cells grown on a Transwell device form a confluent epithelial barrier between two compartments. This in vitro culture system is useful in studying physiology, biochemistry, pharmacology, and toxicology of blood-CSF barrier.

Acknowledgments

The authors gratefully acknowledge the gift of rat TTR antibody from Dr. William S. Blaner in the Institute of Human Nutrition, Columbia University. This research was supported in part by National Institute of Environmental Health Sciences Grant Nos. RO1 ES-07042 and RO1 ES-08146.

References

1. Zheng, W. (2001) Toxicology of choroid plexus: special reference to metal-induced neurotoxicities. *Microsc. Res. Tech.*, **52**, 89–103.
2. Zheng, W. (1996) The choroid plexus and metal toxicities, p. 609–626. In *Toxicology of metals* (Chang, L. W., Magos, L., and Suzuki, T., eds.), CRC Press, New York.
3. Southwell, B. R., Duan, W., Alcorn, D., Brack, C., Richardson, S., Kohrle, J., and Schreiber, G. (1993) Thyroxine transport to the brain: role of protein synthesis by the choroid plexus. *Endocrinology* **133**, 2116–2126.
4. Zheng, W., Zhao, Q., and Graziano, J. H. (1998) Primary culture of rat choroidal epithelial cells: a model for in vitro study of the blood-cerebrospinal fluid barrier. *In Vitro Cell. Biol. Dev.* **34**, 40–45.
5. Zheng, W., Blaner, W. S., and Zhao, Q. (1999) Inhibition by Pb of production and secretion of transthyretin in the choroid plexus: its relationship to thyroxine transport at the blood-CSF barrier. *Toxicol. Appl. Pharmacol.* **155**, 24–31.
6. Mayer, S. E. and Sanders-Bush, E. (1993) Sodium-dependent antiporters in choroid plexus epithelial cultures from rabbit. *J. Neurochem.* **60**, 1304–1316.
7. Dickson, P. W., Howlett, G. J., and Schreiber, G. (1985) Rat transthyretin (prealbumin): molecular cloning, nucleotide sequence, and gene expression in liver and brain. *J. Biol. Chem.* **260**, 8214–8219.
8. Schreiber, G., Aldred, A. R., Jaworowski, A., Nilsson, C., Achen, M. G., and Segal, M. B. (1990) Thyroxine transport from blood to brain via transthyretin synthesis in choroid plexus. *Am. J. Physiol.* **258**, R338–R345.
9. Sambrook, J., Fritsch, E. F., and Maniatis, T. (eds.) (1989) *Molecular cloning,* p. 7.6–7.11. CSH Laboratory Press, Cold Spring Harbor, NY.
10. Crook, R. B., Kasagami, H., and Prusiner, S. B. (1981) Culture and characterization of epithelial cells from bovine choroid plexus. *J. Neurochem.* **37**, 845–854.

11. Kao, W. and Prokop, D. (1977) Proline analogue removes fibroblasts from cultured mixed cell population. *Science* **266,** 63–64.
12. Saito, Y. and Wright, E. M. (1983) Bicarbonate transport across the frog choroid plexus and its control by cyclic nucleotides. *J. Physiol.* **336,** 635–648.
13. Zheng, W., Perry, D. F., Nelson, D. L., and Aposhian, H. V. (1991) Protection of cerebrospinal fluid against toxic metals by the choroid plexus. *FASEB J.* **5,** 2188–2193.
14. Zheng, W., Shen, H., Blaner, S. B., Zhao, Q., Ren, X., and Graziano, J. H. (1996) Chronic lead exposure alters transthyretin concentration in rat cerebrospinal fluid: the role of the choroid plexus. *Toxicol. Appl. Pharmacol.* **139,** 445–450.
15. Aldred, A. R., Brack, C. M., and Schreiber, G. (1995) The cerebral expression of plasma protein genes in different species. *Comp. Biochem. Physiol.* **111B,** 1–15.
16. Herbert, J., Wilcox, J. N., Pham, K. C., et al. (1986) Transthyretin: a choroid plexus-specific transport protein in human brain. *Neurology* **36,** 900–911.
17. Bouille, C., Mesnil, M., Barriere, H., and Gabrion, J. (1991) Gap junctional intercellular communication between cultured ependymal cells, revealed by Lucifer yellow CH transfer and freeze-fracture. *Glia* **4,** 25–36.
18. Peraldi-Roux, S., Nguyen-Than Dao, B., Hirn, M., and Gabrion, J. (1990) Choroidal ependymocytes in culture: expression of markers of polarity and function. *Int. J. Dev. Neurosci.* **8,** 575–588.
19. Strazielle, N., and Ghersi-Egea, J. F. (1999) Demonstration of a coupled metabolism-efflux process at the choroid plexus as a mechanism of brain protection toward xenobiotics. *J. Neurosci.* **19,** 6275–6289.
20. Tsutsumi, M., Skinner, M. K., and Sanders-Bush, E. (1989) Transferrin gene expression and synthesis by cultured choroid plexus epithelial cells. *J. Biol. Chem.* **264,** 9626–9631.
21. Harter, D. H., Hsu, K. C., and Rose, H. M. (1967) Immunofluorescence and cytochemical studies of visna virus in cell culture. *J. Virol.* **1,** 1265–1270.
22. Whittico, M. T., Hui, A. C., and Giacomini, K. M. (1991) Preparation of brush border membrane vesicles from bovine choroid plexus. *J. Pharmacol. Methods* **25,** 215–227.

11

An In Vitro Model of Differentiated Human Airway Epithelia

Methods for Establishing Primary Cultures

Philip H. Karp, Thomas O. Moninger, S. Pary Weber, Tamara S. Nesselhauf, Janice L. Launspach, Joseph Zabner, and Michael J. Welsh

1. Introduction

1.1. The Airway Epithelium

The human airway epithelium forms a barrier between the external and internal environments, separating air from the interstitial space. However, it also serves many other functions. By active transepithelial transport of electrolytes, it controls the composition and quantity of the airway surface liquid covering the epithelium. It secretes numerous agents into the airway surface liquid, including IgA and antimicrobial factors; these form part of the defensive shield that protects the airways and lungs from infection. The activity of its cilia are key to mucociliary clearance. The epithelium participates in the inflammatory response when challenged with environmental factors or infectious agents. It responds to and produces a number of cytokines and other pro- and anti-inflammatory agents. To study and understand the complex and varied functions of human airway epithelia, investigators have developed cell culture models of the epithelium. Compared to in vivo studies, such models have the important advantage of flexibility, control of experimental conditions, and greater opportunities for intervention. They also allow the study of epithelial function in the absence of other cells and tissues such as macrophages, submucosal glands, fibroblasts, and cells of the immune system. Conversely, for some studies, the presence of nonepithelial cells and tissues would be advantageous.

From: *Methods in Molecular Biology, vol. 188: Epithelial Cell Culture Protocols*
Edited by: C. Wise © Humana Press Inc., Totowa, NJ

Importantly, in some cases, these other cell types can be added back to the epithelial culture system.

The surface epithelium lining the large human airways is pseudo-stratified; that is, all cells extend to the basement membrane, but not all cells extend to the luminal surface. Three of the most common cell types are the ciliated epithelial cells, goblet cells, and basal cells. For a description of cell types and morphology see Wheater et al. *(1)*. In the more distal airways, the epithelium is not as tall, it becomes columnar, and Clara cells become prominent. The cartilaginous airways also contain submucosal glands in the connective tissue layer beneath the epithelium.

This chapter describes a protocol to harvest and develop primary cultures of differentiated human airway epithelia from donor lungs and nasal polyps and turbinates. The epithelial cells are enzymatically dissociated from the airway tissue and seeded on permeable membrane supports. The cell culture with at least three different cell types develops into a pseudo-stratified epithelium with columnar cells supported on a collagen-treated membrane. This in vitro airway culture model has polarized epithelial cells with tight junctions and distinct apical and basolateral membranes. The culture is maintained with culture medium only on the basolateral surface, and the apical surface is exposed to air. The apical membrane surface develops microvilli and cilia and a covering of mucus. Thus, this in vitro model exhibits many properties comparable to the in vivo human airway epithelium.

1.2. Morphology of Primary Cultures of Differentiated Human Airway Epithelia

The differentiated human airway epithelial cultures we describe show morphologic properties similar to those of the airways in vivo. To examine the morphology, we have employed scanning electron microscopy (SEM) and transmission electron microscopy (TEM). **Fig. 1** shows an SEM image of the apical surface of a conventionally processed primary culture of human airway epithelia. This view shows the confluent arrangement of ciliated cells (C) and microvilli-covered goblet cells (G), which is characteristic of airway epithelia in vivo.

One limitation of conventional processing methods for electron microscopy (using aqueous-based fixatives and buffers) is that, for the most part, they remove the airway surface liquid (ASL) and mucus that cover the epithelial surface. Application of as little as 10 μL of saline is sufficient to disrupt the ASL of the cultures. To examine better the overall morphology of the unaltered epithelial cultures, including the ASL, we have adopted a processing technique originally described by Thurston et al. and Sims et al. *(2,3)*. This method uses osmium tetroxide dissolved in perfluorocarbon (PFC/OsO$_4$) as the fixative and avoids all aqueous reagents. The PFC is not miscible with water and

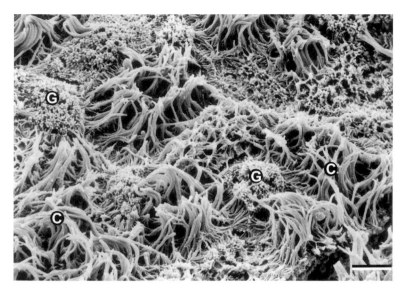

Fig. 1. Scanning electron micrograph of conventionally fixed and processed differentiated human airway epithelia grown on a semipermeable membrane filter. Visible are goblet cells (**G**) and ciliated cells (**C**). Scale bar equals 5 μm.

does not disturb the ASL, leaving the OsO_4 free to diffuse into the ASL and the cells to stabilize the morphology. The cultures are then dehydrated with several changes of 100% ethanol and either transitioned to Eponate 12 epoxy resin and embedded for TEM sectioning or transitioned to hexamethydisilizane and air-dried for SEM observation.

Fig. 2 shows a TEM cross-section of a PFC/OsO_4-processed airway epithelial culture. The morphology shows a classic pseudo-stratified epithelium, overlain by a layer of ASL as found in native human airway tissue. Identifiable cell types include basal cells (B), goblet cells (G), and ciliated cells (C). Cilia are visible within the ASL (arrowheads) some of which are in cross-section. Note the secretory granules contained within the goblet cells, with the cell on left having recently discharged much of its contents. Also visible are extensive interdigitations between the basal and adjacent cells. The 0.4-μm pores in the filter are visible at the bottom of the image.

Fig. 3 shows an SEM image of a PFC/OsO_4-processed airway epithelial culture. This side-on view shows the edge of the epithelial culture, where the membrane was cut for removal. The apical portion of the epithelial cell layer has peeled back, exposing the ruffled surface of the basal cells (B), some of which remain adherent to the filter (F). The 0.4-μm pores in the filter are also visible (arrowheads). Also note the mucus layer (M), which was not visible in **Fig. 1**. The mucus overlays the cilia (C) on the surface of the epithelium (E).

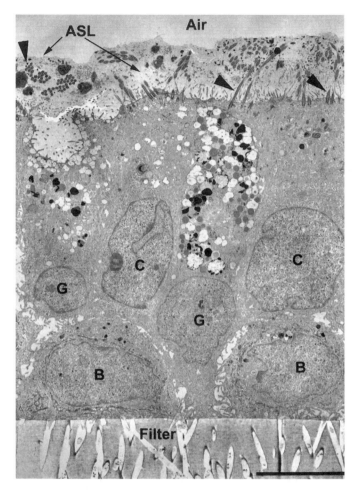

Fig. 2. Transmission electron micrograph of PFC/OsO$_4$-fixed human airway epithelia grown on a semipermeable membrane filter. Labeled structures include air, filter, ASL, cilia (arrowheads), goblet cells (**G**), basal cells (**B**), and ciliated cells (**C**). Scale bar equals 5 µm.

1.3. Applications for Primary Cultures of Differentiated Airway Epithelia

Cultures of airway epithelia have been utilized for many applications. Here we mention several.

1.3.1. Measurement of Transepithelial Electrolyte Transport

Transepithelial transport can be evaluated by using radioisotope fluxes, or the epithelia can be mounted in Ussing chambers (Jim's Instruments, Iowa

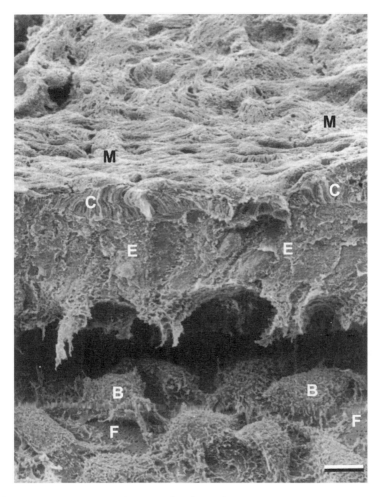

Fig. 3. Scanning electron micrograph of PFC/OsO$_4$-fixed differentiated human airway epithelia. View is from edge of filter where epithelium has separated from membrane filter. Labeled structures are filter (**F**), filter pores (arrowheads), basal cells (**B**), cilia (**C**), epithelia (**E**), and mucus layer (**M**). Scale bar equals 5 µm.

City, IA) to measure electrogenic ion transport *(4)*. **Fig. 4** shows an example of the short-circuit current measured from differentiated airway epithelia. The tracing shows the amiloride-sensitive Na$^+$ current and the cAMP-simulated cystic fibrosis transmembrane conductance regulator (CFTR)-dependent Cl$^-$ current.

1.3.2. Evaluation of Gene Transfer Using Viral And Non-Viral Vectors

Gene transfer offers the potential to be a new treatment for cystic fibrosis (CF) and other genetic and acquired diseases. However, when delivered from

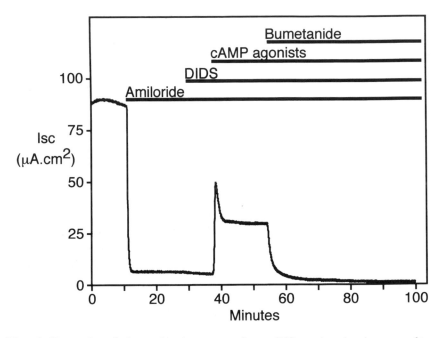

Fig. 4. Example of short-circuit current from differentiated primary culture of human airway epithelia derived from human bronchus. Tracing is from an epithelium mounted in a modified Ussing chamber, in which short-circuit current (Isc) was continuously measured (558C-5 Voltage Clamp System, University of Iowa Bioengineering, Iowa City, IA). Bars at top indicate sequential additions of the indicated compounds. Apical amiloride (100 μM) inhibits apical membrane Na^+ channels. Addition of 4,4'-diisothiocyanato-stilbene-2,2'-disulfonic acid (DIDS; 100 μM) to the apical surface inhibits Ca^{2+}-activated apical membrane Cl^- channels. The cAMP agonists forskolin (10 μM) and 3-isobutyl-2-methylxanthine (IBMX; 100 μM) leads to phosphorylation and activation of apical membrane CFTR Cl^- channels. Basolateral addition of bumetanide (100 μM) inhibits the basolateral Na^+-K^+-2Cl^- cotransporter. Epithelia were bathed in a symmetrical Ringers solution containing 135 mM NaCl, 1.2 mM $CaCl_2$, 1.2 mM $MgCl_2$, 2.4 mM K_2HPO_4, 0.6 mM KH_2PO_4, 10 mM dextrose, and 5 mM HEPES (titrated to 7.2 with 10 N NaOH). The Ussing chamber bath solution was continuously bubbled with 100% O_2.

the apical surface, most current vectors are very inefficient. Differentiated airway epithelia studied in vitro have proven to be an excellent model with which to investigate the underlying mechanisms for the inefficiency. For example, **Fig. 5** shows that the receptor for adenovirus type 2 and 5 vectors, the coxsackie-adenovirus receptor (CAR), is located on the basolateral surface of the epithelium, where it is inaccessible to apically applied vector *(5)*. The epithelia are also proving to be a very useful model for developing improved methods for gene transfer *(6)*.

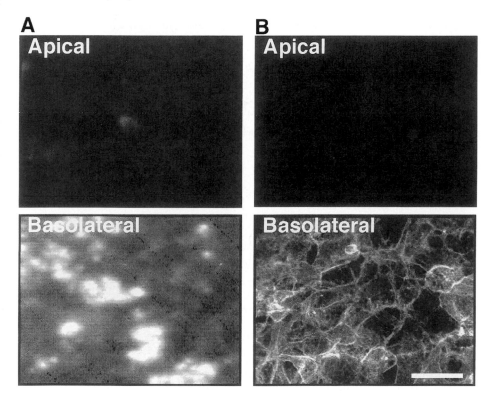

Fig. 5. Expression of the CAR and major histocompatibility complex (MHC) class I in well-differentiated human airway epithelia evaluated by immunoctyochemistry. **(A)** Immunocytochemistry of unpermeabilized epithelia incubated with monoclonal anti-CAR Ab and an fluorescein isothiocyanate (FITC)-labeled secondary antibody applied to either the apical or basolateral side. Top panel shows absence of CAR staining on the apical membrane. Bottom panel shows a low intensity staining on most cells, with higher intensity staining of a small proportion of cells. **(B)** Unpermeabilized epithelia were incubated with an FITC-labeled monoclonal anti-MHC class I antibody applied to either the apical or basolateral side. Top panel shows absence of MHC class I staining on the apical membrane. Bottom panel shows high intensity staining on all cells. Bar represents 50 μm. From **ref. 5** with permission.

1.3.3. Models for Testing and Developing Novel Pharmaceuticals

Many pharmaceuticals are delivered via the airways, often as aerosols. The epithelial cultures can provide a system with which to investigate their effect on the epithelium *(7)*. It can also be used to assess movement of agents across the epithelium to the smooth muscle, the interstitium, and ultimately the circulation. The converse is also true; the epithelium can be used to assess the movement of agents from the basolateral surface to the apical surface. An example is the use of the polymeric immunoglobulin receptor to shuttle agents from the submucosal to the mucosal surface *(8)*.

1.3.4. Models for Disease Pathogenesis

Differentiated airway epithelia provide an excellent model for studying the pathogenesis of acquired and genetic diseases. An example comes from epithelia generated with cells obtained from people with CF. Studies have shown that the epithelia generate a defense system that can kill small numbers of bacteria, and that this system is defective in CF *(9)*.

1.3.5. Models for the Interaction of Airway Epithelia with Environmental Agents

The airways are constantly being exposed to pollutants, toxic agents, and micro-organisms. Differentiated airway epithelia provide an experimentally facile model system with which to evaluate such interactions. For example, they retain receptors and cytokine signaling networks that play key roles in inflammation.

1.4. Development of Primary Cultures of Human Airway Epithelia

Here we describe the methods and techniques required to harvest and culture human airway epithelia as an in vitro model of the airway. We focus on primary cultures, because in our experience, these have proven most reliable in yielding a functional and morphological phenotype that resembles the in vivo airway epithelium. We have not been able to consistently reproduce these features with cell lines originally derived from the airways. Even after very few passages, we find that the phenotype of the cells changes. Thus, at the present time in our hands, we find that a good model system requires the effort associated with primary cultures. Of note to the investigator studying airway epithelia, epithelia like those we describe here can be extremely useful when it is necessary to have a model that mimics airway epithelia. However, some experiments do not require such a model. When that is the case, there are other cells and approaches that may suffice with less work and expense.

The methods and procedures we describe here were adapted and modified from those originally reported in 1992 by M. Yamaya et al. *(10)*. Thus, we owe them a debt of gratitude for their original work. The culture methods have been progressively modified to provide a high volume cell harvest that requires a reduced time investment and provides differentiated airway epithelia that remain viable for months. The adaptations have also enhanced the transepithelial transport properties of this culture method. We view the development of these cultured epithelia as both a science and an art. It is a science for standardization purposes. It is an art because people vary in their technique, experience, and judgment, which produces adequate to excellent cultures. Moreover, the cell culture protocols we describe are a "work in progress". Future research will further improve the methods we describe here. We recommend that a person culturing these epithelia be willing to test a new media supplement, attachment substrate, or membrane support. When doing so, compare the culture results with the standard procedures.

2. Materials

1. Dulbecco's phosphate-buffered saline (PBS), Ca^{2+}- and Mg^{2+}-free (Sigma, cat. no. D5773). Store chilled stock at 4°C for rinsing surgical specimens. Store another stock at room temperature for rinsing Millicell membrane inserts.
2. Dulbecco's PBS with Ca^{2+} and Mg^{2+} (Sigma, cat. no. D5780). Keep chilled at 4°C for transporting surgical specimens.
3. Dissection kit:

   a. Pair of medium size straight edge dissecting scissors.
   b. Tissue forceps, which have jaws with fine teeth (Graefe Tissue Forceps, Biomedical Research Instruments, Rockville, MD, cat. no. 30-1680).
   c. Plasticware pan with a plastic liner, to keep the lung chilled on wet ice and to contain spills during dissection.

4. Minimal essential medium (MEM), Ca^{2+}- and Mg^{2+}-free dissociation solution. This solution is made from scratch and contains (per liter deionized water): 400 mg KCl, 6400 mg NaCl, 3700 mg $NaHCO_3$, 125 mg $NaHPO_4 \cdot H_2O$, 15 mg phenol red, 110 mg sodium pyruvate, 100,000 U penicillin, and 100,000 µg streptomycin. The pH of the solution is adjusted to 7.5 in room air with a few drops of concentrated HCl. Then it is filter-sterilized with a 0.22-µm membrane filter unit using vacuum. This solution can be stored for months at 4°C.
5. Dissociation enzyme solution. The two enzymes used in the dissociation solution are Pronase (Roche/Boehringer Mannheim, cat. no. 165921), which should be stored dry at 4°C and deoxyribronuclease 1 (Sigma, cat. no. DN-25), which should be stored dry at less than 0°C. For 100 mL, dissolve 140 mg pronase and 10 mg DNase in 100 mL MEM.
6. Fetal bovine serum (FBS) (Hyclone, cat. no. SH30070.03). It is not necessary to heat-inactivate the serum to remove complement. Moreover, it is preferable not to heat-inactivate the serum so as not to affect the potency of nutrient factors in the serum. Filter-sterilize the serum with a 0.22-µm filter unit to remove precipitate. Store at 4°C.
7. Dulbecco's modified eagle's medium (DMEM), high glucose (Life Technologies, cat. no. 12800082). Store at 4°C.
8. Ham's F-12 nutrient mixture (Life Technologies, cat. no. 21700091). Store at 4°C.
9. Ultroser G supplement, a serum substitute (Biosepra SA, Cergy-Saint-Christophe, France, cat. nos. 259516 or 259515, USA distributor Crescent Chemical Co., Inc. Islandia, NY 11749). Store at 4°C. (A USDA import permit is required for USA import. The VS Form 16-3 application can be downloaded from web site: http://www.aphis.usda.gov/NCIE/).

10. Airway medium 1: this medium is for cell seeding and the first culture day only. It is composed of a 1:1 ratio of DMEM and Hams F-12 supplemented with 5% FBS (not heat-inactivated) and 1% MEM nonessential amino acids solution (Life Technologies, cat. no. 11140-050).

11. Airway medium 2: this medium is for use after culture d 1 and then continuously. It consists of a 1:1 ratio of DMEM and Ham's F-12 supplemented with 2% Ultroser G.

12. Freezing medium: 40% FBS, 50% airway medium 1, and 10% dimethyl sulfoxide (DMSO).

13. Culture antibiotics: we routinely add penicillin (100 U/mL) and streptomycin (100 µg/mL) (Life Technologies, cat. no. 15140-122), gentamycin (50 µg/mL) (Life Technologies, cat. no. 15750-060), fluconazole (2 µg/mL) (Diflucon; Pfizer), and amphotericin B (1.25 µg/mL) (Sigma, cat. no. A9528) to the two airway medias. The concentrations of antibiotics may be reduced, or the number of antibiotics reduced or eliminated after a few days in culture. For long-term maintenance of cultures, the combination of fluconazole and amphotercin B is especially effective in preventing or keeping in check yeast infection. For airway cultures from CF epithelia, we use additional antibiotics for the first 5 to 6 d of culture. The antibiotics are: 77 µg/mL ceftazidime (Fortaz; GlaxoWellcome), 2.5 µg/mL colistin (Coly-Mycin; Monarch Pharmaceuticals), and 12.5 µg/mL imipenem and cilastin (Primaxin; Merck). Culturing longer with the imipenem and cilastin will injure the epithelial cells.

14. Culture surface substrate for attachment and proliferation.
    a. 60 µg/mL Collagen type VI from human placenta, acid soluble (Sigma, cat. no. C-7521). Store dry at less than 0°C until reconstitution. We routinely use this collagen as the preferred attachment factor for permeable membrane supports and plastic surfaces. We prescreen, in a small quantity, multiple available lots of the Sigma collagen because an occasional lot gives poor culture results on the membrane supports. We will then order a sizable quantity of a desired collagen lot and store it at −20°C for up to 18 mo.
    b. Optional substrate: Vitrogen 100, bovine dermal collagen (Cohesion Technologies, Palo Alto, CA, cat. no. 0701). Prepare according to manufacturer's instructions. This substrate forms a gel surface support on the permeable membrane support.

15. Optional use: 100 ng/mL keratinocyte growth factor (R & D Systems, cat. no. 251KG-010).

16. Permeable membrane supports for culture of epithelia.
    a. Millicell-PCF membrane inserts, 0.4 µm pore size, 12 mm diameter (Millipore cat. no. PIHP 01250). Millipore also makes the same PCF membrane insert with a 30 mm diameter (cat. no. PIHP 03050).
    b. Optional use. A transparent membrane in a culture plate insert can be used as an alternative: Costar Transwell-Clear, 0.4 µm pore size, 6.5 mm diameter (Costar, cat. no. 3470). Costar makes the same clear Transwell membrane with a 12 mm diameter size (cat. no. 3460); our experience has been that different lots vary in terms of their ability to support successful cultures.

17. Falcon Primaria tissue culture dish 100 × 20 mm (Becton Dickinson Labware, cat. no. 353803). Harvested cells are incubated on this plastic surface to remove fibroblasts prior to seeding cells on the permeable membrane supports.
18. Costar 24-well cell culture cluster dishes (Costar, cat. no. 3524). We prefer the Costar brand for uniform distribution of CO_2 to all Millicell inserts in the 24-well cluster dish.
19. Sterile 50- and 15-mL polypropylene conical tubes with screwcaps (Falcon, cat. nos. 352098 and 352097).
20. 150 × 75 mm Crystallizing dish (Fisher Scientific, cat. no. 08-762-9).
21. Hemacytometer counting chamber (Fisher Scientific, cat. no. 02-671-5).
22. Recommended optional equipment for measuring transepithelial resistance of airway epithelia grown on permeable membrane supports is a Millicell-ERS Voltohmmeter (Millipore MERS, cat. no. 00001). Epithelial integrity can be quantitatively assessed with a portable instrument without compromising sterility or damaging the cells on the membrane.

3. Methods

3.1. Preparation and Dissection of Human Airway Tissue

Excellent viability of suitable human airway tissue is critical for the successful harvesting of epithelial cells and their subsequent culturing as polarized epithelia (*see* **Note 1**). We routinely use human donor lungs, but also use nasal polyps and turbinates as fresh specimens. Immediately after surgical removal, specimens should be chilled in either sterile cold physiologic saline, PBS with Ca^{2+} and Mg^{2+}, or DMEM, and then transported in sealed containers on wet ice to the laboratory. Specimens should remain chilled during dissection.

1. For ideal aseptic and safety conditions, the dissection is best done in a laminar flow hood. The person should always wear sterile gloves. Handling human tissue and primary airway cultures may expose the user to bloodborne pathogens; suitable health protection measures should be followed.
2. Transfer all dissected tissue segments directly to 50- or 15-mL sterile polypropylene tubes for convenient processing and storage.
3. Rinse intact nasal polyps and turbinates in chilled sterile Ca^{2+}- and Mg^{2+}-free PBS (antibiotics are optional) in 50- or 15-mL sterile tubes to remove blood, mucus, and debris.
4. If necessary, the nasal tissue specimens can be picked apart from attached mucus and fibrous tissue in a sterile Petri dish. PBS rinsing may be required several times to remove blood clots.
5. Transfer the specimen to sterile 50- or 15-mL tubes containing the dissociation enzymes in chilled Ca^{2+}- and Mg^{2+}-free dissociation solution. The solution without divalent cations facilitates dissociation of cells.
6. Airway tissue from the lung includes the attached trachea, the main stem bronchi, and the lobar bronchi, which divide repeatedly in the pulmonary lobe. We dissect bronchial segments down to the third segmentation (*see* **Note 2**).

7. Intact segments of the trachea and bronchi (containing the epithelium, smooth muscle, and cartilage) should be separated from extraneous connective tissue using scissors and cut into longitudinal 2–4 cm sections. Segments of smaller diameter bronchi are cut longitudinally to maximize lumen exposure.
8. Place the segments in polypropylene tubes with cold DMEM.
9. Rinse with Ca^{2+}- and Mg^{2+}-free PBS multiple times to remove blood, mucus, and purulent material from the lumen.
10. Airway segments can be immersed in cold Ca^{2+}- and Mg^{2+}-free PBS for 1 h to help remove blood clots. The segments can then be transferred to new 50- or 15-mL polypropylene tubes containing the chilled dissociation solution.
11. Segregate segments in different tubes according to airway region and lobe, because of possible variation in viability of the epithelium in the different branches of the airway.
12. It is important to prevent warm and cold temperature changes of airway specimens during processing to prevent epithelial degradation.

3.2. Dissociation and Harvesting

1. On the day of use, prepare the dissociation solution by dissolving the two enzymes, pronase and deoxyribronuclease, in the previously prepared stock of Ca^{2+}- and Mg^{2+}-free MEM (*see* **Subheading 2., step 4.**). In the MEM solution, dissolve 140 mg pronase and 10 mg DNase per 100 mL. Stir to dissolve enzymes and then saturate the solution with 5% CO_2 in either air or 95% O_2 to provide an optimal pH. We use a line from the gas cylinder to bubble the solution for several minutes in a beaker covered with parafilm. Then sterilize the solution with a 0.22-μm filter and transfer to new sterile 50- or 15-mL polypropylene tubes.
2. Store the dissected airway specimens in the tubes with the enzyme dissociation solution at 4°C for 24–96 h. Occasionally invert tubes during dissociation to agitate and break apart cell clumps.
3. Nasal specimens can be dissociated for 24–48 h. Trachea and bronchus tissue require a minimum of 40 h to a maximum 96 h. The time for dissociation depends on the desired degree of separation into single cell vs cell clumps (*see* **Note 3**).
4. Aliquots can be examined with a microscope on a glass slide to assess the degree of clumping over time.
5. To end dissociation, add 10% (v/v) FBS to the dissociation solution. Invert the tube(s) several times to agitate the cell suspension.
6. Transfer the harvested cell suspension to new polypropylene tubes with a pipet.
7. Rinse tissue segments with chilled sterile DMEM or Hams F-12 to collect additional cells.
8. Centrifuge the cell suspension at 120g for 5 min.
9. Resuspend the cell pellet in airway media 1 (5% fetal calf serum [FCS]) with antibiotics at 37°C. Gently break apart the cell pellet by pipeting with a sterile short stem Pasteur pipet. Be careful not to pipet too vigorously. The harvested cell suspension will consist of single cell and multiple-cell clumps.
10. Transfer the cell suspension by pipet to Primaria tissue culture dishes. A cell strainer is optional to filter large clumps and tissue debris (*see* **Note 4**).

11. Incubate the suspension in a CO_2 incubator at 37°C for a minimum of 1 h or longer. This incubation allows fibroblasts within the cell suspension to attach to the plastic surface. Airway epithelial cells will not attach to the plastic surface without collagen pretreatment. We have found that the Falcon Primaria tissue culture plastic works best for enhanced fibroblast cell attachment. The numbers of fibroblasts in the airway cell suspension varies with different lung specimens. Occasionally, a specimen yields densely attached fibroblasts so that a second incubation with a new Primaria dish is required. If too many fibroblasts are present in the seeded suspension, and they attach with the epithelial cells to the permeable membrane support, the fibroblasts will prevent the cells from forming an intact epithelium with a good transepithelial resistance, because there will be intermixed colonies of fibroblasts that do not form tight junctions.

12. Total epithelial cell yield will vary depending upon tissue viability and size. An adult lung with trachea and 2 to 3 generations of bronchi will yield in the range of 5×10^7 to 2×10^8 epithelial cells.

3.3. Substrate Preparation

Primary human airway epithelial cells will not attach to the Millicell membranes without surface pretreatment. We coat the top of the Millipore PCF membrane insert with a solution of human placental collagen (60 µg/mL) for a minimum of 18 h. The collagen solution can be stored on the membrane supports (12 mm diameter) for several days in 24-well cluster dishes at room temperature.

1. Use a ratio of 30 mg collagen with 50 mL deionized water and 100 µL glacial acetic acid.

2. Cover the holding beaker with parafilm and stir moderately at about 37°C until collagen strands are dissolved. We use a crystallizing dish containing warm (up to 37°C, changed approx every 5 min) tap water as a make-shift water bath and place it on a magnetic stirrer. The time required for the collagen to dissolve varies significantly. Fifteen to twenty minutes is usually sufficient.

3. Dilute the filtered collagen stock 1:10 with deionized sterile water. This diluted collagen stock (60 µg/mL) is the working solution for coating plastic and membrane surfaces. The working collagen stock can be stored in a glass bottle at 4°C for several weeks.

4. Filter-sterilize with a 0.2-µm membrane. If the filter membrane quickly plugs, the collagen strands have not fully dissolved.

5. Collagen-coat the surface of the membrane for a minimum of 18 h at room temperature. The collagen improves cell attachment efficiency and proliferation. Shorter times may work in an emergency. The liquid collagen can remain at room temperature on the membrane for several days.

6. On the day of cell seeding, remove the liquid collagen from surface and air-dry the membrane surface.

7. Rinse at least twice with sterile PBS or DMEM on both sides of membrane support. It is important to remove all trace of the liquid collagen. Residual liquid collagen can be toxic to cells.

8. An alternative substrate is a Vitrogen gel, which is prepared on top of the membrane before seeding. This substrate has advantages and disadvantages. One advantage is that the columnar cells appear taller. One disadvantage is that it is more difficult to work with and maintain stable airway cultures because the gel is fragile (*see* **Note 5**).

3.4. Seeding Cells on the Membrane

1. After collecting the nonattached cell suspension from the incubation dish in airway medium 1 (5% FCS), the cells are counted to determine cell density.
2. We recommend manual counting with a hemacytometer counting chamber and viewing the cell suspension under a microscope. By looking under higher magnification (400×) at an aliquot from the cell suspension, one can make judgements about the viability and homogeneity of the airway epithelia cells. The hemacytometer count will underestimate the number of cells if there are sizable cell clumps present in suspension; the cover glass prevents large clumps uniformly covering the grid area. A complementary approach is to also use an aliquot thinly smeared onto a glass slide; this allows viewing of the representative degree of clumping in the cell suspension. We include a "fudge factor" for larger clumps when calculating cell suspension density. The greater the degree of clumping, the lower the calculated seeding volume derived from the hemacytometer count. The cell suspension may be heterogeneous, ranging from single cells to multiple-cell clumps. There may occasionally be other nonepithelial cells in the suspension, including red blood cells.
3. Follow the instructions of the hemacytometer manufacturer. Count at 400× magnification only the epithelial cells that have a distinctly dark cell membrane appearance and that are noncolumnar in shape. Cells that are pale in appearance, cells with a broken cell membrane, or cells that appear empty are not counted. Nonmotile ciliated cells are also not counted. Smaller cells that have a halo appearance are red blood cells and are not counted. Estimate the number of cells per clump and include that in the total cell count.
4. Our experience with using the Trypan blue exclusion assay with the primary cultures of human airway epithelial cells is that it is inadequate for assaying nonviable cells. Except when counting viable cells thawed from cryostock, we recommend not depending upon the dye assay for an accurate determination of cell viability.
5. It is best to try a range of seeding densities based upon your manual count method until you are comfortable with the accuracy of your counts and can correlate the counts with the later successful confluence of the airway culture on the membrane support. The seeding range that we use is 2.5×10^5 to 5×10^5 epithelial cells/cm^2 on the Millicell insert. Cell harvest suspensions that have more clumps than "average" can be seeded at the lower density range. There is a higher efficiency of attachment with cell clumps than single cells, especially with ciliated cells (*see* **Note 3**). Confidence with the appropriate seeding density of primary epithelial cells requires trial-and-error experience. The presence of red blood cells in the cell suspension will not interfere with epithelial cell attachment.

6. The cell suspension seeded onto the top of the permeable membrane insert (12 mm diameter) should be of sufficient volume, 100–400 µL, to insure a uniform distribution of cells settling upon the membrane surface. The volume of medium under the membrane insert should be sufficient (250–500 µL) to immerse the membrane bottom without floating the insert.

7. After seeding, make sure that the membrane supports are level to insure uniform cell attachment during the first 12 h. We use 24-well cluster dishes to maintain the 12-mm membrane inserts. The 6-well cluster dish can be used with the larger 24- to 30-mm inserts.

8. Leave the cluster dishes with the seeded membrane supports undisturbed for a minimum 18–24 h in a CO_2 incubator at 37°C and 8 to 9% CO_2 (*see* **Note 6**). The higher CO_2 increases successful achievement of confluence, especially with CF airway cultures.

9. The day after seeding, change the airway medium 1 (5% FCS) on both sides of the membrane to airway medium 2 (2% Ultroser G).

10. Remove the top medium with vacuum suction and rinse the top of the membrane surface once with airway medium 2 to remove unattached cells.

11. Then remove the medium from the top of the membrane surface (air interfacing) so that medium is present only on the bottom of the membrane insert. When cells grow at the air interface, they form a confluent sheet with tight junctions and no visible fluid on top. The air interface allows the confluent sheet to better differentiate as a barrier separating air on top from the liquid media immersing the bottom. This air interface condition is comparable to the air-covered surface of the airway epithelium in vivo.

12. Remove any liquid from the top surface once daily until the membrane culture remains visibly dry on top; which usually occurs 3–6 d after seeding in 8 to 9% CO_2. Media seepage will occur through the membrane and the nonconfluent cell cultures for several days until the cells replicate to confluence.

13. Maintain the airway medium 2 on the bottom side of the membrane insert for the entire culture duration to prevent the culture from drying and the cells dying.

14. After the cells achieve confluence, the polarized sheet of epithelial cells will regulate the minimal fluid level and content on top. The amount of liquid is so small that it is not visible to the eye.

15. For cryopreservation of primary airway epithelial cells, resuspend cells in freezing medium. Cryovials are frozen at –70°C for 4–24 h and then transferred to liquid nitrogen for long-term storage.

16. At the time of later use, thaw the cryovial in a 37°C water bath and rinse with airway medium 1.

17. Centrifuge and resuspend the cell pellet in airway medium 1. Up to 70% cell viability is possible.

3.5. Routine Culturing and Long-Term Maintenance

Two cell culture conditions facilitate the long-term viability of polarized human airway epithelial cells on membrane supports. The combination of the airway medium 2, which contains 2% Ultroser G, and the apical air interface allow the epithelium to remain viable for months. Our data suggest that the epithelium probably does not continue to differentiate past approx d 14 in culture. Long-term culture maintenance is most economical and allows for time flexibility in use of the epithelium in experiments. We have maintained viable airway epithelia on membrane supports for up to 15 mo. During this time, the epithelia maintain an air interface and a transepithelial resistance. Such long-term preservation can be especially valuable for studies designed to evaluate the persistence of transgene expression following viral or nonviral vector-mediated gene transfer.

1. After the first 4–6 d of culture and once the air interface can be maintained by the cells, keep the cultures in a 5% CO_2 humidified atmosphere at 37°C for the remainder of their time in culture.

2. Beginning the day after seeding, any liquid on the top surface must be removed daily until the epithelium becomes confluent and can maintain the air interface. Long-term viability requires an air interface at the apical membrane.

3. We estimate that between 50–70% of the seeded airway cells will attach to the collagen-coated membrane within 12 h after seeding. Cell replication continues until 7–9 days after seeding. By the ninth day there will be on average 650,000–750,000 airway epithelial cells on a 0.6-cm² membrane surface. Cell numbers will then remain relatively constant unless a growth factor such as the keratinocyte growth factor (KGF) is introduced into the basolateral cell culture medium to initiate cell replication *(11)*.

4. The rate of medium acidification by the cell culture varies depending upon the age of the culture. Younger cultures will require more frequent medium changes every 2 to 3 d. Older cultures require a medium change every 5–7 d. Change the medium whenever it becomes too acidic, as indicated by a yellow appearance. It is critical that the membrane surface not be touched by a pipet tip when changing media to prevent damage to the epithelium and a reduction in transepithelial resistance.

5. The greatest challenge to maintaining cultures for weeks and months will be preventing infection by opportunistic pathogens, especially yeast. We have found the combination of two fungicides, fluconazole and amphotericin B, are especially effective in preventing infection or limiting exponential growth after initial infection. Decreased antibiotic concentrations or complete elimination of antibiotics is also feasible for extended periods of time if required by an experimental protocol. We pre-incubate culture medium in filter-top flasks in the CO_2 incubator prior to use in order to screen for any contamination of media stocks. Especially for long-term culturing of up to a year, we will "spread the risk" of loss due to incubator failure or mechanical problems by using two or more CO_2 incubators for different trays of epithelia from the same specimen. Before every change of media, we inspect each multiwell tray of epithelia for signs of media discoloration and turbidity that would indicate contamination. We also alternate days for media changes of different airway cultures to reduce the chances of cross-contamination from one contaminated culture.

6. Airway epithelia are maintained long-term with airway medium 2 present only on the bottom surface. If the experimental protocol requires supplement depletion, the epithelia can remain viable without the Ultroser G supplement for several days in the 50/50 DMEM and Ham's F-12 medium.

7. Additional medium supplements can be added for special needs. For example, to reinitiate cell replication following confluence, we use keratinocyte growth factor for 24–48 h during days 8–10 post-seeding.

3.6. Evaluation of Airway Epithelia

1. The evaluation of the cultures is critically important to determine that they have the phenotype associated with airway epithelia. During the process of culturing, they must be continuously examined in several ways.

2. For example, check to see if the apical surface appears dry. Routinely check the transepithelial electrical resistance (Rt) and the morphology on every set of cultures.

3. We also study several epithelial cultures from every airway specimen in Ussing chambers to measure Rt, transepithelial voltage, the amiloride-sensitive Na^+ current, and the CFTR-dependent Cl^- current.

3.6.1 Transepithelial Resistance.

Here, we briefly describe the measurement of Rt and evaluation of morphology. Measurement of transepithelial electrical properties in Ussing chambers will not be described. To learn more about those procedures, the reader may consult other references (*12,13*).

1. Rt can be conveniently monitored using a portable ohmmeter. We use the Voltohmmeter attached to dual "chopstick" electrodes.

2. Each of the two electrode stems contains at their tip a Ag/Ag Cl^- electrode for measuring voltage and a concentric spiral of silver wire for passing current across the epithelium.

3. Presterilize the electrode tips in 70% alcohol before use to maintain cell culture sterility.

4. To measure electrical properties, place 300–400 µL of airway media 2 on the apical surface. It is removed after measurement.

5. Using a culture membrane insert such as the Millipore PCF, place the shorter electrode tip into medium on top of the apical surface, and place the longer electrode tip into the external bathing medium.

6. Current can then be passed across the epithelium to measure Rt. Rt values higher than the background fluid resistance indicate a confluent airway epithelium with tight junctions.

7. In our experience, we have found that Rt measured in this way is consistently higher than that obtained with the more accurate measurements obtained when the epithelia are studied in Ussing chambers. This difference is probably due, at least in part, to the fact that the distribution of current across the epithelium is more uniform in Ussing chambers. In contrast, with the chopstick electrodes, the

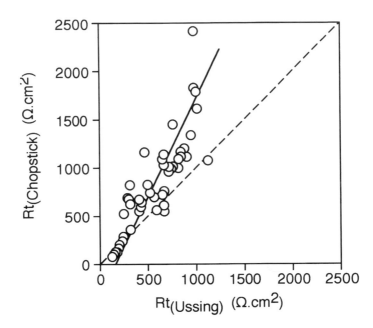

Fig. 6. Comparison of measurements of transepithelial electrical resistance in primary cultures of human airway epithelia using a chopstick ohmmeter, Rt(chopstick), and measured in Ussing chamber, Rt(Ussing). Both measurements were made on the same epithelia. Measurements made with the chopstick ohmmeter consistently overestimate the true Rt. The dashed line is the line of identity, and the solid line is the linear fit to the data.

distribution of current flow may be influenced by spatial constraints independent of the permeability of the epithelium. We have compared Rt values measured by the Millipore ERS Voltohmmeter with Rt values measured by voltage-clamp in Ussing chambers. The data are shown in **Fig. 6**. In both cases, the electrical resistance of the fluid and the filter were subtracted, and the measurements were corrected for the area of the epithelium.

The relationship is described by the formula:

$$Rt(Ussing\ chamber) = (0.492 \times Rt[chopstick]) + 158$$

When area and fluid resistance are not corrected for measurements taken with the chopstick electrodes, the relationship is described by the formula:

$$Rt(Ussing\ chamber) = (0.295 \times Rt[chopstick]) + 107$$

3.6.2. Morphology

1. On every set of cultures you should use SEM to evaluate the morphology of the apical surface. As the epithelia mature and differentiate, apical surface morphol-

ogy changes. **Fig. 7** shows SEM photomicrographs taken at increasing durations after seeding epithelial cells from a human bronchial specimen *(14)*.

2. Three days after seeding, the cells appear confluent (**Fig. 7A,B**). The cells vary in size and most appear to have short microvilli. However, there are very few ciliated cells. Six days after seeding, most of the cells appear to have immature cilia (**Fig. 7C,D**). On d 10 (**Fig. 7E,F**) and 14 (**Fig. 7G,H**) after seeding, the surface of the monolayers is covered completely by cilia, making it difficult to identify individual cells. In some areas, there is also amorphous material mixed in with the cilia.

3. In our experience, by 14 d in culture, the epithelium has fully differentiated and is ready for use in experiments. Airway specimens can vary greatly in the percentage of epithelia cells that develop cilia in culture. This may reflect, in part, the history of the human donor. For example, chronic exposure to cigarette smoke or other insults or disease, which damages the airway epithelium in vivo, may influence in vitro results. Increasing the degree of clumping of ciliated cells by shortening the dissociation time may increase the proportion of ciliated cells that attach to the membrane within the first 12 h.

4. Notes

1. Development of successful primary airway epithelial cultures depends on the viability of the original tissue. The harvested cells need to be viable and in sufficient quantity to ensure an equitable distribution of viable cells seeded on the permeable membrane supports. This should then later produce confluent epithelia with intact tight junctions. With these requirements, it can be problematic to obtain viable human airway specimens in a quantity to yield a significant cell harvest. We have obtained human airway nasal tissue and lung from several sources. They include nasal polyps and turbinates following endoscopic polypectomy or endoscopic sinus surgery. The polyps need to be harvested intact, using a scissors or sharp manual dissection, and not minced by a mechanical microdebrider, which is increasingly popular for polypectomy. We have obtained poor viability of epithelial cells harvested from minced specimens.

   We have also tried to use tracheas and lung specimens obtained postmortem. This source is problematic due to the time between death and harvesting the tissue and the greater risk for bacterial and yeast contamination. Rinsing airway epithelium with water at the postmortem surgery site is to be avoided. Our experience has been that we had occasional success with cells obtained from the trachea, but the viability of cells of lower airway was poor.

   Our best success in obtaining high quality cultures has come when we used viable trachea and bronchus segments from human donor lungs. These lungs have been prepared and harvested aseptically according to transplant standards, but have then been rejected for human transplantation. The lungs are immersed in sterile saline and sealed in sterile bags, which are then chilled by immersion in wet ice. Lung specimens usually arrive in the laboratory within 6–18 h following removal. These lungs come from donors of all ages and medical histories. The donor lungs have been rejected for human transplantation due to donor age older

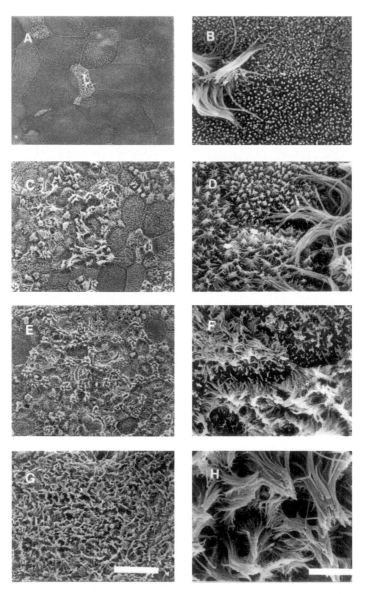

Fig. 7. Scanning electron photomicrographs of primary cultures of human airway epithelia grown at the air–liquid interface. Photomicrgraphs of monolayers are shown at the following times after seeding: 3 d **(A,B)**, 6 d **(C,D)**, 10 d **(E,F)**, and 14 d **(G,H)**. In panels **A**, **C**, **E**, and **G**, the scale bar indicates 37.5 µm, and in panels **B**, **D**, **F**, and **H**, the scale bar indicates 5 µm. On d 3, sporadic ciliated cells can be observed surrounded by undifferentiated cells with short microvilli. By d 6, most of the cells have cilia (thin arrows in panel **D**) or immature cilia (thick arrows). By d 10 and 14, most of the cells are ciliated. From **ref. *14*** with permission.

than 60, presence of sepsis, chronic smoking exposure, or lung damage due to bruising and bleeding. We dissect and segregate tissue segments according to the airway region and lobe because of possible variation in epithelial viability. Airway epithelium from CF lungs are especially variable in viability from area to area due to chronic inflammation and infection.

A commercial source for cryofrozen primary or first passage human airway cells is Clonetics (Walkersville, MD). This source is economical when the cells are serially passaged to expand cell numbers. However, based upon comparative studies using primary and passaged airway cells, our laboratory prefers the morphology and functional properties of the primary cells, because they more closely resemble those of the airway epithelium in vivo.

2. The lobar bronchi divide repeatedly with each branch, becoming progressively smaller in diameter. Our experience has been that the smaller airway segments are less likely to yield viable cells, and the yield will be smaller. In considering the trade-offs of time and cost vs viable cell yield, we routinely end dissection after the third bronchial branching. However, special needs and protocols may require harvesting cells from smaller bronchi.

3. Dissociation time can vary depending upon requirements. The longer the dissociation time, the finer the single-cell dissociation. Aliquots removed at staggered times from the dissociation tubes and microscopically examined on a glass slide can be used to assess the degree of dissociation. It is important to determine by experience what will work best for you. Small clumps of cells (approx 4–10 cells/clump) have a higher efficiency of attachment than single cells and provide cluster seeds for cell division. We usually harvest cells about 60–72 h after starting the dissociation.

4. For certain protocols, it may be desirable to remove or segregate large-size clumps of airway cells from the cell harvest suspension. A sterile 100-μm nylon cell strainer (Falcon, cat. no. 2360) can be used for this purpose.

5. Vitrogen gel substrate. According to the manufacturer's insert, mix in an 8:1:1 ratio of the cold Vitrogen 100, sterile cold 10× DMEM, and cold 0.1 N NaOH. Using pH indicator strip paper, adjust the solution pH to 7.4 with 0.1 HCl and 0.1 NaOH. The collagen solution is then aliquoted onto the top surface of the membrane support (150–200 μL/0.6 cm^2). Then warm the coated membrane surface to 37°C (not in CO_2), for a minimum of 1 h to gelate the collagen. Then use the gel for cell seeding within 3 h. Rinse the collagen surface with medium prior to seeding cells. Do not use vacuum suction on the collagen gel surface. Use a hand-held suction pipet bulb to avoid damage to the collagen gel. This gel substrate is fragile during culturing. Our experience has been that there is a steady attrition rate. Therefore, we always cultured more than we needed for a particular experiment.

6. For the first 4–6 d, we routinely culture the airway cells on the membrane in a high CO_2 atmosphere (8 to 9%) until the culture can maintain an air interface. Then the cultures are transferred to a 5% CO_2 atmosphere for long-term maintenance. Not all airway specimens require this enhanced CO_2 condition. But there

is a critical time window during the first several days of culture for the cells to grow to confluence and form acceptable transepithelial resistances. If the cells have not become confluent by d 6 after seeding, the rate of later confluence success is low. We have observed a higher success rate using an initially higher CO_2 atmosphere for our airway cultures.

References

1. Wheater, P. R., Burkitt, H. G., and Daniels, V. G. (1987) Respiratory system, p. 178–190. In *Functional Histology*. Churchill Livingston, London.
2. Thurston, R. J., Hess, R. A., Kilburn, K. H., and McKenzie, W. N. (1976) Ultrastructure of lungs fixed in inflation using a new osmium-fluorocarbon technique. *J. Ultrastruct. Res.* **56,** 39–47.
3. Sims, D. E., Westfall, J. A., Kiorpes, A. L., and Horne, M. M. (1991) Preservation of tracheal mucus by nonaqueous fixative. *Biotech. Histochem.* **66,** 173–180.
4. Zabner, J., Smith, J. J., Karp, P. H., Widdicombe, J. H., and Welsh, M. J. (1998) Loss of CFTR chloride channels alters salt absorption by cystic fibrosis airway epithelia *in vitro*. *Mol. Cell* **2,** 397–403.
5. Walters, R. W., Grunst, T., Bergelson, J. M., Finberg, R. W., Welsh, M. J., and Zabner, J. (1999) Basolateral localization of fiber receptors limits adenovirus infection from the apical surface of airway epithelia. *J. Biol. Chem.* **274,** 10219–10226.
6. Drapkin, P. T., O'Riordan, C. R., Yi, S. M., Chiorini, J. A., Cardella, J., Zabner, J., and Welsh, M. J. (2000) Targeting the urokinase plasminogen activator receptor enhances gene transfer to human airway epithelia. *J. Clin. Invest.* **105,** 589–596.
7. Zabner, J., Seiler, M. P., Launspach, J. L., et al. (2000) The osmolyte xylitol reduces the salt concentration of airway surface liquid and may enhance bacterial killing. *Proc. Natl. Acad. Sci. U.S.A.* **97,** 11614–11619.
8. Ferkol, T., Eckman, E. A., Swaidani, S., Silski, C., and Davis, P. (2000) Transport of bifunctional proteins across respiratory epithelial cells via the polymeric immunoglobulin receptor. *Am. J. Respir. Crit. Care Med.* **161,** 944–951.
9. Smith, J. J., Travis, S. M., Greenberg, E. P., and Welsh, M. J. (1996) Cystic fibrosis airway epithelia fail to kill bacteria because of abnormal airway surface fluid. *Cell* **85,** 229–236.
10. Yamaya, M., Finkbeiner, W. E., Chun, S. Y., and Widdicombe, J. H. (1992) Differentiated structure and function of cultures from human tracheal epithelium. *Am. J. Physiol.* **262,** L713–L724.
11. Wang, G., Slepushkin, V. A., Bodner, M., et al. (1999) Keratinocyte growth factor induced epithelial proliferation facilitates retroviral-mediated gene transfer to distal lung epithelia *in vivo*. *J. Gene Med.* **1,** 22–30.
12. Cotton, C. U. and Reuss, L. (1996) Characterization of epithelial ion transport, p. 70–92. In *Epithelial transport: a guide to methods and experimental analysis* (Wils, N. K., Reuss, L. and Lewis, S. A., eds.). Chapman & Hall, London.
13. Lewis, S. A. (1996) Epithelial electrophysiology, p. 93–117. In *Epithelial transport: a guide to methods and experimental analysis* (Wills, N. K., Reuss, L. and Lewis, S. A., eds.). Chapman & Hall, London.

14. Zabner, J., Zeiher, B. G., Friedman, E., and Welsh, M. J. (1996) Adenovirus-mediated gene transfer to ciliated airway epithelia requires prolonged incubation time. *J. Virol.* **70,** 6994–7003.

12

Primary Mouse Keratinocyte Culture

Kairbaan Hodivala-Dilke

1. Introduction

The use of human neonatal keratinocyte cultures has provided a valuable tool in understanding the cellular and molecular mechanisms in skin growth, maintenance, and disease *(1,2)*. With the onset of transgenic studies in mice, a new level of understanding development and disease has become apparent. Recently, several transgenic mouse models for skin diseases, such as the suprabasal integrin-expressing mouse model for psoriasis *(3)*, and the bullous pemphigoid and integrin knock-out mice for blistering disorders *(4–6)* have shed light on direct molecular mechanisms underlying the onset of these disorders.

Although the mouse models are of vital importance, it is also imperative that cell biology be carried out on epidermal keratinocytes isolated from such transgenic mice. Here, I describe the isolation of epidermal keratinocytes from neonatal mice, which is based on the protocol of Dlugosz et al. *(7)*. Briefly, neonate mouse skin is trypsinized overnight, and the resulting epidermal sheet is dissociated, and the single-cell suspension of keratinocytes is cultured in low calcium conditions on collagen-coated tissue culture plastic. This method is the easiest method to grow mouse keratinocytes, with a quick yield of large numbers of cells. The method produces epidermal keratinocyte monolayers that can be used for almost all cell and molecular biological investigations ranging from immunohistochemistry to transfections *(8,9)*.

2. Materials

1. Flask-coating medium: 30 µg/mL Vitrogen (Nudacon, cat. no. P99E131C); 10 µg/mL fibronectin. Immediately before coating the plates, dilute the Vitrogen (concentrated stock 3 mg/mL) and fibronectin (concentrated stock 1 mg/mL) 1:100 in phosphate-buffered saline (PBS) (*see* **Notes 2** and **3**).

From: *Methods in Molecular Biology, vol. 188: Epithelial Cell Culture Protocols*
Edited by: C. Wise © Humana Press Inc., Totowa, NJ

2. Sterile dissecting instruments.
3. Tissue culture plastic.
4. Sterile PBS.
5. 10% Iodine (Sigma) in PBS.
6. 70% Ethanol.
7. 0.25% Trypsin (Life Technologies).
8. Sterile Pasteur pipets. Prepare all of the following stock reagents and sterilize them in advance. Store solutions either as frozen aliquots or at 4°C as specified.
9. Chelex-treated fetal calf serum (FCS): FCS contains high levels of calcium. For this method of primary mouse keratinocyte culture, it is important to remove all free calcium by treating FCS with Chelex-100 resin (BioRad, cat. no. 142-2832). Chelex resin (100 g) should be used to chelate 500 mL fetal bovine serum (FBS).
   a. Swell 100 g chelex resin in 400–500 mL distilled water for approx 1 h.
   b. Titrate to pH 7.4 with concentrated HCl while stirring (*see* **Note 1**).
   c. Filter the chelex through Whatman no. 1 paper.
   d. Scrape the resin slurry off the filter into 500 mL FCS and stir using a magnetic stirrer at room temperature for 3 h or at 4°C overnight.
   e. Filter the chelated FCS through Whatman no. 1 paper and discard the resin slurry.
   f. Finally, filter-sterilize the chelated FBS through a 0.2-μm bottle filter. Store in 20-mL aliquots at –20°C.
10. 0.1 M CaCl$_2$ (Sigma): prepare 15 mL of 0.1 M calcium chloride (0.24 g in 15 mL) in sterile water. Filter-sterilize with a 0.2-μm filter and store at 4°C.
11. 0.2 mg/mL Hydrocortisone (Sigma): prepare a concentrated stock of 5 mg/mL by dissolving 50 mg hydrocortisone in 10 mL 95% ethanol. Store the concentrated stock at –20°C in 0.4-mL sterile aliquots. Prepare a 0.2 mg/mL stock by adding 0.4 mL of concentrated stock to 9.6 mL of sterile serum-free EMEM. Store 1.0-mL aliquots at –20°C.
12. 5 mg/mL Insulin (Sigma): dissolve 100 mg insulin in 20 mL of 0.005 M HCl (prepared by adding 10 μL concentrated HCl to 20 mL water) to prepare a 5-mg/mL insulin solution. Filter-sterilize using a 0.2-μm filter and store 0.5-mL aliquots at –20°C.
13. 10 μg/mL Epidermal growth factor (EGF) (Life Technologies):
    a. Dissolve 100 μg EGF in 1 mL 0.1% BSA (10 mg ultrapure BSA in 10 mL water).
    b. Bring volume to 10 mL with 0.1% BSA to make a 10-μg/mL solution.
    c. Filter-sterilize using a 0.2-μm filter and store 0.5-mL aliquots at –20°C.
14. 10^{-7} M stock cholera toxin (Sigma):
    a. Prepare a concentrated stock of 10^{-5} M by dissolving 1 mg (1 vial) cholera toxin in 1.18 mL distilled water. Store the stock at 4°C (do not freeze the concentrated stock).
    b. Prepare a 10^{-7} M cholera toxin solution by adding 0.1 mL of the concentrated stock to 10 mL EMEM containing 4% chelated FBS. Filter-sterilize with a 0.2-μm filter and aliquot at 0.5 mL/tube; store at –20°C.

15. Growth medium: EMEM, Ca^{2+}-free (Biowhittaker), 500 mL supplemented with the following:
    a. 8% Chelated FCS; 20 mL chelex-treated stock.
    b. 0.05 mM $CaCl_2$; 250 µL of 0.1 M stock.
    c. 0.4 µg/mL Hydrocortisone; 1.0 mL of 0.2 mg/mL stock.
    d. 5 µg/mL Insulin; 0.5 mL of 5 mg/mL stock.
    e. 10 ng/mL EGF; 0.5 mL of 10 µg/mL stock.
    f. 10^{-10} M cholera toxin; 0.5 mL of 10^{-7} M stock.
    g. 100 U/mL Penicillin, 100 µg/mL streptomycin; 5.0 mL of 100× pen–strep stock.
    h. 2 mM L-Glutamine; 5.0 mL of 200 mM stock.
    Store sterile 500 mL bottles at 4°C.
16. 70-µm Cell strainers (Becton Dickinson).

3. Methods

3.1. Preparation of Collagen-Coated Dishes

1. Prepare fresh flask-coating medium and apply approx 5 mL/25 cm² of tissue culture plastic.
2. Incubate at 33°C for several hours or at 4°C overnight.
3. Aspirate collagen from the dish before adding cells (*see* **Note 4**).

3.2. Preparation of Keratinocyte Cultures

1. Sacrifice newborn mice (*see* **Note 5**) and keep them wrapped in cling film on ice until beginning the procedure (*see* **Note 6**). Carry out the rest of the procedure in a laminar flow hood and work under sterile conditions.
2. Place the carcasses into a 100-mL beaker and submerge them in 10% iodine for 10 min to sterilize them. Decant the iodine solution and discard it.
3. Rinse carcasses with 2 changes of sterile PBS.
4. Submerge the carcasses in 70% ethanol for 10 min on ice. Decant the ethanol and discard it.
5. Rinse carcasses with 2 changes of sterile PBS and then submerge them in sterile PBS at 4°C.
6. Using a sterile scalpel, remove and discard the legs and tail (*see* **Note 7**).
7. To remove skin from the torso and head, place the carcass on a sterile tissue culture dish, and using sterile scissors, make a longitudinal incision from tail to snout, then peel the skin from the carcass using 2 pairs of sterile curved forceps (*see* **Note 8**).
8. Lay the skin onto the bottom of a clean dish, with the dermis facing down, and spread out all edges using the curved edges of the forceps. Allow the skin to dry for approx 5–10 min (*see* **Note 9**).
9. Using curved forceps, pick up the skin carefully by the corners and place each skin, dermis facing down, onto 5 mL of sterile 0.25% trypsin solution in a 60-mm tissue culture dish.

10. Use the tips of the forceps to tease out the folded edges of the skin, so that it floats flat with most of the epidermis above the surface of the trypsin solution.
11. If individual mice are of differing genotypes, the Petri dishes should be clearly labeled to match the tail sample.
12. Incubate at 4°C for 15 to 24 h (*see* **Note 10**).
13. Transfer each skin to a dry sterile tissue culture plate and spread it out with the epidermis facing down. Drag the dermis away from the epidermis using a sterile Pasteur pipet and discard it (*see* **Note 11**).
14. Mince the epidermis using a crosswise action of 2 scalpels on the Petri dish.
15. With a 10-mL pipet, suspend the skin in 6 mL of growth medium, transfer to a 15-mL Falcon tube, and agitate to create a single-cell suspension (*see* **Note 12**).
16. Pass the suspension through a sterile 70-μm nylon cell strainer into a fresh 50-mL Falcon tube in order to remove any sheets of dead cells.
17. To ensure that the maximum number of cells are harvested, rinse the initial tube with 5 mL fresh growth medium, and rinse it through the same filter into the same 50-mL tube (cells will be in a final volume of 10 to 11 mL).
18. Plate 10 mL of keratinocyte suspension from each skin onto a 10-cm tissue culture dish coated with flask-coating medium.
19. Culture mouse keratinocytes at 33 to 34°C, 8% CO_2, for 5 to 7 d before use in experiments.
20. The cultures can be passaged once or twice for expansion by splitting 90% confluent monolayers in a 1:3 ratio.
21. The keratinocytes should become confluent within 5–7 d and have a cobblestone appearance.
22. Once confluent, the cells may begin to differentiate, and individual cells will appear large and flattened. If more than 20% of the culture has a differentiated appearance, the cells may not passage well so it is always best to passage or use the cells before they reach confluency.
23. Cells should be fed by the replacement of old medium every 2 d.
24. The epidermis from a single newborn mouse should yield approx $5–10 \times 10^6$ cells.

4. Notes

1. pH adjustment of swollen chelex resin takes several hours. Keep the resin solution stirring continuously throughout and allow the pH to stabilize fully between additions of approx 200 μL HCl until pH 7.4 is reached.
2. Vitrogen should be kept at 4°C at all times. Do not freeze the stock solution and do not allow it to warm while preparing the flask-coating medium.
3. Fibronectin is not necessary for the coating medium. Most keratinocytes will grow well without it, but some, especially those with adhesion defects, may benefit from the addition of fibronectin to the coating medium.
4. Vitrogen solution is very acidic, and it is important to aspirate the dish after the coating incubation, since any residual acidity may kill the cells.
5. When sacrificing newborn mice for keratinocyte preparation, it is vital that the skin be damaged as little as possible. It is, therefore, preferable to either sacrifice the animal by CO_2 inhalation or decapitation using very sharp scissors.

6. It is possible to store the carcasses wrapped in cling film on ice for up to 6 h before beginning the cell isolation procedure. Longer storage may result in a lower yield and viability of cells.

7. If necessary, the tail can be processed for genotyping the pup. When removing the legs and tail, ensure that the dissection is made as close to the body as possible. It is often easiest to place round-ended forceps around the limb near the body and draw a scalpel against the forceps to remove the limb. This gives a clean cut without destroying the torso skin.

8. Avoid puncturing the gut to maintain sterility.

9. When several pups are being processed simultaneously, the skins should be allowed to dry on chilled Petri dishes. This is an important step, not only because it gives time to process all the skins in the same session, but it also helps stiffen the skin slightly, which aids in the proceeding steps. It should be noted that the skins should not be allowed to dry out completely.

10. When laying the skins onto trypsin, the skins should be free to float, and the epidermal surface should appear to be above the level of the trypsin. It is important to uncurl the free edges of the skin, since this can inhibit the trypsinization procedure.

11. When the trypsinization procedure has worked well the skins should appear very flat and dry on the epidermal surface. When dragging the dermis (with a gelatenous cloudy appearance) off the epidermis (with a thin chiffon appearance), the dermis should come away very easily. Any difficulty in removing the dermis is indicative of a poor trypsinization, and the skin should be discarded.

12. At this stage, avoid creating bubbles that would destroy the cells.

References

1. Rheinwald, J. G. (1980) Serial cultivation of normal human keratinocytes. *Methods Cell Biol.* **21A,** 229–254.

2. Rheinwald, J. G. and Green, H (1975) Serial cultivation of strains of human epidermal keratinocytes: the formation of keratinizing colonies from single cells. *Cell* **6,** 331–343.

3. Carroll, J. M., Romero, M. R., and Watt, F. M. (1995) Suprabasal integrin expression in the epidermis of trasngenic mice results in a phenotype resembling psoriasis. *Cell* **83,** 957–968.

4. Van der Neut, R., Krimpenfort, P., Calafat, J., Nissen, C. M., and Sonnenberg, A. (1996) Epithelial detachment due to absence of hemidesmosomes in integrin b4 null mice. *Nat. Genet.* **13,** 366–369.

5. Georges-Labouesse, E., Messaddeq N., Yehia G., Cadalbert., L., Dierich A., and Le Meur M. (1996) Absence of integrin α6 leads to epidermolysis bullosa and neonatal death in mice. *Nat. Genet.* **13,** 370–73.

6. Guo, L., Degenstein, L., Dowling, J., Yu, Q. C. Wollmann, R. Perman, B., and Fuch, E. (1995) Gene targeting of BPAG1: abnormalities in mechanical strength and cell migration in stratified epithelia and neurologic degeneration, *Cell* **81,** 233–243.

7. Dlugosz, A. A., Glick, A. B., Tennenbaum, T., Weinberg, W. C., and Yuspa, S. H. (1995) Isolation and utilization of epidermal keratinocytes for oncogene research. *Methods Enzymol.* **254,** 3–20.

8. DiPersio, M., Hodivala-Dilke, K., Jaenish, R., Kreidberg, J., and Hynes, R. O. (1997) α3β1 integrin is required for normal development of the epidermal basement membrane. *J. Cell Biol.* **137,** 729–742.

9. Hodivala-Dilke, K. M., DiPersio, C. M., Kredberg, J. A., and Hynes, R. O. (1998) Novel roles for alpha3beta1 integrin as a regulator of cytoskeletal assembly and as a trans-dominant inhibitor of integrin receptor function in mouse keratinocytes. *J. Cell Biol.* **142,** 1357–1369.

13

Analyzing Apoptosis in Cultured Epithelial Cells

Andrew P. Gilmore and Charles H. Streuli

1. Introduction

This chapter will outline a number of assays in use in the authors' laboratory for the quantification of apoptosis in cultured mammary epithelial cells. These assays are each directed at particular stages of apoptosis, which are outlined below. There are a number of commercial assays available, utilizing such reagents as fluorescent caspase substrates, which determine an average level of apoptosis throughout a population of cells. However, we find a considerable use for assays that identify individual apoptotic cells, and it is chiefly these that will be described here.

Cells are constantly dying through the normal wear and tear of cellular turnover and through the consequences of differentiation. In most cases, they die by apoptosis, a defined pathway in which damaged cells are removed by mechanisms inherent to the cell (*1,2*). This is in contrast to passive cell death, or necrosis, which results in cell lysis with the risk of inflammation and subsequent tissue damage. Indeed, the purpose of apoptosis is to remove cells without inducing a damaging inflammatory response (*3*). Inhibiting the normal function of the apoptotic program can have serious implications. Uncontrolled apoptosis can contribute to degenerative conditions, and conversely, the inability to carry out apoptosis can contribute to the development of neoplasia (*4*). Under normal conditions, a cell requires the constant presence of survival signals to prevent the activation of the apoptotic program. Survival signals can consist of growth factors, cell–extracellular matrix adhesion, and cell–cell adhesion.

To kill without inducing any inflammatory response, the cell is dismantled in a series of ordered steps, each of which can provide a set of markers diagnostic for apoptosis (*5,6*). These steps include: (*i*) a decision phase; (*ii*) activation of the apoptotic program and commitment of the cell to die; (*iii*) the execution

From: *Methods in Molecular Biology, vol. 188: Epithelial Cell Culture Protocols*
Edited by: C. Wise © Humana Press Inc., Totowa, NJ

phase, during which intracellular proteases (the caspases) cleave a wide range of specific substrates; and (*iv*) phagocytic clearance. The boundaries between these steps are somewhat arbitrary and unclear, if they exist as boundaries at all, but they are useful in how to view the process. The key event is activation of the caspase proteases, which exist within a normal cell as inactive proenzymes. The process of cellular commitment to death involves caspases being activated by the cleavage of a prodomain and their subsequent dimerization to form an active enzyme. There are two pathways by which caspases can become activated. One is through the release of cytochrome c from mitochondria *(7)*, which acts as a cofactor for the formation of a large multiprotein complex, the apoptosome *(8)*, which recruits and activates a subset of caspase family members. The second is through the activation of death receptors on the cells surface, such as Fas or TNF-R, which recruit a different subset of caspases and activate them. Downstream of either event, further caspase members are activated in a proteolytic cascade, and the cleavage of cellular proteins ensues. This activation of caspases provides one of the key diagnostic features of apoptosis, and one that can be readily viewed in a number of assays. Following caspase activation, the end is swift. The nucleus condenses, and caspase-activated nucleases cleave DNA into nucleosomal fragments. The plasma membrane begins to bleb, and the cell breaks up into contained fragments, preventing the release of inflammatory agents. The plasma membrane of these fragments has also changed, with the exposure of phosphatidylserine on the outer surface *(9)*. This acts as a ligand for a specific receptor present on macrophages, allowing the rapid removal of these potentially hazardous corpses.

For the researcher interested in examining apoptosis in their cell system, the precisely controlled nature of apoptosis provides a number of ideal endpoints for initially determining if apoptosis has indeed occurred, and then to quantify it. However, a certain amount of caution is required, and it may be necessary to examine a number of the possible markers to be confident that cells are dying by apoptosis. Some markers for apoptosis appear relatively late in the process. Once a cell has committed itself to apoptosis, the process is extremely rapid and can occur within minutes *(10)*. However, in many situations, the time leading to commitment can be extensive. For example, death following application of DNA damaging agents can take 48 to 72 h. Indeed, cells that are ultimately going to apoptose may look perfectly normal for quite some time. Also, the use of epithelial cell lines is likely to affect the extent to which apoptosis occurs, as by their very nature they have been selected for their ability to survive. In our hands, mammary tumor cell lines (MCF-7, MDA-MB-231) are completely resistant to insults that result in 90% of primary cells apoptosing in 24 h. Indeed, carcinoma cell lines are more resistant than primary cultures of carcinoma cells.

A further point of caution concerns the very transient nature of apoptosis. In vivo, macrophages remove apoptotic cells and any traces of them very rapidly. In culture, there may not be any macrophages to clear away the corpses, but the fragmentation of the cell does result in a considerable amount of debris, and often there is little to indicate what was once a cell, making quantification of apoptosis difficult. Cells that are apoptotic are identifiable as such for a brief window of time, and it is difficult to identify either those cells that have completed the program or those that are about to commence upon it. Thus, any count of the number of apoptotic cells within a population provides a snapshot of an event that probably affects a greater number of cells than the numbers might suggest. One way of taking this into account is simply to determine the number of cells the population has to start with and repeat this at the end.

2. Materials
2.1 Analysis of Apoptosis in Adherent Cultured Cells by Activation of Caspase 3 and Nuclear Morphology

1. 13-mm Glass coverslips (Merck).
2. 12-Well tissue culture plates (TCS).
3. Phosphate-buffered saline (PBS) (Life Technologies).
4. Freshly made 3.7% paraformaldehyde in PBS (*see* **Note 1**).
5. 0.5% Triton X-100 in PBS.
6. Horse blocking buffer: 150 mM NaCl, 25 mM Tris-HCl, pH 7.6, 0.1% Triton X-100, 0.05% Tween 20, 0.1% horse serum, 0.05% sodium azide.
7. Anti-caspase 3 antibody (*see* **Note 2**), and fluorescent secondary antibody (Jackson Immunoresearch Laboratories).
8. 4 µg/mL Hoechst 33258 (Sigma).
9. Fluorescent mounting medium (*see* **Note 3**).
10. Glass slides (Merck).

2.2. Cytospinning of Detached Apoptotic Cells for Immunohistochemistry

1. Cytospin centrifuge (Shandon).
2. Polysine slides (Merck).
3. Wax pen (DAKO).

2.3. Analysis of Membrane Polarity by Annexin V Staining

1. Annexin V binding buffer: 10 mM HEPES/NaOH, pH7.4, 140 mM NaCl, 2.5 mM CaCl$_2$.
2. Biotin-conjugated annexin V (BD Pharmingen).
3. Fluorescein isothiocyanate (FITC)-labeled streptavidin (BD Pharmingen).
4. Freshly made 3.7% paraformaldehyde in PBS.
5. PBS.

2.4. Fractionation of Adherent Cells into Cytosolic and Mitochondrial Compartments

1. PBS.
2. Hypotonic buffer: 10 mM NaCl, 1.5 mM MgCl$_2$, 10 mM Tris-HCl, pH 7.6, 1 mM NaF, 100 µM sodiumorthovanadate, 1× protease inhibitor cocktail (Calbiochem).
3. Dounce homogenizer, with glass pestel (Wheaton).
4. 5× Isotonic buffer: 525 mM mannitol, 172 mM sucrose, 12.5 mM Tris-HCl, pH 7.6, 2 mM EDTA.
5. Beckman TL 100 ultracentrifuge, or equivalent, with rotor capable of accomodating samples of 0.5 mL (TLA 100 or TLA 100.1).

2.5. Bax Activity—Translocation to Mitochondria by Immunohistochemistry

1. 13-mm Glass coverslips (Merck).
2. 12-Well tissue culture plate (TCS).
3. Mitotracker green-fm (Molecular Probes).
4. Cell fixation and staining reagents as in **Subheading 2.1.**
5. Anti-Bax antibody (*see* **Note 4**).
6. Cy3 or tetramethylrhodamine isothiocyanate (TRITC)-conjugated secondary antibody (Jackson Immunoresearch Laboratories).

3. Methods

3.1. Analysis of Apoptosis in Adherent Cultured Cells by Activation of Caspase 3 and Nuclear Morphology

Caspase activation is a central event for apoptosis. There are a number of biochemical assays for examining caspase activation in cell populations, although these are not as useful for looking at apoptosis in single cells within a population. Recently, antibodies have become available that only recognize activated caspase 3, an isoform which is found in most cell types and which becomes activated in response to most apoptotic insults. Nuclear degradation is another hallmark of apoptosis, and here there are a plethora of methods for identifying the nuclei of apoptotic cells. Many of these are quite complex and can be prone to artefacts. A simple and straightforward way is simply to examine nuclear morphology following staining with a DNA stain such as Hoescht or 4'6-diamidine-2-phenylindole (DAPI). Both these methods together provide a near foolproof way of accurately quantifying apoptosis in adherent cultures of epithelial cells and are particularly useful for experiments involving transient transfections.

1. Cells should be grown on glass coverslips in a 12-well plate (*see* **Note 5**). We use 13-mm coverslips that fit into a 12-well plate, which allows for easy washing and processing of multiple samples.
2. Following an experiment, wash cells at room temperature once in 1 mL PBS.

3. Fix in 3.7% paraformaldehyde for 10 min at room temperature (*see* **Note 1**).
4. Wash twice with 1 mL PBS.
5. Permeabilize cells with 0.5% Triton X-100 in PBS for 5 min at room temperature.
6. Wash in PBS.
7. Place 20 µL of anti-active caspase 3 antibody (1:1000 dilution in horse block buffer) on a piece of parafilm spread on a glass plate (*see* **Note 2**).
8. Place the coverslip, cell side down, onto the drop of diluted antibody and place in a humidified incubator at 37°C for 1 h.
9. Place coverslip in 12-well plate and wash 3 times with PBS.
10. Repeat staining with diluted secondary fluorescent antibody for 30 min at 37°C in the dark.
11. Wash 3× in PBS.
12. Stain cells with Hoescht 33258 (4 µg/mL in PBS) for 1 min at room temperature.
13. Wash once in PBS.
14. Coverslips should be mounted on a drop of fluorescent mounting medium with a suitable anti-bleaching agent (*see* **Note 3**).
15. Prior to mounting coverslips, briefly rinse them in distilled water (a few seconds is sufficient).
16. Leave mounting medium to set for 2 to 3 h before viewing.
17. Apoptosis can be scored both by caspase staining and by nuclear morphology. Caspase staining is straightforward, but nuclear morphology requires some knowledge of what an apoptotic nucleus looks like. In tissue culture, this is quite clear, and examples are shown in **Fig. 1**. The important characteristics to look for are the loss of detail within the nucleus, condensation with intense staining, and a smooth appearance to the surface. During the early stages of nuclear degradation, it will appear as a single brightly stained structure, but cells in the later stages of apoptosis will show an increasing degree of fragmentation. These are clearly shown in the figure.

3.2. Cytospinning of Detached Apoptotic Cells for Immunohistochemistry

A major problem associated with looking at apoptosis in adherent cells is that the apoptotic cells detach and float into the culture medium. Examination of just the adherent cells at the end of an experiment can give a significant underestimation of the degree to which cell death has occurred. It is therefore important to collect any cells that have detached and to take these into account using the above methods. This method is a simple procedure by which our laboratory collects apoptotic cells from the culture medium for further study.

1. Collect supernatant from cell culture and transfer to tube suitable for centrifugation (we use 1.5-mL Eppendorf tubes and a refrigerated microfuge).
2. Centrifuge cells at 1300g for 5 min and aspirate supernatant. To avoid aspirating the cells, leave about 100 µL of medium in the tube.
3. Wash the remaining adherent cells with 1 mL PBS and add this to the cell pellet and centrifuge again.

A

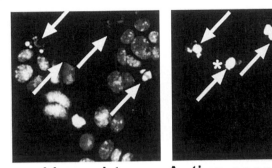

Hoescht   Active caspase 3

B

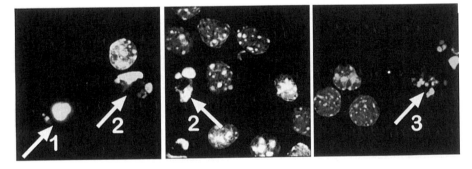

Fig. 1. Mammary epithelial cells maintained in the absence of adhesion to extracellular matrix undergo apoptosis over several hours. (**A**) Cells were maintained on a nonadhesive substrate for 6 h before cytospinning onto polysine slides. Cells were fixed and stained as described with Hoescht and a polyclonal anti-caspase 3 antibody specific for the activated form of the enzyme. Apoptotic cells have been indicated with arrows. Note the cell indicated by the asterix. Though this cell stains positively for caspase 3, there is no detectable nucleus. This is often seen, presumably because the cell has fragmented, and the nucleus has been lost. In vivo, this debris would be removed by phagocytic cells, but in culture, these corpses often remain. (**B**) Mammary epithelial cells treated as in panel **A**, but just stained for nuclei with Hoescht. Three separate forms apoptotic cells have been indicated with arrows. These show the range of different appearances of apoptotic nuclei from condensed (1), starting to fragment (2), and very fragmented (3).

4. Cytospin cells onto Polysine slides. These have a charged surface to aid attachment of the cells. Spin cells in a total of 50 μL of PBS at 1300*g* for 10 min (*see* **Note 6**).

5. View under a phase contrast microscope to check cell density and respin if necessary (*see* **Note 6**).
6. Cells can then be fixed and stained following the above protocols.

3.3. Analysis of Membrane Polarity by Annexin V Staining

Cells that are undergoing apoptosis demonstrate a loss of polarity with regard to their plasma membrane. This results in the exposure of phosphatidylserine, usually restricted to the cytoplasmic face, on the extracellular side. Phosphatidylserine has been shown to act as a ligand for receptors on macrophages, targeting fragments of apoptotic cells for phagocytosis *(11)*. Annexin V binds phosphatidylserine with high affinity, and, in nonpermeabilized cells, provides a method for determining which cells have lost membrane polarity. Normal cells will not stain with annexin V, but staining should increase in apoptotic cells.

1. Grow cells for experiment on glass coverslips (*see* **Note 5**).
2. Following an experiment, wash live cells twice with PBS at room temperature.
3. Add 1:20 dilution of biotin-conjugated annexin V (in annexin V dilution buffer) at room temperature for 15 min.
4. Wash once 5 min in annexin V buffer at room temperature.
5. Incubate cells with 1:100 dilution of FITC-labeled streptavdin for 15 min at room temperature.
6. Wash for a further 5 min in annexin V buffer.
7. Cells can now be viewed live or fixed in 3.7% paraformaldehyde to allow counterstaining with antibodies to transfected or microinjected proteins (*see* **Note 7**).

3.4. Fractionation of Adherent Cells into Cytosolic and Mitochondrial Compartments

The translocation of the pro-apoptotic member of the Bcl-2 family, Bax, from the cytosol to mitochondria and the subsequent release of cytochrome c have been observed during apoptosis in a number of systems *(5,12,13)*. In nonapoptotic epithelial cells, Bax would be expected to be predominantly cytosolic and cytochrome c mitochondrial, and in an apoptotic population, this may be reversed.

1. Wash cells once in PBS on ice, before addition of ice-cold hypotonic lysis buffer (0.5 mL for a 35-mm dish).
2. Scrape cells into hypotonic buffer with a rubber policeman, and leave on ice to swell for 2 min.
3. Transfer to a glass prechilled Dounce homogenizer, and lyse with 10–20 strokes of the pestle (*see* **Note 8**).
4. Lysis can be checked by placing a few microliters of the lysate under a coverslip and viewing under a phase contrast microscope (*see* **Note 9**). If lysis is efficient, most of the nuclei should appear as smooth isolated structures.
5. Add 100 µL of ice-cold 5× isotonic buffer.

6. Centrifuge (in a refrigerated microfuge with 1.5-mL Eppendorf tubes) at 1000_g for 1 min at 4°C to pellet unlysed cells and nuclei. Save the pellet.

7. Centrifuge supernatant at $100,000g$ (Beckman TL 100 ultracentrifuge, TLA 100 rotor or similar) for 30 min at 4°C to pellet internal membranes, including mitochondria (*see* **Note 10**).

8. Each of the fractions (the pellet from **step 4.**, as well as the pellet and supernatant from **step 6.**) can be analyzed by Western blotting for marker proteins for each fraction, along with antibodies for Bcl-2 family proteins and cytochrome c (*see* **Note 11**).

3.5. Bax Activity—Translocation to Mitochondria by Immunohistochemistry

A number of workers have shown that the translocation of Bax to the mitochondria is accompanied by a conformational change in the molecule, and that this can be detected by the exposure of otherwise cryptic epitopes in the N terminus of the molecule *(12–14)*. This can be visualized by immunohistochemistry. A number of commercial antibodies are available that detect these epitopes (*see* **Note 4**). This method provides a way of examining Bax translocation and activation in individual cells rather than within a population.

1. Grow cells on glass coverslips prior to experiment (*see* **Note 5**).

2. During the last 30 min of the experiment, add mitotracker green-fm to the culture medium to a final concentration 500 n*M* (*see* **Note 12**).

3. Wash briefly in PBS and fix the cells in 3.7% paraformaldehyde in PBS for 10 min at room temperature (*see* **Note 12**).

4. Wash cells twice in 1 mL PBS following fixation.

5. Permeabilize cells for 5 min in PBS/0.5% Triton X-100, followed by 2 washes in PBS.

6. Incubate with primary antibody (*see* **Note 4**) diluted to 10 µg/mL in horse block buffer for 1 h at 37°C. We place 20 µL of diluted antibody on a piece of parafilm stretched over a glass plate. The coverslip is then placed cell side down on the antibody drop in a humidified incubator.

7. Wash 2 to 3 times in 1 mL of PBS for 5 min each.

8. Repeat staining with a Cy3- or TRITC-conjugated secondary antibody at 37°C for 30 min in the dark.

9. Wash 3 times in PBS.

10. Rinse coverslip briefly in distilled water before mounting on a drop of mounting medium containing an antifading agent (*see* **Note 3**).

4. Notes

1. Paraformaldehyde should always be made fresh by dissolving it in PBS (pH 7.6) at 55–60°C. This takes 1 to 2 h.

2. There are a number of suitable antibodies. However, choice must be restricted to those that have been raised specifically against the activated form of the enzyme, and not the pro-form. We use a rabbit polyclonal from R & D Systems (cat. no.

AF835), although Cell Signaling Technology, among others, have similar reagents available. For detection, we use a Cy3-conjugated Donkey anti-Rabbit antibody (Jackson). Some care must be taken, however, if no activation of caspase 3 is seen. There are many caspase isoforms, and examples exist where caspase 3 is not activated or even present (in MCF-7 cells, for example). A variety of similar reagents are now becoming available to other caspase family members, such as caspase 7 and caspase 9, although we have not tried these.

3. Use of an antifading agent is important when viewing some of the reagents mentioned later (for example mitotracker green-fm), as we have found them to bleach very quickly. We use fluorescent mounting medium from DAKO (cat. no. S3023).
4. During apoptosis, Bax undergoes a conformational change concomitant with its insertion into mitochondria. A number of antibodies are available, chiefly against epitopes at the aminoterminus of the molecule, which only recognize Bax in its activated, "open", conformation. These are ideal markers for cells in which Bax has been activated as part of the apoptotic response. We have had good results with a rat monoclonal anti-Bax from BD Pharmingen (clone G206-1276) and also a mouse monoclonal from Zymed (clone 5B7).
5. Some cell types do not adhere well to glass coverslips, and upon application of damaging stimuli, they may all detach. It may, therefore, help to either acid wash the coverslips and/or treat them with a suitable adhesive coating such as collagen or gelatin. To acid wash, make up a few hundred milliliters of 2 parts nitric acid and 1 part HCl in a large beaker. Add a number of coverslips, making sure that they are all separated from each other, and leave them for 2 to 3 h, swirling them occasionally. Decant the acid carefully into a receptacle and rinse the coverslips in running tap water until the pH reaches normal. Rinse the coverslips in distilled water and the leave them in a container of 70% ethanol. To coat coverslips, there are a number of possibilities. We typically use collagen I, coated at 100 µg/mL in PBS overnight at 4°C. Alternatively, gelatin, fibronectin, or poly-L-lysine can be used, since all promote adhesion. The choice of substrate could affect the experimental outcome, and so should receive some consideration. In normal mammary epithelial cells, integrin-mediated adhesion is required for inhibition of apoptosis. Nonphysiological substrata, such as poly-L-lysine or gelatin may not provide survival signals for cultured epithelial cells.
6. It is important to obtain cytospun cells at the correct density. If they are too dense, then it will be difficult to determine one from another following staining. Cells (200–300) per slide give a good density. If the cells are too dense, spend the extra few minutes to respin them at a lower density. To stain cytospun cells, draw around the circle of cells with a wax pen (DAKO) while the slide is dry. This will then allow the addition of small volumes (20–30 µL) of antibody.
7. As with mitotracker, the intensity of annexin V staining is decreased upon fixation and permeabilization.
8. There are a number of types of homogenizer available. To achieve sufficient lysis of the cells, it is important to use a Dounce homogenizer with a glass pestel. These have been made with a more precise fit between the pestle and the mortar

than the glass Teflon varieties and are available from Wheaton. We use one with a 5-mL volume for 0.5 mL of lysate. Good homogenization can also be obtained by drawing the cells through a small (19 gauge) needle with a syringe. Alternatively, cells can be repeatedly freeze/thawed using a dry ice/ethanol bath or liquid nitrogen, and it may be useful to try a number of methods to see which works best with your cell type, as there can be a degree of variation.

9. Whichever method is used for homogenization, it is important to check that it has been effective. Using a phase contrast microscope is quick and can be used during the homogenization procedure to determine when it is sufficiently complete. The nuclei should appear as a clean smooth structure, and there should be no large aggregates of cytoplasm. These clumps can often occur if the cells have been over homogenized, when the nuclei can be disrupted and release DNA. The best way to assay for the effectiveness of homogenization is to analyze each fraction by Western blotting for suitable markers (*see* **Note 11**).

10. The protocol here will provide a pellet that contains all of the internal cell membranes and does not distinguish between mitochondria and endoplasmic reticulum (ER). The protocol can be modified to further separate fractions such as the mitochondria (which pellet at 14,000g) and the lighter ER. However, for the purposes of examining the release of cytochrome c or the translocation of Bcl-2 family proteins, this is not necessary.

11. There are a number of useful markers for identification of ER, mitochondria, nuclear fractions, and cytoplasmic fractions. We use the following: nucleus, poly ADP ribose polymerase (BD Transduction Laboratories, cat. no. 65196E); ER, calnexin (StressGen, cat. no. SPA-860); mitochondia, cytochrome-oxidase subunit I (Molecular Probes, cat. no. A-6403); the cytoplasm, caspase 3 (Santa Cruz, cat. no. sc-1224), which also provides a marker for apoptosis, as it will be cleaved from its 30 kDa pro-form to 11- and 18-kDa fragments. To assay cytochrome c release, we use an antibody from BD Transduction Laboratories (cat. no. 65981A).

12. Molecular Probes market a number of fluorescent dyes that are taken up by live mitochondria. In our studies, we have utilized these along with conventional immunohistochemistry, in which case your choice of mitochondrial stain is quite important. Most of the dyes are not fixed by paraformaldehyde and, therefore, are lost following permeabilization prior to staining. Mitotracker green-fm (cat. no. M-7514) is fixed, although it loses some of its intensity. This can be compensated for by using it at 500 nm, which is higher than the concentration normally recommended.

Acknowledgments

A.P.G. is a Wellcome Trust Career Development Fellow. C.H.S. is a Wellcome Trust Senior Fellow in Basic Biomedical Science.

References

1. Jacobson, M.D, Weil, M., and Raff. M. C. (1997) Programmed cell death in animal development. *Cell.* **88,** 347–354.

2. Raff, M. (1998) Cell suicide for beginners. *Nature.* **396,** 119–122.
3. Savill, J. (2000) Corpse clearance defines the meaning of cell death. *Nature* **407,** 784–788.
4. Nicholson, D. W. (2000) From bench to clinic with apoptosis-based therapeutic agents. *Nature* **407,** 810–816.
5. Gross, A., Jockel, J., Wei, M. C., and Korsmeyer, S. J. (1998) Enforced dimerization of BAX results in its translocation, mitochondrial dysfunction and apoptosis. *EMBO J.* **17,** 3878–3885.
6. Hengartner, M. O. (2000) The biochemistry of apoptosis. *Nature* **407,** 770–776.
7. Desagher, S. and Martinou, J. C. (2000) Mitochondria as the central control point of apoptosis. *Trends Cell Biol.* **10,** 69–77.
8. Cain, K., Bratton, S. B., Langlais, C., Walker, G., Brown, D. G., Sun, X. M., and Cohen, G. M. (2000) Apaf-1 oligomerizes into biologically active approximately 700-kDa and inactive approximately 1.4-MDa apoptosome complexes. *J. Biol. Chem.* **275,** 6067–6070.
9. Green, D. R. and Beere, H. M. (2000) Gone but not forgotten. *Nature* **405,** 28–29.
10. Green, D. R. (2000) Apoptotic pathways: paper wraps stone blunts scissors. *Cell* **102,** 1–4.
11. Fadok, V. A., Bratton, D. L., Rose, D. M., Pearson, A., Ezekewitz, R. A. B., and Henson, P. M. (2000) A receptor for phosphatidylserine-specific clearance of apoptotic cells. *Nature* **405,** 85–90.
12. Wolter, K. G., Hsu, Y. T., Smith, C. L., Nechushtan, A., Xi, X. G., and Youle, R. J. (1997) Movement of Bax from the cytosol to mitochondria during apoptosis. *J. Cell Biol.* **139,** 1281–1292
13. Gilmore, A. P., Metcalfe, A. D., Romer, L. H., and Streuli, C. H. (2000) Integrin-mediated survival signals regulate the apoptotic function of Bax through its conformation and subcellular localization. *J. Cell Biol.* **149,** 431–446.
14. Desagher, S., Osen-Sand, A., Nichols, A., et al. (1999) Bid-induced conformational change of Bax is responsible for mitochondrial cytochrome c release during apoptosis. *J. Cell Biol.* **144,** 891–901.

14

Keratins as Markers of Epithelial Cells

David L. Hudson

1. Introduction

Epithelial tissues, whether protective (such as skin or gut), or secretory (glandular linings) are required to withstand both physical and chemical stress, while at the same time maintaining normal tissue turnover. Much of this stress resistance is provided by a specialized cytoskeleton formed, as in all human cells, from three types of cytoplasmic filaments: actin filaments, microtubules, and intermediate filaments. The actin cytoskeleton is responsible for changes in cell shape and motility, the tubulin cytoskeleton for orientation and cytoplasmic polarization, and the intermediate filament cytoskeleton provides structural resilience *(1)*. Intermediate filaments are 10-nm diameter cytoplasmic structures that, unlike the other two classes, show tissue-specific expression. The five main groups are the keratin filaments (epithelia), vimentin filaments (mesenchyma), desmin filaments (muscle), glial filaments (astrocytes), and neurofilaments (nerve).

Epithelial cells show a pattern of keratin expression that defines not only the epithelial tissue type, but also the differentiation status of the cells. The keratin family, originally cataloged by Moll et al. *(2)*, currently consists of 20 different polypeptides. These are divided into two major subgroups, the basic, type I keratins (1–9), and the acidic, type II keratins (10–20), according to their mobility in 2-dimensional gel electrophoresis. Filaments are assembled from parallel heterodimers, containing one polypeptide of each type, which are bundled into mature filaments. The minimum number of keratins an epithelial cell expresses is therefore two, one each of type I and type II. Although, in vitro, any type I keratin can form heterodimeric complexes with any type II keratin *(3)*, specific pairs are expressed in different epithelial tissues. Basal layer cells

From: *Methods in Molecular Biology, vol. 188: Epithelial Cell Culture Protocols*
Edited by: C. Wise © Humana Press Inc., Totowa, NJ

in all multilayered epithelia express K5 with K14 *(4,5)*, but this expression is down-regulated during differentiation and switched to new tissue-specific heterodimers as cells migrate into suprabasal layers (*see* **Table 1**). These newly expressed keratins include K1 and K10 in cornified epithelia, such as epidermis, K4 and K13 in noncornifying squamous epithelia, and K3 with K12 in cornea. In glandular tissues, such as breast and prostate, the basal layer also expresses K5/14, while luminal secretory cells express K8/18 *(2)*.

Primary cells from epithelial tissues also express keratin patterns similar to the proliferative population from which they were derived and, under the right growth conditions, will also express differentiation-specific keratins *(6–8)*. Epithelial keratins are relatively abundant and stable and are readily detected immunologically. This means that they are ideal for use as markers in the characterization of cultured epithelial cells and for monitoring cell differentiation.

Although, as a family, they share a high degree of homology, there are enough differences between members for mono-specific antibodies to have been raised against most of them, and many are commercially available (*see* **Table 1**). Some antibodies, such as LP34, recognize several different keratins and will stain virtually all cells of epithelial origin. These are termed pan-keratin antibodies.

The protocols presented here describe methods for the preparation and staining of cultured cells to identify keratin expression and include two different detection methods. The first method is immunocytochemical, where a color reaction is used to detect bound antibody, and the second method involves the use of immunofluorescence, whereby the primary antibody is detected with a fluorescently conjugated secondary antibody and visualized on an epifluorescence or confocal microscope. The basic principles for the two procedures are similar but, while use of fluorescence-tagged secondary antibodies is simpler, it depends on the availability of specialized fluorescence microscope equipment which may not be available to all researchers. In this case, immunocytochemistry is the only option. Another advantage of using fluorescence is that, with a suitable combination of primary antibodies differing in species or Ig type, it is possible to stain for two or more antigens simultaneously and to detect them with differently labeled secondary antibodies. The two most commonly used fluorophores are fluorescein isothiocyanate (FITC; green emission) and tetramethyl rhodamine isothiocyanate (TRITC; red emission). Additionally, there are also aminomethylcoumarin (AMCA; blue emission) and

---

(*see* Table 1 *right*) Keratins listed as commonly expressed type I/type II pairs with typical tissue locations. The specificity of each antibody is described in the reference listed and each has been chosen for minimal nonspecific cross-reactivity.

[a]These antibodies may also be available from other suppliers.

[b]This antibody also recognizes keratin 10.

Table 1
Keratin Expression in Epithelial Tissues

Keratin	Typical tissue expression pattern	Antibody clone	Supplier[a]
5	Basal cells in all stratified epithelium	None commercially available.	
14		LL002 (*5*)	Novocastra Serotec
15	Patchy staining of basal cells in stratified epithelia.	LHK15 (*9*)	Novocastra
1		34βb4 (*10*)	Novocastra
2	Suprabasal cells in stratified epithelium.	None commercially available	
10		LHP1 (*11*)	Novocastra
11		K8.60[b] (*12*)	Sigma
9	Suprabasal palmoplantar epidermal layers.	None commercially available	
3	Corneal epithelium.	AE5 (*13*)	Biogenesis
12		None commercially available	
4	Suprabasal cells of non-cornifying epithelium.	6B10 (*14*)	Novocastra/Dako
13		1C7 (*14*)	ICN
6	Hyperproliferative epidermis, oral mucosa.	LHK6B (*15*)	Novocastra
16		LL025 (*16*)	Novocastra
7	Simple epithelium and some basal prostate cells.	RCK105 (*17*)	ICN/Dako
17		E3 (*18*)	Sigma/Dako Novocastra
8	Simple epithelium and luminal cells in breast and prostate.	35βH11 (*10*)	Dako
18		RGE53 (*19*)	ICN
19	Hair follicle keratinocytes, simple epithelium, some basal and luminal prostate epithelial cells, luminal breast epithelial cells.	RCK108	Dako
20	Umbrella cells of urothelium and merkel cells.	Ks20.8 (*21*)	Novocastra/Dako
Pan-Keratin	Keratin 1, 5, 6, and 18	LP34 (*11*)	Novocastra/Dako

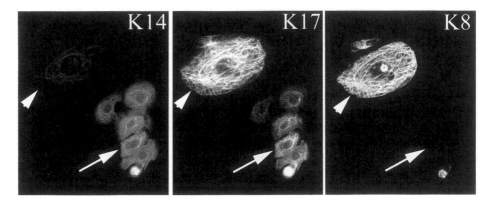

Fig. 1. Keratin staining of cultured epithelial cells. Triple immunofluorescent staining of prostate epithelial cells with antibodies recognizing keratins 14 (LLOO2, IgG3),
17 (E3, IgG2b), and 8 (35βH11, IgM). Cells were plated onto coverslips and allowed
to grow for 48 h. After this time, the cells were fixed and stained as described in
Subheading 3.4. Primary antibodies were detected with secondary antibodies conjugated to Cy5, anti-IgG3, TRITC (anti IgG2b), and FITC (anti IgM). Note K14 staining
of small "basal"-like cells (arrows) and K8 staining of larger more differentiated "luminal"-like cells (arrowheads). K17 is expressed by almost all prostate epithelial cells in
culture. Images were captured on a Hg-arc Zeiss axiophot fluorescence microscope
and stored separately as data files. Images were processed using Adobe Photoshop
(v5.0, Adobe Systems, San Jose, CA, USA).

indocarbocyanine 5 (Cy5; far-red emission). With a suitable filter block, all of
these can be used simultaneously, and separate images captured for each can
be viewed either overlaid or singly (*see* **Fig. 1**).

2. Materials

1. Subconfluent cultures of epithelial cells grown on coverslips (*see* **Notes 1** and **2**)
   or trypsin-harvested cells air-dried onto clean coverslips (*see* **Note 3**).
2. 7×-PF Laboratory detergent (ICN Biomedicals).
3. Phosphate-buffered saline (PBS) (Life Technologies).
4. 10 µg/mL Rat tail collagen type I (Vitrogen 100) (Nutacon, Postbus 94, 2450 AB
   Leimuiden, Netherlands) in PBS.
5. 1:1 (v/v) Acetone (Merck):methanol (Merck).
6. Peroxidase blocking solution: 100 µL 30% hydrogen peroxide (Sigma) in 100 mL PBS.
7. Antibody diluent: L15 medium (Life Technologies) containing 10% fetal calf
   serum (FCS) (Sigma).
8. 140-mm Petri dishes or 500-cm^2 square Petri dish.
9. Primary antibodies raised against keratins of interest (*see* **Table 1**).
10. Fluorochrome-conjugated secondary antibodies (Southern Biotechnology Asso-
    ciation, Birmingham, AL, USA) (*see* **Notes 16** and **17**).

11. Vectastain® Elite ABC kit (anti-mouse or rabbit) (Novocastra).
12. DAB substrate kit (Novocastra) (or 3,3'-Diaminobenzidine (DAB) tablets [Sigma]) (*see* **Note 4**).
13. 1 µg/mL bisBenzamidine Hoechst No. 33258 trihydrochloride (Sigma) in deionized water.
14. Tween-20 (Sigma).
15. Vectashield® aqueous mounting medium (Novocastra).
16. VectaMount™ (Novocastra) or DPX permanent mounting medium (Merck).
17. Clear nail polish.
18. Gills hematoxylin (Merck).
16. Filter paper squares or 15-cm rounds (i.e., Whatman No. 1).
17. 13-mm Coverslips, No. 1 size (prewashed and sterilized as described in **Note 1**).
18. Fine watchmaker's forceps, size No. 5.

3. Methods

3.1. Fixing and Permeabilizing Epithelial Cell Cultures Grown on Coverslips

1. Select coverslips with evenly distributed cells and few confluent areas. If air-dried cells are being used these should also be distributed evenly over the coverslip (*see* **Note 3**).
2. Wash wells with 3 changes of PBS, removing as much liquid as possible after the final rinse.
3. Fix and permeabilize the cells by adding 1 mL of a 1:1 mixture of acetone and methanol per well and incubating at room temperature for 2 min (*see* **Note 5**). Air-dried cells should be fixed and permeabilized in the same way, but without prior PBS washing.
4. Remove methanol:acetone (*see* **Note 6**) and wash coverslips with 3 changes of PBS.
5. The coverslips are now ready to stain immediately or can be stored at –70°C by freezing the plates immediately after stage 4, omitting the PBS washing stage (*see* **Note 7**).

3.2. Immunocytochemical Staining of Cells for Keratins

1. After fixation or thawing coverslips, add peroxidase-blocking solution and incubate for 15–30 min at room temperature (*see* **Note 8**).
2. Wash coverslips with PBS, either by dipping into beakers of PBS and draining onto filter paper or by flooding the coverslips 3 times with PBS and incubating for 5 min.
3. Block nonspecific antibody binding by incubating the coverslips with antibody diluent solution for 30 min at room temperature.
4. To set up a moist incubation chamber, line the lid of an inverted 140-mm diameter round or 500-cm² square Petri dish with filter paper.
5. Using a pencil, mark a 2-cm grid on the filter paper consisting of numbered squares. The numbers are used as a code to identify the coverslips during the

staining procedure. Add sufficient water to moisten the filter paper without flooding the surface.

6. Using fine watchmaker's forceps, pick up the coverslips one at a time and transfer them, from the plate or Petri dish, to the grid. Use at least 2 coverslips per antibody or dilution, and additionally include extra coverslips as controls (*see* **Note 9**).

7. Dilute the primary antibodies in labeled Eppendorf tubes with diluent solution. 30–50 μL/13-mm coverslip should be sufficient (*see* **Note 10**).

8. Tip the blocking solution off each coverslip in turn and replace it with diluted antibody. Ensure at this point to make careful notes of the cell type, any treatment, and antibody used along with the grid number.

9. Incubate the cells in diluted primary antibody or control solution for a minimum of 45 min and a maximum of 2 h. If more convenient, this incubation can be carried out overnight at 4°C (*see* **Note 11**).

10. At the end of the incubation period tip off the primary antibody and wash the coverslips as in stage 2 (*see* **Note 12**).

11. Add diluted horseradish-conjugated secondary antibody and incubate for 45 min.

12. Prepare a DAB substrate solution following the manufacturer's instructions. Add 50 μL of DAB solution per coverslip and incubate for 2–5 min until a color reaction develops (*see* **Note 13**). This can be monitored under a microscope, but care must be taken not to contaminate the stage with DAB solution (*see* **Note 14**).

13. Transfer the used DAB solution into a universal tube for neutralization with bleach and wash the coverslips 3× in distilled water.

14. If counterstaining is required, add 50 μL of hematoxylin solution and incubate for between 30 s and 5 min (*see* **Note 15**).

15. Wash the coverslips in distilled water, allow to air-dry, and mount in a nonaqueous mountant, such as DPX or VectaMount, cell side down onto microscope slides. Mark the microscope slides with the identification number of each coverslip.

16. The coverslips are now ready for examination, and the staining will be stable for long periods if kept cool and dark.

3.3. Immunofluorescent Staining of Cells for Keratins

1. Following fixation of cells or thawing of frozen coverslips, block nonspecific antibody binding by incubating coverslips in 50 μL of antibody diluent solution for 30 min.

2. Follow stages 4 to 10 in **Subheading 3.2.** for immunocytochemical staining.

3. Add diluted fluorophore-conjugated secondary antibody and incubate for 45 min (*see* **Note 16**). From this point onwards, the secondary antibody will be sensitive to light, and therefore, all incubations should be in the dark. Wrapping foil around the humid box should provide sufficient protection from light.

4. Wash coverslips as before and, after a final rinse in distilled water, mount coverslips face down onto aqueous mounting medium containing bleaching retardant (such as Vectashield mounting medium).

5. For long term storage, seal the coverslip around the edge with nail polish and store in the dark at 4°C.

6. The slides are now ready to view on a confocal or epifluorescence microscope and, if sealed, will keep in the dark for several weeks.

3.4. Simultaneous Immunofluorescent Staining of Cells for Multiple Keratins

1. Carry out coverslip preparation in exactly the same way as for single antibody staining.
2. Select a range of primary antibodies that are either different species or different Ig class or subclass (*see* **Note 17**).
3. Dilute all primary antibodies in appropriate combinations in antibody diluent solution in Eppendorf tubes to the desired dilution.
4. Incubate coverslips with primary antibody for 45 min to 2 h at room temperature. If convenient, this step can be carried out at 4°C overnight (*see* **Note 11**).
5. Wash as described in **Subheading 3.2.**
6. Incubate coverslips in appropriate combinations of secondary antibodies (*see* **Note 17**) in antibody diluent for 35 min to 2 h.
7. Wash coverslips and incubate with the DNA stain, Hoechst, for 5 min.
8. Wash coverslips as before and, after a final rinse in distilled water, mount coverslips cell side down onto aqueous mounting medium containing bleaching retardant (such as Vectashield mounting medium).

4. Notes

1. As part of the manufacturing process, coverslips are silicon-treated to prevent them from sticking together. This can interfere with the attachment of some cells, and therefore, it is preferable to wash coverslips before sterilization. The coverslips are boiled for 15 min, either over a Bunsen burner or in a microwave oven, in a weak solution (0.3%) of 7× detergent. If using a Bunsen burner, gently stir at regular intervals with a glass rod to resuspend the coverslips. If boiling in a microwave, stir at 5-min intervals. The coverslips will "bump" in the solution, so a beaker over a flame should not be left unattended. It is possible to wash 300–500 coverslips at a time in 1 L of detergent solution in a 2-L beaker. After heating, allow to cool to room temperature, stirring every 10 min. Rinse by gently running tap water into the beaker for 15 min. Run the water at a speed that keeps the coverslips moving without washing them over the edge of the beaker. Rinse with 10 changes of distilled water and finally 2 changes of 70% ethanol. Separate and spread the coverslips out on tissue paper to dry before transferring into glass Petri dishes or heat-resistant boxes for oven sterilization.
2. To grow the cells on coverslips, place 13-mm coverslips (treated as in **Note 1**) into either 24-well plates or evenly distributed over the surface of 6-cm Petri dishes. Seed the epithelial cells of interest at low density (10^3–10^4 per well, 10^5 per 6-cm dish) in growth medium and allow to grow for a minimum of 24 h. The cells will have attached and spread sufficiently in this time for the detection of keratins. Either fix the cells at this point or leave longer to allow the formation of small colonies. Avoid confluent cultures, as stratification of the cells can impair

antibody access to the underlying cells. In the event that the cells do not attach to the coverslips, it may be necessary to precoat them with an extracellular matrix protein such as collagen. To do this, dilute collagen type I to 10 µg/mL in PBS and add sufficient to cover the coverslips. Incubate at 37°C for 1 h, then remove the solution, wash coverslips 3 times with PBS, and seed the cells as before.

3. An alternative to growing cells on coverslips is to harvest cells from cultures by trypsinization and transfer aliquots to washed coverslips onto which they are air-dried and fixed before staining. Prepare a suspension of epithelial cells at 3×10^5/mL in culture medium containing 10% FCS. Add 50 µL to each of 10–15 coverslips in a 90-mm Petri dish. Gently spread the cell suspension over the coverslip surface and place in a dry oven at 37°C for 15–30 min, until only the very center of the coverslip remains damp.

4. While there are several different substrates available, DAB gives a strong dark brown color reaction that is insoluble in water, alcohol, and xylene. It contrasts well with the blue nuclear counterstain obtained with hematoxylin. Although it can be purchased as a powder, it is also available in tablet form, allowing a 1-, 5-, or 15-mL solution to be made from a single fast dissolving tablet. The third and easiest of all options is liquid substrate kits, which provide separate DAB, buffer and hydrogen peroxide solutions in dropper bottles with easy-to-follow instructions.

5. Some protocols recommend the use of 1:1 methanol:acetone at –20°C for 5–10 min. While this also works well, it has the added complication that storage of solvents in non-spark-free freezers presents a serious fire hazard and should be avoided. Therefore, the methanol:acetone will need to be chilled immediately prior to carrying out the staining.

6. As acetone is highly inflammable, used solution should be stored as solvent waste and disposed of following laboratory safety protocols.

7. The samples must be thawed slowly, by taking them from –70°C and allowing them to reach room temperature before rinsing in PBS and proceeding with the staining protocol.

8. As the detection system for immunocytochemistry relies on a reaction involving peroxidase-conjugated secondary antibodies, it is advantageous to block endogenous peroxidase activity in the cells.

9. Wherever possible, a positive control should be included to check the staining procedure. This could be cultures of cells, or tissue sections containing cells, which are known to be positive for the antigen of interest. Additionally, negative controls should be included for each secondary antibody type used. Where possible, negative controls should be irrelevant antibodies (recognizing proteins not expressed by the cells under analysis) of the same species, source (purified antibody, supernatant, or acites), and Ig subclass. If such an antibody is not available, a minimum control should be incubation with antibody diluent alone.

10. If the optimal concentrations of primary and secondary antibodies are unknown, it is possible to set up a checkerboard of positive control samples and use a range of primary antibody concentrations of 1:10, 1:100, 1:1000, and 1:10,000 in conjunction with a range of secondary antibody concentrations over the same range.

After establishing the best dilution from this range, the concentration can be optimized further with smaller changes in dilution, until maximal staining with the lowest background is obtained. To avoid microbial contamination of the antibodies, dilutions should be carried out under sterile conditions, such as in a class II laminar flow hood.

11. It is vital that, once the primary antibody has been added, the coverslips do not dry out until the staining process is complete. For this reason, if incubations are carried out at 4°C, care should be taken not to disturb the coverslips when moving the incubation chamber.

12. If background staining is a problem, it is possible to increase the efficiency of the washing solution by the inclusion of detergents such as 0.2% Tween-20.

13. At this stage, the negative control coverslips are used to check the maximum incubation time before background staining appears in the negative controls. If positive control samples are available, some idea of the minimum time required to develop a positive reaction can be determined.

14. DAB is a carcinogen and therefore should be handled with caution at all times. Used and excess solutions should be collected and neutralized with a bleach solution, such as chloros, before disposal with plenty of water down a sink.

15. Gill's hematoxylin formula allows for a slow progressive increase in intensity of staining with time. The optimal time can be determined beforehand. A light stain is required, which allows the nuclei to be visible without masking the brown DAB color.

16. Secondary fluorescent antibodies should be selected to suit the filter sets on the available epifluorescent or confocal microscope. The most commonly used secondary antibodies are conjugated to fluorescein or rhodamine. Fluorescein emits a green signal that is easily detected visually, but fades easily by photobleaching, so bleaching retardant is used in the mounting media. Rhodamine emits a red signal, but, while being less prone to bleaching, tends to produce higher background fluorescence.

17. Detection of more than one epitope is possible as long as the primary antibodies differ either in the species in which they were raised (such as mouse, rabbit, or sheep) or in immunoglobulin class (IgG, IgM) or subclass (IgG1, IgG2a, IgG2b, or IgG3). It is important that there is no cross reactivity between chosen sets and that commercial suppliers of secondary antibodies provide details of their specificity. For example, in a simultaneous staining with a rabbit and a mouse primary antibody, the goat anti-mouse secondary antibody must not recognize rabbit immunoglobulins, and the goat anti-rabbit must not bind mouse immunoglobulins. The most common coupling used is that of an antibody raised in rabbit together with one raised in mouse. These are then detected with a mixture of anti-rabbit and anti-mouse, one FITC- and one TRITC-conjugated. Since the majority of commercially available antibodies are raised in mice, it is often difficult to find antibodies from different species for particular antibody combinations. The recent introduction of mouse Ig subclass-specific secondary antibodies has improved this situation, and it is now possible to use several mouse antibodies at the same

time as long as they are of different subclasses. For example, the triple staining shown in **Fig. 1** was carried out using LL002, anti-keratin 14 (IgG3), E3, anti-keratin 17 (IgG2b), and 35βH11, anti-keratin 8 (IgM), and detected with Ig-type-specific secondary antibodies conjugated to far-red, rhodamine, and FITC.

References

1. Morley, S. M. and Lane, E. B. (1994) The keratinocyte cytoskeleton, p. 293–321. In *The keratinocyte handbook* (Leigh, I., Lane, E. B., and Watt, F. M., eds.). Cambridge University Press, Cambridge.
2. Moll, R., Franke, W. W., Schiller, D. L., Geiger, B., and Krepler, R. (1982) The catalog of human keratins: patterns of expression in normal epithelia, tumors and cultured cells. *Cell.* **31,** 11–24.
3. Hatzfeld, M. and Franke, W. W. (1985) Pair formation and promiscuity of cytokeratins: formation *in vitro* of heterotypic complexes and intermediate-sized filaments by homologous and heterologous recombinations of purified polypeptides. *J Cell Biol.* **101,** 1826–1841.
4. Nelson, W. G. and Sun, T. T. (1983) The 50- and 58-kdalton keratin classes as molecular markers for stratified squamous epithelia: cell culture studies. *J. Cell Biol.* **97,** 244–251.
5. Purkis, P. E., Steel, J. B., Mackenzie, I. C., Nathrath, W. B., Leigh, I. M., and Lane, E. B. (1990) Antibody markers of basal cells in complex epithelia. *J. Cell Sci.* **97,** 39–50.
6. Krueger, G. G., Jorgensen, C. M., Matsunami, N., et al. (1999) Persistent transgene expression and normal differentiation of immortalized human keratinocytes *in vivo. J. Invest. Dermatol.* **112,** 233–239.
7. Stingl, J., Eaves, C. J., Kuusk, U., and Emerman, J. T. (1998) Phenotypic and functional characterization *in vitro* of a multipotent epithelial cell present in the normal adult human breast. *Differentiation* **63,** 201–213.
8. Hudson, D. L., O'Hare, M., Watt, F. M., and Masters, J. R. W. (2000) Proliferative heterogeneity in the human prostate: evidence for epithelial stem cells. *Lab. Invest.* **80,** 1243–1250.
9. Waseem, A., Dogan, B., Tidman, N., et al. (1999) Keratin 15 expression in stratified epithelia: downregulation in activated keratinocytes. *J. Invest. Dermatol.* **112,** 362–369.
10. Gown, A. M. and Vogel, A. M. (1984) Monoclonal antibodies to human intermediate filament proteins. II. Distribution of filament proteins in normal human tissues. *Am. J. Pathol.* **114,** 309–321.
11. Lane, E. B., Bartek, J., Purkis, P. E., and Leigh, I. M. (1985) Keratin antigens in differentiating skin. *Ann. N.Y. Acad. Sci.* **455,** 241–258.
12. Huszar, M., Gigi-Leitner, O., Moll, R., Franke, W. W., and Geiger, B. (1986) Monoclonal antibodies to various acidic (type I) cytokeratins of stratified epithelia. Selective markers for stratification and squamous cell carcinomas. *Differentiation* **31,** 141–153.
13. Rodrigues, M., Ben-Zvi, A., Krachmer, J., Schermer, A., and Sun, T. T. (1987)

Suprabasal expression of a 64-kilodalton keratin (no. 3) in developing human corneal epithelium. *Differentiation* **34,** 60–67.

14. Van Muijen, G. N., Ruiter, D. J., Franke, W. W., Achtstatter, T., Haasnoot, W. H., Ponec, M., and Warnaar, S. O. (1986) Cell type heterogeneity of cytokeratin expression in complex epithelia and carcinomas as demonstrated by monoclonal antibodies specific for cytokeratins nos. 4 and 13. *Exp. Cell Res.* **162,** 97–113.

15. Markey, A. C., Lane, E. B., Macdonald, D. M., and Leigh, I. M. (1992) Keratin expression in basal cell carcinomas. *Br. J. Dermatol.* **126,** 154–160.

16. Lane, E. B., Wilson, C. A., Hughes, B. R., and Leigh, I. M. (1991) Stem cells in hair follicles. Cytoskeletal studies. *Ann. N.Y. Acad. Sci.* **642,** 197–213.

17. Ramaekers, F., Huysmans, A., Schaart, G., Moesker, O., and Vooijs, P. (1987) Tissue distribution of keratin 7 as monitored by a monoclonal antibody. *Exp. Cell Res.* **170,** 235–249.

18. Troyanovsky, S. M., Guelstein, V. I., Tchipysheva, T. A., Krutovskikh, V. A., and Bannikov, G. A. (1989) Patterns of expression of keratin 17 in human epithelia: dependency on cell position. *J. Cell Sci.* **93,** 419–426.

19. Ramaekers, F., Huysmans, A., Moesker, O., Kant, A., Jap, P., Herman, C., and Vooijs, P. (1983) Monoclonal antibody to keratin filaments, specific for glandular epithelia and their tumors. Use in surgical pathology. *Lab. Invest.* **49,** 353–361.

20. Kwaspen, F. H. L., Smedts, F. M. M., Broos, A., Bulten, H., Debie, W. H. M., and Ramaekers, F.C.S. (1997) Reproducible and highly sensitive detection of the broad spectrum epithelial cell marker keratin 19 in routine cancer diagnosis. *Histopathol.* **31,** 503–516.

21. Moll, R., Lowe, A., Laufer, J., and Franke, W. W. (1992) Cytokeratin 20 in human carcinomas. A new histodiagnostic marker detected by monoclonal antibodies. *Am. J. Pathol.* **140,** 427–447.

15

Epithelial Cell Integrins

Joachim Rychly

1. Introduction

Integrin receptors mediate the adhesion of cells to the extracellular matrix and to other cells. They play a significant role in a variety of biological functions including growth, differentiation, survival, and tissue organization. Integrins are heterodimeric transmembrane proteins consisting of a β and an α subunit, and their different combinations determine the binding specificity *(1)*. In epithelial cells, for example keratinocytes, different β1-integrins like β1α2, β1α3, and β1α5 are expressed. In addition, β4α6 is an integral part of hemidesmosomes which are specialized adherence junctions linked to the basement membrane *(2)*. Epithelial cells are generally polar and in a single-layered epithelia basolateral and apical cell surfaces are separated by tight junctions. This polarity also concerns the localization of integrins in the basolateral domains, which are detectable in a confluent culture of epithelial cells *(3–5)*. To study the role of different integrin receptors in biological functions, both the expression density and the distribution on the cell surface, including polarity, clustering or colocalization with other proteins in the cell surface, may be significant *(6)*. Techniques based on immunofluorescence are a suitable tool to analyze integrin expression and localization in epithelial cells. A variety of antibodies to different β- and α-integrin subunits are available and are distributed by a number of companies. In contrast to the basolateral integrin expression in a confluent culture, subconfluent cells express, in addition to the basal expression, integrins on the dorsal surface. Fixation is used to analyze integrins in cells with an intact membrane, or fixation is combined with permeabilization of the membrane to detect integrins in lateral or basal sites, for example, in surface domains that are not accessible in unpermeabilized cells. To examine the distribution of the receptors in the various domains of the cell surface, confocal

From: *Methods in Molecular Biology, vol. 188: Epithelial Cell Culture Protocols*
Edited by: C. Wise © Humana Press Inc., Totowa, NJ

laser scanning microscopy is recommended because of the possibility to perform horizontal and vertical optical sections through the cell. A quantitative evaluation of the integrin receptors can be carried out in the monolayer as well as by flow cytometric measurements of suspended epithelial cells *(7,8)*. The procedures and notes we describe here are mainly based on experiences with an simian virus 40 (SV40) immortalized epithelial cell line, which was derived from hepatocytes *(3)*.

2. Materials

1. Plastic Petri dishes.
2. Glass slides and glass coverslips (8 × 25 mm or 8 × 60 mm).
3. Cell culture medium: Dulbecco's Modified Eagle's medium (DMEM) supplemented with 10% fetal calf serum (FCS).
4. CO_2 incubator.
5. Phosphate-buffered saline (PBS), pH 7.2–7.4: 137 mM NaCl, 2.7 mM KCl, 4.3 mM Na_2HPO_4, 1.4 mM KH_2PO_4.
6. Humid chamber: use a glass Petri dish with a cover. This should be larger than the culture dish that the cells are grown on. Lay a filter paper on the bottom of the chamber and soak with distilled water to maintain the humidity. The culture dish should sit on top of the filter paper.
7. Adjustable pipets with tips.
8. Paraformaldehyde (PFA) solution (1, 2, and 4%): the solution should be freshly prepared. Add the required amount of PFA to 2 mL of PBS in a test tube. To dissolve the PFA, add some drops of 1 M NaOH and slightly heat the solution. Then add 8 mL of PBS and adjust the pH again to 7.2–7.4.
9. Glutaraldehyde.
10. Monoclonal antibodies to integrin subunits (β1, α1, α2, α4, α5).
11. Secondary fluorochrome-labeled antibody: fluorescein isothiocyanate (FITC)-labeled anti-mouse antibody.
12. Secondary ^{125}I-labeled antibody: sheep anti-mouse IgG, 19–74 Bq/mmol (Amersham).
13. Mounting medium: 30 g glycerol, 12 g polyvinylic alcohol (Mw 30–70 kDa), 30 mL distilled water, 0.5 g phenol. Mix glycerol, water, and phenol. Add polyvinylic alcohol under constant stirring. Keep the solution for 12 h in the water bath at 40–45° C. Add 60 mL of 0.1 M Tris, pH 8.5. The medium should be stored at 4°C.
14. Triton X-100.
15. 2 mM EGTA in Ca^{2+}-free DMEM.
16. 96-Well culture plates.
17. 0.05% Trypsin, 0.02% EDTA solution.
18. Pasteur pipets.
19. Water-jet vacuum pump.
20. Low-speed centrifuge.
21. Polystyrene round-bottom tubes (12 × 75) (Falcon, cat. no. 2052).
22. Facsflow solution (Becton Dickinson).
23. Vortex mix.

24. Confocal laser scanning microscope (LSM 5; Carl Zeiss).
25. Flow cytometer (Facscan; Becton Dickinson).
26. Multicrystal gamma counter (Berthold, cat. no. LB 2111-R).

3. Methods

3.1. Cell Subculture for Microscopic Examinations

To analyze integrin receptors for microscopic examinations, cell cultures are prepared on a coverslip.

1. Place a coverslip into a 35-mm (for 8 × 25 mm slips) or 60-mm (for 8 × 60 mm slips) plastic cell culture dish (*see* **Note 1**).
2. Add 2 mL of cell culture medium.
3. The number of cells you add to the Petri dish depends on the growth rate of the cells. With our immortalized epithelial cells, to obtain a subconfluent culture, we add 500 µL cell suspension containing 5×10^5 cells. For a confluent culture, we add 4×10^6 cells (*see* **Note 2**).
4. Culture the cells at 37°C in a CO_2 incubator for 24 h.
5. The density of the cell monolayer has to be controlled. For the analysis of a subconfluent culture, most of the cells should adhere as single cells. To analyze a confluent culture, the whole monolayer should form cell–cell contacts. If the cells do not reach a confluent monolayer, the cells should be cultured for a further day.

3.2. Cell Preparation to Detect Integrins in Nonpermeabilized Cells

To analyze integrins, which are accessible for antibodies, for example, on the dorsal surface of subconfluent cells, fixation is performed, which leaves the membrane intact.

1. After culturing the cells on a coverslip (confluent or nonconfluent), carefully remove the cell culture medium from the Petri dish using a pipet.
2. Rinse the Petri dish 3 times with 1 mL PBS.
3. For further preparation, the coverslip should remain in the Petri dish. Do not allow the cells to dry out at any step during the preparation.
4. Place the Petri dish, which contains the coverslip, into a humid chamber.
5. To fix the cells, add 100 µL of 1% PFA/0.025% glutaraldehyde and incubate for 10 min at room temperature (*see* **Note 3**).
6. Rinse 3 times with 1 mL PBS.
7. Incubation with antibodies: monoclonal mouse antibodies are available to detect a wide variety of integrin subunits. The concentration of these antibodies should be adjusted. When we use commercially available antibodies (for example, from Immunotech), with a protein concentration of 0.2 mg/mL, in general a dilution of 1:6 is appropriate. Add 50 µL of the diluted antibody onto the coverslip and incubate for 30 min at room temperature in the humid chamber.
8. Rinse twice with 1 mL PBS.

9. Incubate the cells with a secondary fluorochrome-labeled antibody. For example, FITC-labeled sheep-anti mouse IgG fragments can be used. Add 50 µL of the secondary antibody, diluted 1:16, for 30 min at room temperature.
10. Rinse with PBS.
11. Postfix with 2% PFA (*see* **Note 5**)
12. Embed the cells on the coverslip with mounting medium. The embedding medium that we use becomes solid within 24 h. Add 50 µL of mounting medium on a clean glass slide and place the coverslip on the slide with the cell monolayer towards the mounting medium (*see* **Note 6**).

3.3. Cell Preparation to Detect Integrins in Permeabilized Cells

Integrins interact at the basal surface with the extracellular matrix and laterally in cell–cell contacts in a confluent monolayer. In these sites, they are not accessible to antibodies. Fixation combined with permeabilization is necessary prior to antibody incubation.

1. Culture cells on coverslips in Petri dishes.
2. Rinse the cells with PBS and use a humid chamber for the following incubation steps.
3. Add 200 µL of 4% paraformaldehyde for 10 min at room temperature.
4. Wash the cells twice with 1 mL PBS.
5. Incubate the cells with 0.1% Triton X-100 for 1 h at room temperature (*see* **Note 7**).
6. Wash the cells twice with 1 mL of PBS.
7. Incubate with antibodies and follow the procedure further as described above (*see* **Subheading 3.2.**).

3.4. Accessibility of Integrins in Lateral Sites

For the interaction of integrins in lateral domains of confluent cells with different ligands to stimulate cells via integrins or perform specific analyses, it is necessary to make them accessible. Therefore, a dissection of cell–cell contacts without detaching the cells from the substrate is required.

1. Prepare a confluent cell culture on coverslips that are placed in a Petri dish.
2. Wash the cells twice with PBS.
3. Incubate the cell monolayer with Ca^{2+}-free DMEM containing 2 mM EGTA for 20 min at 4°C (*see* **Note 4**).
4. Incubate with anti-integrin antibodies to detect integrins or incubate with other ligands in the EGTA-containing medium.

3.5. Quantitative Analysis of Integrin Expression

3.5.1. Analysis of Integrins in a Monolayer

For quantitative analysis of the expression of integrins, which are accessible in a monolayer, it is possible to use radiolabeled secondary antibodies. To detect integrins in cell–cell contacts, dissolve the cell contacts prior to the incubation with integrin antibodies as described.

1. Prepare a culture in single wells of 96-well cell culture plates (2 wells for each condition).
2. Incubate with a monoclonal antibody to integrins as described in **Subheading 3.2.**
3. Wash the cells in PBS.
4. Incubate with 20 µL of ^{125}I-labeled sheep anti-mouse IgG, diluted 1:40, for 20 min at room temperature.
5. Wash 3× with PBS.
6. Measure the radioactivity in a multicrystal gamma counter. At least triplicate measurements should be performed.

3.5.2. Analysis of Integrins in Suspended Epithelial Cells

To measure the overall quantitative expression of integrins in epithelial cells, the flow cytometric analysis of suspended cells is a suitable technique.

1. Prepare a confluent or subconfluent culture of epithelial cells in plastic Petri dishes (35 mm size) or in a 10-mL cell culture flasks.
2. Wash the cell monolayer with PBS.
3. Detach the cells from the substrate using 0.05% trypsin-0.02% EDTA (*see* **Notes 8** and **9**). Add an appropriate volume of trypsin solution to cover the cell monolayer completely.
4. Leave the cells for 3 min in an CO_2 incubator.
5. Collect the detached cells in a test tube by rinsing the Petri dish or cell culture flask with PBS.
6. Wash the cells in the test tube twice with PBS by adding 2 mL PBS and centrifuging the cells at 400*g* for 10 min. Remove the supernatant and resuspend the cells in PBS with a pipet. Centrifuge again and resuspend in PBS (*see* **Note 10**)
7. To incubate with anti-integrin antibodies, use 20 µL of the cell suspension containing about 5×10^5 cells and add 20 µL undiluted anti-integrin antibodies (*see* **Note 11**).
8. Incubate for 30 min at room temperature.
9. Wash the cells once in PBS.
10. Add 20 µL of undiluted FITC-labeled sheep-anti mouse antibody to the cell sediment and mix carefully.
11. Incubate the cells for 30 min at room temperature in the dark.
12. Add 2 mL of PBS and wash the cells twice in PBS.
13. For the flow cytometric measurement add 0.5 mL Facsflow solution and measure the cells in a flow cytometer.

3.6. Confocal Laser Scanning Microscopy

The main techniques we use to analyze integrins in epithelial cells after fluorescence staining are confocal laser scanning microscopy and flow cytometry.

For detailed information of these techniques, we refer to handbooks (*9–12*). Here, and in **Subheading 3.7.**, we give some principal remarks concerning integrin analyses in epithelial cells using these techniques.

1. Most confocal laser scanning microscopes consist of an inverted fluorescence microscope, which is useful for both analysis of living cells in cell culture wells as well as coverslip preparations. For the analysis of coverslips embedded on a slide you turn the slide around to analyze the preparations through the coverslip.
2. In general, for analysis of the integrin distribution, use a 63× objective. We recommend a 63×/1.25 oil Plan-neofluar objective, which can be used for detailed analyses of integrin expression on individual cells.
3. To analyze the distribution of integrins in subconfluent cells, which express integrins on the whole cell surface, it is useful to perform optical sections in three horizontal planes: on the top, in the middle, and on the base of the cell. The distances between the planes will be about 3 μm, provided that the total cell height is 6 μm. Use the confocal version with a pinhole size of about 20 μm. You will obtain images of the integrin expression on the dorsal cell surface of the cell margin and of the basal adhesion site of the cell.
4. Despite permeabilization with acetone or Triton X-100, the fluorescence of receptors on the basal side is rather weak. Therefore, to demonstrate the receptor distribution, an enhanced brightness and contrast of the digital signals is required.
5. For analysis of confluent cultures, optical sections in the vertical direction are useful to demonstrate the expression of integrins in lateral cell–cell contacts. First, you perform a horizontal scan of the dorsal surface, then you set a cut line in the xy-plane, which crosses a number of cell–cell contacts. At this line, you scan in z-direction to obtain an image of the vertical area of the cell.

3.7. Flow Cytometry

1. Flow cytometric measurements require single cells in suspension. In general, epithelial cells can be measured by flow cytometry in the same way as separated blood cells. Nevertheless, normally adherent cells, like epithelial cells, tend to clump in suspension. Therefore, perform the measurement within 2 h after cell preparation. Resuspend carefully with a pipet or with vortex mixing before the measurement. If you observe clumps, filter the cells through gauze before the measurement.
2. For flow cytometric measurements, you first adjust the instrument settings to see the forward/sideward scatter of the cells on the monitor. Normally, you will have a relatively homogeneous population, which will be separated by some debris and clumps which differ in the scatter. Note that epithelial cells have a bigger size than blood cells. Therefore, the instrument setting for the level of the forward scatter detector may be very different compared with blood cell measurements.
3. The fluorescence measurement in the flow cytometer is identical to other cells. You measure first the control cells that are incubated only with the secondary fluorochrome-labeled antibody. You adjust the detector for the fluorescence that

the dot plot is set on the base line. Measure, then, all the samples with the same instrument settings (in general 10,000 cells are measured).

4. For the analysis, the cells are first gated in the forward/sideward scatter. The fluorescence intensities, which represent the expression of integrins, are presented as histograms.

4. Notes

1. Usually, before culturing the cells, coverslips are precoated with a matrix protein. Collagen I (from rat tail; Harbor Bio-Products, Norwood, USA) is a suitable protein for coating. Collagen has to be diluted in acetic acid (1:1000 v/v). Use a concentration of 0.2 mg/mL and add 20 µL onto the coverslip (8 × 25 mm) (50 µL for a 8 × 60 mm coverslip). Dry the collagen on the coverslips under the sterile box for 2 h.

2. For preparation of the culture on coverslips, seed the cells directly on the coverslip with a pipet, so that the cells adhere mainly to the coverslip and not to the bottom of the Petri dish. Usually, for analysis of a confluent cell culture, the culture is used on the first day of confluency. When the confluent monolayer is cultured longer, the cells change their morphology and may adhere more strongly. Therefore, for flow cytometric measurements, the detachment of the cells with trypsin may take longer and may injure the cell membrane.

3. A 4% PFA solution can also be used.

4. Breaking the cell–cell contacts with the calcium-free medium leads to an opening of the contacts without losing the adherence to the substrate. Labeling of the integrins after breaking the contacts show that the integrins remain relatively stably localized in the lateral sites without moving to the apical surface.

5. When the cell preparation is to be microscopically examined within the next few days, a postfixation with PFA is not necessary, but we recommend it for stabilizing the fluorescence for later examination of the specimens.

6. Avoid air bubbles during embedding the coverslips on the slides, by placing the coverslip with the edge into mounting medium and then drop it slowly.

7. As an alternative to the procedure we describe for permeabilization of the cells with PFA and Triton X-100, it is also possible to use acetone to fix and permeabilize the cells. Add 50 µL of cold acetone (–20°C) to the cell monolayer for 5 min. Then wash the cells 3 times with PBS.

8. For the detachment of cells from the substrate to perform flow cytometric analysis, trypsin-EDTA was most suitable. We tested other enzymatic and also mechanical approaches. Collagenase and dispase were less effective to detach the adherent cells. Mechanical detaching revealed that a great number of cells were impaired.

9. We found that integrin receptors are resistent to enzymatic treatment like trypsinization with 0.05% trypsin. To prove this, we tested whether trypsinization might reduce the density of integrin receptors. A possible loss of receptors due to trypsinization should be reconstituted by subsequent culturing of the cells in complete medium with serum. Therefore, epithelial cells were trypsinized,

washed in PBS, and the receptor expression then measured by flow cytometry. For comparison, an aliquot of these cells were cultured in complete medium with 10% of serum for a further 4 h at 37°C. The expression of integrins in cells cultured in complete medium after trypsinization was identical compared with the cells that were analyzed immediately after trypsinization. These results showed that trypsinization did not impair the expression of integrins.

10. Washing of the cells in the test tube is a very simple step of the procedure, but we have often observed that beginners lose a great number of cells during these washing steps. After centrifugation of the cells, removal of the supernatant is critical. The use of a water-jet vacuum pump appears most suitable. A pasteur pipet connected with the pump is placed at the inner wall of the test tube, some millimeters above the cell sediment, to suck off the PBS.

11. The concentration of the antibody used for flow cytometry has to be tested. In general, for the commercially available antibodies, 10 or 20 µL of undiluted antibodies are appropriate.

References

1. Hynes, R. O. (1992) Integrins: versatility, modulation, and signaling in cell adhesion. *Cell* **69,** 11–25.
2. Watt, F. M. and Hertle, M. D. (1994) Keratinocyte integrins, p. 156–164. In *The keratinocyte handbook* (Leigh, I. M., Lane, E. B., and Watt, F. M., eds.). Cambridge University Press, Cambridge.
3. Henning, W., Bohn, W., Nebe, B., Knopp, A., Rychly, J., and Strauss, M. (1994) Local increase of beta 1-integrin expression in cocultures of immortalized hepatocytes and sinusoidal endothelial cells. *Eur. J. Cell Biol.* **65,** 189–199.
4. Carter, W. G., Wayner, E. A., Bouchard, T. S., and Kaur, P. (1990) The role of integrins alpha 2 beta 1 and alpha 3 beta 1 in cell-cell and cell-substrate adhesion of human epidermal cells. *J. Cell Biol.* **110,** 1387–1404.
5. Marchisio, P. C., Bondanza, S., Cremona, O., Cancedda, R., and De Luca, M. (1991) Polarized expression of integrin receptors (alpha 6 beta 4, alpha 2 beta 1, alpha 3 beta 1, and alpha v beta 5) and their relationship with the cytoskeleton and basement membrane matrix in cultured human keratinocytes. *J. Cell Biol.* **112,** 761–773.
6. Nebe, B., Sanftleben, H., Pommerenke, H., Peters, A., and Rychly, J. (1998) Hepatocyte growth factor enables enhanced integrin-cytoskeleton linkage by affecting integrin expression in subconfluent epithelial cells. *Exp. Cell Res.* **243,** 263--273.
7. Nebe, B., Bohn, W., Sanftleben, H., and Rychly, J. (1996) Induction of a physical linkage between integrins and the cytoskeleton depends on intracellular calcium in an epithelial cell line. *Exp. Cell Res.* **229,** 100–110.
8. Nebe, B., Bohn, W., Pommerenke, H., and Rychly, J. (1997) Flow cytometric detection of the association between cell surface receptors and the cytoskeleton. *Cytometry* **28,** 66–73.
9. Jaroszeski, M. J. and Heller, R., eds. (1998) *Flow cytometric protocols.* Humana, Totowa, NJ.

10. Ormerod, M. G. (ed.) (2000) *Flow cytometry: a practical approach, 3rd ed.* Oxford University Press, Oxford.
11. Paddock, S. W., ed. (1999) *Confocal microscopy methods and protocols.* Humana, Totowa, NJ.
12. Pawley, J. B., ed. (1995) *Handbook of biological confocal microscopy, 2nd ed.* Olenum Press, New York.

16

Isolation, Cultivation, and Differentiation of Normal Human Epidermal Keratinocytes in Serum-Free Medium

Sebastian Zellmer and Dieter Reissig

1. Introduction

The outer layer of human skin is the epidermis. More than 90% of the epidermal cells are keratinocytes, which originate from stem cells, located in the basal cell layer (*Stratum basale*). Keratinocytes in the basal layer divide, differentiate, and migrate to the outer layer of the epidermis, the horny layer (*Stratum corneum*). The horny layer consists of terminally differentiated keratinocytes (corneocytes) embedded in multilamellar lipid sheets *(1)*. Finally, corneocytes are shed from the surface of the skin by desquamation. Keratinocytes are an ideal target for gene therapy *(2,3)* to treat desquamation disorders *(4,5)*. In addition, keratinocytes are secretory cells *(6)*, which opens the possibility for systemic delivery *(7,8)*.

The pioneering work of Rheinwald and Green *(9)* showed that human epidermal keratinocytes can be isolated and cultivated ex vivo. Therefore, the physiology and biochemistry of keratinocytes, as well as epidermal differentiation, can be studied *(10–14)*. In addition, the cultivation of keratinocytes from epidermal stem cells allows the generation of a reconstructed human epidermis. The latter can be used to study the development of the epidermis *(13)*, for pharmacological studies as an in vitro model system of the epidermis *(15–17)*, or as autografts in clinical applications *(18)*.

Here, we describe a rapid and simple method to isolate and cultivate normal human epidermal keratinocytes in serum-free medium and to generate a reconstructed human epidermis.

From: *Methods in Molecular Biology, vol. 188: Epithelial Cell Culture Protocols*
Edited by: C. Wise © Humana Press Inc., Totowa, NJ

2. Materials

2.1. Solutions

1. Betaisodona® solution (Mundipharma, Limburg, Germany), which is a polyvinylpyrrolidone-iodine complex used for decontamination. Use undiluted.
2. Keratinocyte growth medium (KGM): 500 mL keratinocyte basal medium supplemented with 0.1 μg/mL human epidermal growth factor (hEGF), 5 μg/mL insulin, 0.5 μg/mL hydrocortisone, 50 μg/mL gentamycin, 50 μg/mL amphotericin-B, and 30 μg/mL bovine pituitary extract (BPE). This is purchased ready-made (KGM® Bulletkit®, Clonetics, cat. no. CC-3111) to make up the KGM medium.
3. Sterile phosphate-buffered saline (PBS).
4. Dulbecco's modified Eagle's medium (DMEM) with GlutaMAX I™, 1 g/L glucose, sodium pyruvate. This is purchased ready-made. (Life Technologies) (*see* **Note 1**).
5. Ultroser® G (Life Technologies) (*see* **Note 2**), which is a fetal calf serum (FCS) substitute. Add 1 mL Ultroser G to 50 mL DMEM immediately before use.
6. 2.5 mg/mL Dispase II (Boehringer Mannheim) dissolved in KGM. The solution can be stored at 4°C for 1 to 2 wk, before losing its activity.
7. 0.25% EDTA in PBS. Store the solution at –18°C.
8. 0.25% Trypsin (4 U/mg) (Serva, Heidelberg, Germany) in PBS. Store the solution at –18°C.
9. Trypan blue solution
10. 15 mmol/L $CaCl_2$ stock solution and sterile, dissolved in KGM. Store the solution at 4°C.

2.2. Equipment

1. Incubator with 37°C, 5% CO_2 and 95% air.
2. Laminar air flow cabinet (biohazard).
3. Centrifuge (for example, Sigma 3–12) with 666g and low brake (deceleration 2).
4. Hemocytometer.
5. Inverse microscope with 5- and 20-fold magnification.
6. Cell culture flasks (25 cm²).
7. Transparent cell culture inserts for 24-well plates with 0.45 μm pore size (Falcon).
8. 24-Well plates (Falcon).
9. Sterile forceps and scissors.
10. 40-μm Pore cell strainer for filtration (Falcon).

3. Methods

3.1. Skin Preparation

1. For safe transportation, immediately after circumcision, place foreskin in sterile PBS (4°C) (*see* **Note 3**).
2. Remove, if necessary, the cutaneous fat layer using scissors.
3. Incubate the skin for 15 min at room temperature in Betaisodona® solution.
4. Rinse 3 times in sterile PBS.

5. Place the skin in a sterile Petri dish and cut the tissue in small pieces (approx 5×5 mm).
6. Incubate skin in 15 mL dispase solution at 4°C overnight (*see* **Note 4**).

3.2. Isolation of Human Epidermal Keratinocytes

1. Place skin piece in a sterile Petri dish and add PBS to prevent drying.
2. Detach the epidermis from the dermis using sterile forceps (*see* **Note 5**). Always keep skin and epidermis submerged in PBS.
3. Incubate the epidermis for 15 min at 37°C in 5 mL trypsin-EDTA (1:1; v:v) solution.
4. Shake the suspension every 5 min to increase the amount of dissociated basal keratinocytes.
5. Add 10 mL of Ultroser G in DMEM (*see* **Note 1**).
6. Centrifuge for 5 min at 666*g*.
7. Resuspend the keratinocytes in 5 mL KGM.
8. Filter the cell suspension through a cell strainer (*see* **Note 6**).
9. Count the keratinocytes, determine the viability with Trypan blue solution, and seed 1.25×10^5 cells in 25-cm^2 culture flasks (this corresponds to 5000/cm^2) with 4 mL KGM.
10. Change the medium 3× a wk (every second day) (*see* **Note 7**).

3.3. Subcultivation of Human Epidermal Keratinocytes

1. Use only keratinocyte clones that are highly proliferative (*see* **Note 8**).
2. Rinse cells twice with sterile PBS.
3. Rinse the cells twice with sterile trypsin-EDTA (1:1; v:v) solution. Remove the surplus of trypsin-EDTA solution from the flask.
4. Incubate cells for 5 min at 37°C.
5. Add 10 mL of Ultroser G in DMEM (*see* **Note 1**) and centrifuge for 5 min at 666*g*.
6. Resuspend the keratinocytes in 5 mL KGM, determine the total number of cells, and seed 1.25×10^5 cells in 25-cm^2 culture flasks (this corresponds to 5000/cm^2). The final volume of KGM in the flask should be 4 mL.
7. Change the medium 3× a wk (every second day).
8. Within a few days, a monolayer of normal human epidermal keratinocytes will develop in the culture flask, which can be used for further experiments (*see* **Note 9**).

3.4. Differentiation of Highly Proliferative Normal Human Epidermal Keratinocytes into a Reconstructed Human Epidermis

1. Harvest cells as described above (*see* **Subheading 3.3., steps 2–6.**).
2. Place cell culture inserts into a 24-well plate filled with approx 500 μL KGM per well.
3. Seed the keratinocytes at a density of 5.5×10^5/cm^2 onto the inserts, making sure that the cells are submersed (*see* **Note 10**).
4. Remove the medium from the insert after 3 d and transfer the insert to a fresh plate filled with KGM, supplemented with 1.5 m*M* CaCl$_2$ (*see* **Note 11**).

5. Within 3–4 d, the keratinocytes will differentiate into a cellular multilayer (3-dimensional reconstructed epidermis), which can be used, for example, in pharmacological studies *(16)*.

6. Daily inspection of the culture is recommended, since contamination of these air–liquid interface cultures can occur. Always remove infected inserts.

7. Change the medium once a week (*see* **Note 12**).

4. Notes

1. We use DMEM, supplemented with Ultroser (*see* **Subheading 2.1., step 5.**) to inactivate trypsin after the detachment of the cells (*see* **Subheading 3.2., step 5.** and **Subheading 3.3., step 3.**), since it is less expensive than KGM.

2. Ultroser G (2 g) is reconstituted in 20 mL sterile distilled water, and this stock solution is stored in aliquots of 1 mL at –18°C.

3. We recommend the isolation of keratinocytes from the foreskins of children aged between 3–10 yr. This skin is free of hair follicles, has no cutaneous fat layers, and the keratinocytes will show a high proliferation rate. Do not use foreskin with signs of inflammation, since the cell preparations will contain a high proportion of other cells.

4. The skin can also be incubated for 2 h at 37°C. However, this results in a lower yield of cells.

5. The incubation in dispase II results in a destruction of the hemisdesmosomes. While holding the skin with one pair of forceps, you can easily remove the epidermis with a second pair of forceps, in a similar manner as you would detach a label from a piece of paper.

6. The filtration step results in the separation of the cells and epidermal pieces. In addition, it increases the number of small keratinocytes, which are derived from the stem cells of the epidermis *(19)*.

7. The keratinocytes will attach within 0.5–2 h to the bottom of the flask and start to spread. Within 2–3 d, the cells start to divide. This depends on the age of the skin donor and the body part from where the skin originated. Only small keratinocytes will start to divide and produce clones *(19)*. Larger keratinocytes will cease to divide quite quickly *(20)*. In order to obtain a large number of colonies, you should seed at the indicated density. One can increase the number of keratinocytes from the stem cell population by replacing the medium 30 min after seeding, since the basal cells will attach rapidly *(21)*.

8. After 4–5 d, several clones or colonies are present. When the colonies consist of 50–60 keratinocytes, the cells should be harvested.

9. Close inspection of the culture is important. The culture will consist of 3 different types of keratinocytes clones: holoclones, meroclones, and paraclones *(20)*. The holoclones exhibit a low rate of mitosis in combination with a large growth potential. After 1 wk of cultivation, the individual keratinocytes start to differentiate.

10. The cell density must be high enough to result in confluent culture conditions when the keratinocytes attach to the bottom of the insert.

11. Prepare KGM, supplemented with 1.5 mM $CaCl_2$, using the $CaCl_2$ stock solution (*see* **Subheading 2.1.**). The high $CaCl_2$ concentration will promote the differ-

entiation of the keratinocytes. It is important that the insert is empty and that the level of the medium in the well is not above the cell layer in the insert. The development of the cellular multilayer will be disturbed if the medium in the well creates a hydrostatic pressure. However, if there is not enough medium in the well, the cells will dry out and die. We found that 200 µL KGM in a 24-well plate is sufficient.

12. At this stage of cultivation, growth has ended, and the keratinocytes differentiate. A stratified epithelium develops. This requires less frequent changes of medium, which also decreases the risk of contamination.

Acknowledgments

We thank J. Salvetter for carefully reading the manuscript. This work has been supported in part by the Deutsche Forschungsgemeinschaft through Grant Nos. Re 1426/1-1 and Ze 376/1-1.

References

1. Landmann L. (1988) The epidermal permeability barrier. *Anat. Embryol.* **178,** 1–13.
2. Hengge U. R., Walker P. S., and Vogel J. C. (1996) Expression of naked DNA in human, pig, and mouse skin. *J. Clin. Invest.* **97,** 2911–2916.
3. Levy, L., Broad, S., Zhu, A. J., Carroll, J. M., Khazaal, I., Peault, B., and Watt, F. M. (1998) Optimised retroviral infection of human epidermal keratinocytes: long-term expression of transduced integrin gene following grafting on to SCID mice. *Gene Ther.* **5,** 913–922.
4. Choate, K. A., Kinsella, T. M., Williams, M. L., Nolan, G. P., and Khavari, P. A. (1996) Transglutaminase 1 delivery to lamellar ichthyosis keratinocytes. *Hum. Gene Ther.* **7,** 2247–2253.
5. Vailly, J., Gagnoux-Palacios, L., Dell'Ambra, E., et al. (1998) Corrective gene transfer of keratinocytes from patients with junctional epidermolysis bullosa restores assembly of hemidesmosomes in reconstructed epithelia. *Gene Ther.* **5,** 1322–1332.
6. Katz, A. B. and Taichman, L. B. (1999) A partial catalog of proteins secreted by epidermal keratinocytes in culture. *J. Invest. Dermatol.* **112,** 818–821.
7. Meng, X., Sawamura, D., Tamai, K., Hanada, K., Ishida, H., and Hashimoto, I. (1998) Keratinocyte gene therapy for systemic diseases. Circulating interleukin 10 released from gene-transferred keratinocytes inhibits contact hypersensitivity at distant areas of the skin. *J. Clin. Invest.* **101,** 1462–1467.
8. White, S. J., Page, S. M., Margaritis, P., and Brownlee, G. G. (1998) Long-term expression of human clotting factor IX from retrovirally transduced primary human keratinocytes *in vivo. Hum. Gene Ther.* **9,** 1187–1195.
9. Rheinwald, J. G. and Green, H. (1975) Serial cultivation of strains of human eipidermal keratinocytes: the formation of keratinizing colonies from single cells. *Cell* **6,** 331–344.
10. Vicanova, J., Boelsma, E., Mommaas, A. M., et al. (1998) Normalization of epidermal calcium distribution profile in reconstructed human epidermis is related to improvement of terminal differentiation and stratum corneum barrier formation. *J. Invest. Dermatol.* **111,** 97–106.

11. Ponec, M. (1991) Reconstruction of human epidermis on de-epidermized dermis: expression of differentiation-specific protein markers and lipid composition. *Toxicol. In Vitro* **5,** 597–606.

12. Vecchini, F., Mace, K., Magdalou, J., Mahe, Y., Bernard, B. A., and Shroot, B. (1995) Constitutive and inducible expression of drug metabolizing enzymes in cultured human keratinocytes. *Br. J. Dermatol.* **132,** 14–21.

13. Gibbs, S., Boelsma, E., Kempenaar, J., and Ponec, M. (1998) Temperature-sensitive regulation of epidermal morphogenesis and the expression of cornified envelope precursors by EGF and TGF alpha. *Cell Tissue Res.* **292,** 107–114.

14. Harris, I. R., Farrell, A., Memon, R. A., Grunfeld, C., Elias, P. M., and Feingold, K. R. (1998) Expression and regulation of mRNA for putative fatty acid transport related proteins and fatty acyl CoA synthase in murine epidermis and cultured human keratinocytes. *J. Invest. Dermatol.* **111,** 722–726.

15. Michel, M., L'Heureux, N., Auger, F. A., and Germain, L. (1997) From newborn to adult: phenotypic and functional properties of skin equivalent and human skin as a function of donor age. *J. Cell. Physiol.* **171,** 179–189.

16. Zellmer, S., Reissig, D., and Lasch, J. (1998) Reconstructed human skin as model for liposome-skin interaction. *J. Contr. Rel.* **55,** 271–279.

17. Ponec, M. (1992) *In vitro* cultured human skin cells as alternatives to animals for skin irritancy screening. *Int. J. Cosm. Sci.* **14,** 245–264.

18. Pellegrini, G., Bondanza, S., Guerra, L., and de Luca, L. M. (1998) Cultivation of human keratinocyte stem cells: current and future clinical applications. *Med. Biol. Eng. Comput.* **36,** 778–790.

19. Barrandon, Y. and Green, H. (1985) Cell size as a determinant of the clone-forming ability of human keratinocytes. *Proc. Natl. Acad. Sci. U.S.A.* **82,** 5390–5394.

20. Barrandon, Y. and Green, H. (1987) Three clonal types of keratinocytes with different capacities for multiplication. *Proc. Natl. Acad. Sci. U.S.A.* **84,** 2302–2306.

21. Watt, F. M. (1998) Epidermal stem cells: markers, patterning and the control of stem cell fate. *Philos. Trans. R. Soc. Lond. B Biol. Sci.* **353,** 831–837.

17

Clinical Application of Autologous Cultured Epithelia for the Treatment of Burns and Disfigurement of Skin Surfaces

Norio Kumagai

1. Introduction

In patients who sustain large burns, it is difficult to cover the wounds with the patient's own skin. Therefore, various materials such as allo-skin, porcine skin, and artificial skin have been used as biological dressings. However, only the patient's own skin can survive permanently and succeed in covering the wounds. O'Connor et al. (*1*) first succeeded in the grafting of cultured autologous epithelium for the coverage of burn wounds. Autologous cultured epithelium grafting is effective for permanent coverage of the wounds and is widely used as one of the useful methods for covering wide burn wounds. We have been carrying out cultured epithelium grafting since 1985. We have used autologous or allogenic cultured epithelium grafts for the coverage of excised wounds, such as large burns, burn scars, meshed skin scars, tattoo, nevi, donor sites of split thickness skin (STS), and dermatological diseases, in over 400 cases.

From these grafting experiments, it has been shown that cultured epithelium grafting is a useful technique in the treatment of wide burn wounds and skin disfigurement. In this chapter, we describe the methods and results of cultured epithelial autografting for the treatment of various diseases.

2. Materials and Methods
2.1. Patients

During the past 15 yr, we have treated a total of 276 cases with autologous cultured epithelial grafting and 126 using allogenic cultured epithelial grafting. Out of the 276 autologous cultured grafts, 34 were for fresh burn wounds, 114

From: *Methods in Molecular Biology, vol. 188: Epithelial Cell Culture Protocols*
Edited by: C. Wise © Humana Press Inc., Totowa, NJ

were for burn scar wounds, 12 were for meshed scar wounds, 28 were tattoo wounds, 6 were color mismatch after conventional skin grafting, and 13 were for donor site wounds. We also carried out 69 cases of grafting for various dermatological diseases.

2.2. Human Epidermal Cell Culture

Donor skin was taken from the healthy skin of each patient. Pieces (3 × 1 cm) were taken from each patient. The epidermal cells were cultured according to Green's method, as described previously *(2,3)*. The cells were inoculated into 100-mm culture dishes (60 cm^2 surface area) (Falcon) or culture flasks (600 cm^2 surface area) (Nunc) containing lethally irradiated 3T3 J2 feeder layers. After 2 to 3 wk of cultivation, the epidermal cells became confluent and formed a multilayered epithelium. At this stage, the epithelium was detached from the dish with 300 U/mL dispase (Godo shusei).

2.3. Surgical Techniques

The lesions were abraded using a free-hand dermatome or motor-driven abrasive serrated wheel. When the bleeding had subsided completely, fresh cultured autografts were then applied to the wounds. The grafts were covered with hydrocolloid dressing (Geliperm; Geistlich-Pharma, Switzerland), saline soaked gauze, and dry gauze for 1 or 2 wk. When the grafted site had healed completely, silicone gel sheets (Cica-Care; Smith & Nephew, Hull, England) were applied as a pressure dressing for several months to prevent hypertrophic scarring. The grafted sites were inspected at regular intervals.

2.4. Histological Examination

DOPA-positive melanocytes in the cultured grafts were studied by DOPA staining and by electron microscopy. Punch biopsies (3 mm) were taken from the grafted areas of the cultured epithelia at various stages. The sections were examined by hematoxylin and eosin (H & E), DOPA, and Fontana-Masson staining. Immunohistochemical studies were carried out to study the reconstitution of basement membrane components (type VII collagen, laminin-5) after grafting to the partial skin wounds, deeply excised skin wounds, and dermabraded wounds of burn scars.

3. Results

3.1. Cultured Epithelium

Fig. 1 shows both a 60 and a 600 cm^2 cultured epithelium. The epithelium was approx 7–10 layers thick (**Fig. 2**). The scanning electron microscopy (SEM) micrograph shows that the basal layer and suprabasal layers were almost normal. In addition to keratinocytes, the melanocytes (marked with ←) were seen, as shown

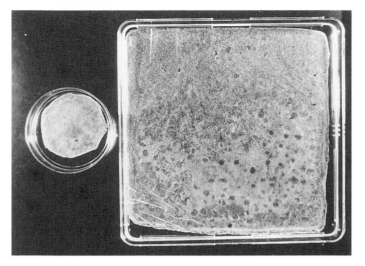

Fig. 1. Cultured epithelium graft (left, 60 cm^2 cultured epithelium; right, 600cm^2 cultured epithelium).

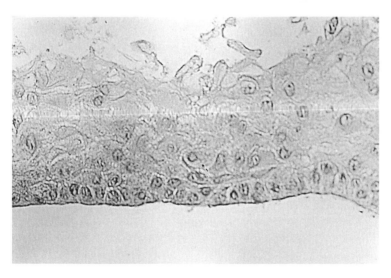

Fig. 2. Vertical section of the cultured graft.

by DOPA staining (**Fig. 3**). The electron micrograph showed that melanocytes were forming melanin granules, which were then transferred to the keratinocytes.

3.2. The Take of the Graft

The take and differentiation of the cultured grafts was influenced by several factors. When the grafting was done on thick STS donor sites, the wounds

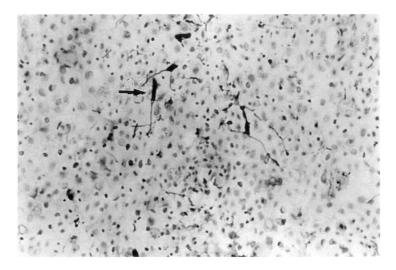

Fig. 3. DOPA-positive melanocytes (→) growing with epidermal cells on the culture dish.

healed within 5 d, at which point rete ridges and basement membranes had reformed (**Fig. 4, left panel**). The tissue structure was almost normal after 1 wk, and elastic fibers were present as in normal skin *(4)*. This indicated that the residual dermal components at the site of the wound play an important role in the success of cultured epithelium grafting. The presence of adipose tissue and granulated tissue in the recipient sites were not good factors for graft take. In cases where deep excisions were needed, such as in the case of tatoos, in which almost the entire thickness of the skin was removed, the normalization of the epidermal thickness can only be seen after 2 to 3 wk. The basement membranes were formed by laminin 5, but it was flat (**Fig. 4, right panel**). Compared to the superficially abraded wound scar, where the dermal components were present, the normalization process within the basement membrane occurs after 1 mo.

3.3. Operative Results

3.3.1. Treatment of Fresh Burn Wounds with Autologous Cultured Epithelium Grafting

In extensive burns, it was very important to prepare the wound beds carefully, so as to make them as sterile as possible. The reason for this is that the results of grafting to poorly granulated and severely infected third degree burn wounds was disappointing. In cases treated with only cultured auto grafts, the average graft take was 15%. Cuono et al. *(5)* reported that, in their hands, if the

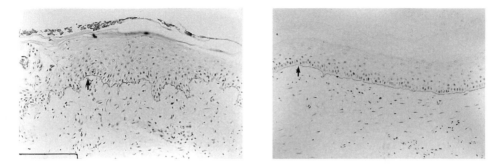

Fig. 4. Reconstitution of the basement membrane after autologous cultured epithelium grafting to the various wounds Left: 1 wk after grafting of the STS wounds. Type VII collagen immunohistochemical staining (↑). Right: 2 wk after grafting of the deeply excised tattoo wounds. Laminin 5 immunohistochemical staining (↑)

wound bed was prepared with allografts followed by cultured autologous epidermal grafting, then the "take rate" on third degree burn wounds was 85%. In our hands, the take rate in these cases was 73%.

3.3.1.1. CASE REPORTS

A 2-yr-old boy with 95% of his body surface burned by hot water. Biological dressings, such as amniotic membranes and frozen cultured epidermal allografts were applied, as soon as possible after the burning occurred, to cover the wounds. The parent's skin was then meshed and grafted. Subsequently, the surfaces were abraded, and autologous cultured epithelium was applied to the allogenic dermis. The graft take was acceptable, and almost all of the wounds healed one and a half months after grafting (**Fig. 5**).

3.3.2. Treatment of Burn Scar Disfigurement and Grafted Sites

For the treatment of skin surface disfigurements by burn scars, irregular scars, hypopigmentation or hyperpigmentation scars, meshed skin scar disfigurements, and conventional skin grafts, the donor skin for epidermal culture was taken from an area adjacent to the recipient sites. The disfigured areas were abraded superficially, and the grafts were applied to the dermabraded wounds. The graft takes were almost complete. The grafted area became soft, and the disfigurement improved remarkably 2 yr after grafting (**Figs. 6–8**). The skin tension and moisture became nearly normal. The softness of the grafted site was measured by cutometer. We have measured 17 cases where the grafted site had 93% elasticity compared to normal skin, whereas untreated scars had only 53% of normal skin elasticity (*6*). The moisture retention of the epidermis was identified by looking at the water absorption and disabsorption ratio. Fifty cases

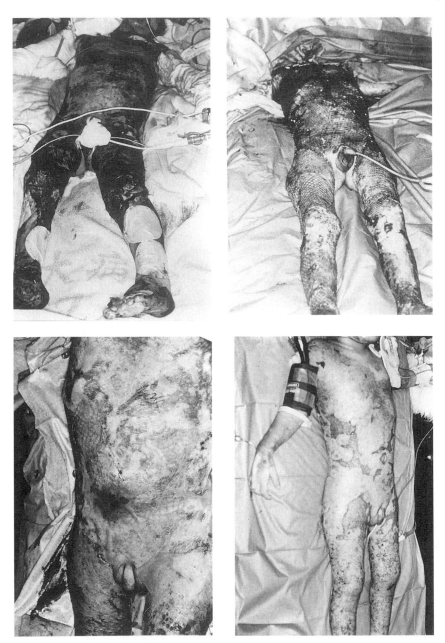

Fig. 5. Treatment of large burn wounds with allo-skin and cultured autografts Above, left: the wounds were covered with amniotic membranes and cultured allografts on the second day after burn injury. Above, right: the wounds were later covered with meshed allo-skin. Below, left: cultured autografts were applied to the allogenic dermis. Below, right: 19 d after grafting. Almost all of the wounds have healed.

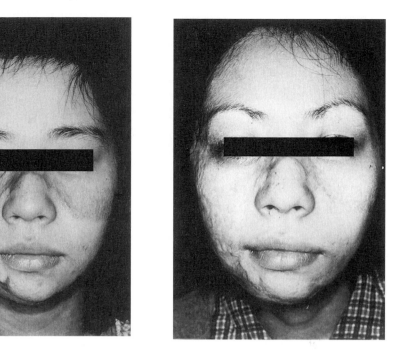

Fig. 6. Treatment of burn scar with hyperpigmentation on the face. Left: preoperative. Right: 4 yr postoperative.

were studied after grafting (6–54 mo: average 18 mo). We have found that the hydration state of the stratum corneum treated with cultured epithelium recovered to normal within 1 yr *(7)*.

3.3.3. Treatment of Dermatological Diseases

We have treated 69 cases of various dermatological diseases such as hypomelanosis, congenital giant nevi, nevus of Ota, ichiocytosis, and so on with cultured autografts.

3.3.3.1. HYPOMELANOSIS

UV light irradiation with psoralens (PUVA) treatment is a photometric therapy routinely used by dermatologists for the treatment of vitiligo. Twenty patients with wide areas of hypomelanosis, who have failed extensive PUVA treatments, were treated with autologous cultured epithelium. Of these 20 patients, 18 had vitiligo, 1 had piebaldism, and 1 had albinism. The donor skin for cultivation was taken from a site adjacent to the lesion. The hypomelanotic lesions were superficially abraded using hand-held motor-driven abrasive serrated wheels. The cultured epithelium was applied to the wound. Corticosteroid

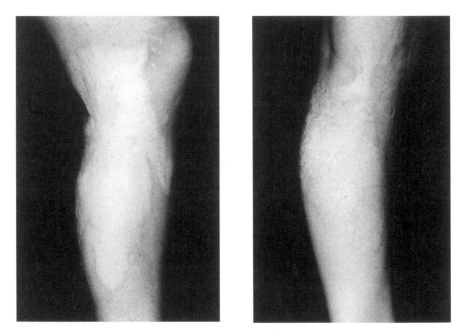

Fig. 7. Treatment of burn scar with hypopigmentation on the leg. Left: preoperative view. Right: 3 yr after grafting.

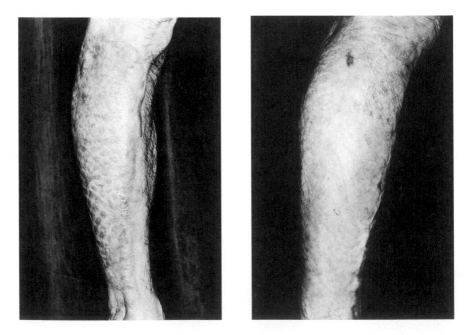

Fig. 8. Treatment of meshed scar. Left: preoperative view. Right: 3 yr after grafting.

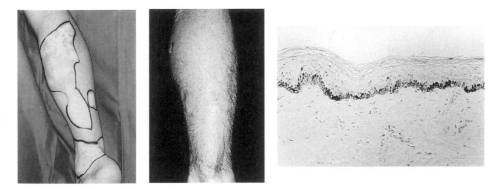

Fig. 9. Treatment of vitiligo vulgaris. Left: preoperative view. Center: 3 yr after grafting. Right: histology of the grafted site 3 yr after grafting (Fontana Masson staining).

ointments were applied to the site for a few months after re-epithelialization. The patients were advised to expose the grafted site to sunlight.

1. Clinical course of the grafted sites. The grafted sites healed completely after 1 wk with minimal scarring. Reddening of the grafted sites was noticed during the first few months. This was replaced by spotty or uniform pigmentation, which can be seen clearly 3 mo after grafting. The grafted sites appeared to be slightly hyperpigmented temporarily, but then returned to normal skin color as time passed, usually more than 6 mo. (**Fig. 9, right, center panels**). There is no recurrence of hypomelanosis after a long follow-up *(8)*.
2. Histology of the grafted site. Preoperative histology showed a complete absence of DOPA-positive melanocytes and melanin in the epidermis. Histochemical studies showed a few DOPA-positive melanocytes in the basal layer of the epidermis and dermis 12–17 d after grafting, even though Fontana-Masson staining failed to show melanin. DOPA-positive melanocytes and melanin were seen in the basal layer of the epidermis one and a half months after grafting. However, these numbers are still lower when compared to normal skin. It takes 6–8 mo after grafting for the site to have near normal skin histology (**Fig. 9, left panel**).

3.3.3.2. Giant Congenital Nevi

Twenty-one patients with very extensive giant congenital nevi were treated with autologous cultured epithelium grafting. Large areas on the trunk and extremities were treated with autologous cultured epithelium grafting combined with cryopreserved allogenic skin. The lesions were totally removed and allogenic skin was grafted to the wounds. Ten days later, the allo-skin was superficially abraded, and fresh cultured autografts were applied to the allogenic dermis *(9)*. The grafts took very well, as shown in **Fig. 10**.

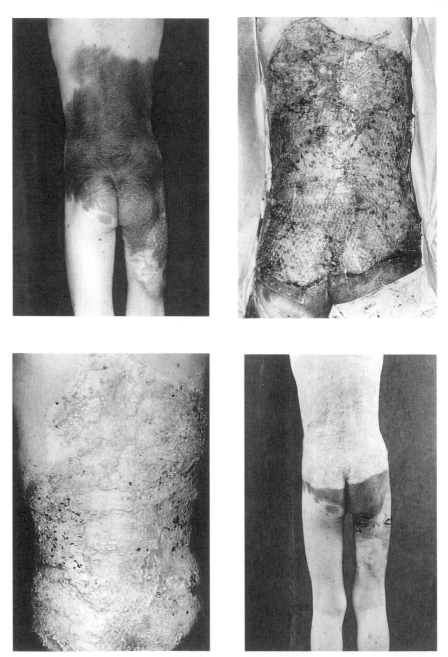

Fig. 10. Treatment of giant nevi with cryopreserved allo-skin and fresh cultured autografts. Above, left: preoperative view. Above, right: excised wounds were covered with allo-skin. Below, left: 1 mo after cultured epithelium grafting. Below, right: 1 yr after grafting.

4. Notes

1. Cultivation of human epidermal cells. The success of the cultivation is mostly due to the condition of the 3T3 J2 cells. As the passage number of the 3T3 J2 cells increases, the growth rate of the epidermal cells on the feeder cells declines. It is necessary to use 3T3 cells, which are of a low passage number.

2. Several factors influence whether or not the Graft takes, although quite why the success of the graft take, as well as the basement formation and the differentiation of the epidermis, is reliant on the condition of the wound bed is still unclear. Firstly, the quality of cultured grafts is important. Secondly, the condition and the quality of the wound bed is important; for example, whether it is infected or not. Thirdly, whether or not we need a dermal component is important. These were some of the factors that were particularly important in deciding the survival of the cultured graft. As described above, Cuono's method was reliable in the treatment of extensive third degree burn wounds. The immune response to the allo-skin is depressed in patients with severe burns. However, patients with giant congenital nevi have normal immune function. The antigenicity of the allogenic skin decreases a little during cryopreservation. We applied the cryopreserved allo-skin for temporary coverage of the wounds and anchoring to the cultured grafts. The average take rates was not so good when compared with burn wounds. Working out how to depress the immunogenicity of the allo-skin is a key factor in the treatment of full thickness skin wounds.

3. Treatment of skin surface disfigurement. We found that in addition to burn treatment, disfigurement of skin surfaces, hyperpigmentation, depigmentation or hypopigmentation, irregular contour scars, meshed scars, and unmatched skin color after conventional skin grafting are good indications for cultured epithelium grafting. This procedure enabled us to treat a wide range of disfigurements, which would have been difficult to treat with conventional skin grafting. In the treatment of burn scar disfigurement, the question of the best donor skin for epithelial culture always arises, in order to get the best color and texture match. We have investigated 38 patients with disfigurement of the skin surfaces 2 yr after the initial grafting. Cultured cells from buttock, the sole of the foot, and normal adjacent skin were applied. The most favorable results were obtained in the patients who had grafts obtained from skin adjacent to the grafted sites. This revealed that cultured epithelium has site specificity.

4. Importance of the melanocytes. Cultured epithelium has DOPA-positive melanocytes distributed in the basal layer of the epidermis. The distribution of the melanocytes is dispersed and not uniform within the graft. Incomplete repigmentation after cultured epithelial grafting might be due partly to the graft take, but mainly to the graft itself. Good appearance and complete repigmentation can be obtained by applying shrunken cultured grafts containing melanocytes to the area.

References

1. O'Connor, N. E., Mulliken, J. B., Banks-Schlegel, S., et al. (1981) Grafting of burns with cultured epithelium cells. *Lancet* **1**, 75–81.

 2. Rheinwald, J. G. and Green, H. (1975) Serial cultivation of strains of human epidermal keratinocytes: the formation of keratinizing colonies from single cells. *Cell* **6,** 331–344.
 3. Kumagai, N., Fukushi, S., Matsuzaki, K., et al. (1995) Treatment of nevus of Ota with autologous-cultured epithelium grafting. *Ann. Plast. Surg.* **34,** 180–186.
 4. Kumagai, N., Nishina, H., Tanabe, H., et al. (1988) Clinical application of autologous cultured epithelia for the treatment of burn wounds and burn scars. *Plast. Reconstr. Surg.* **82,** 99–108.
 5. Cuono, C. B., Langdon, R., and McGuire, J. (1986) Use of cultured epidermal autografts and dermal allografts as skin replacement after burn injury. *Lancet* **1,** 1123–1124.
 6. Matsuzaki, K., Kumagai, N., Fukushi, S., et al.(1995) Cultured epithelial autografting on meshed skin grafts scars: evaluation of skin elasticity. *J. Burn Care Rehabil.* **16,** 496–502.
 7. Oshima, H., Kumagai, N, Matsuzaki, K., et al. (1996) The state of hydration in the stratum corneum after a cultured epithelium graft: a clinical study. *Jap. J. Plast. Reconstr. Surg.* **39,** 47–55.
 8. Kumagai, N. and Uchikoshi, T. (1997) Treatment of extensive hypomelanosis with autologous cultured epithelium. *Ann. Plast. Surg.* **39,** 68–73.
 9. Kumagai, N., Oshima, H., Tanabe, M., et al. (1997) Treatment of giant congenital nevi with cryopreserved allogeneic skin and fresh autologous cultured epithelium. *Ann. Plast. Surg.* **39,** 483–488.

18

Transplantation of Cultured Epithelial Cells

Minoru Ueda, Yukio Sumi, Yoshitaka Hibino, and Ken-Ichiro Hata

1. Introduction

Cultured human epithelium (autografts) have been used su+ccessfully since 1980 as a permanent cover for large full skin thickness burn wounds *(1,2)*. They were also applied successfully to treat traumatic scars, giant nevi, and tattoo *(3,4)*. The use of allogenic cultured epithelium (allografts) in deep partial and full thickness skin burns has also been used successfully as temporary covering material *(5,6)*. However, the data on the permanent coverage of full thickness skin lesions with allografts are particularly controversial.

Although cultured autogenic and allogenic epithelial grafts are very useful for the treatment of skin defects (*see* **Notes 1** and **2**), if a hospital does not have both culture equipment and specialized skills to manipulate the living cells, then they cannot make use of the cultured epithelium techniques. In order to overcome these problems, Bio-Skin Bank has been established for the production of cultured epithelium in Nagoya *(7,8)*. Since January 1995, the Bio-Skin Bank, which is organized to fabricate and supply cultured epithelium, has provided cultured epithelium to 1 burn unit, 4 plastic surgery departments, and 1 oral surgery department in a medical school. The availability of standardized, quality cultured epithelium to different hospitals led us to draw some general conclusions regarding the applications of this therapeutic approach. In this chapter, the technique for cultured epithelial grafting and the clinical results of the graft are described.

In our laboratory, the size of a skin or mucosal specimen can multiply at least 1,000 times in culture within 3 wk, and the resulting grafts can be successfully applied to patients with large epidermal and mucosal defects. Our laboratory provides cultured epithelium for several plastic surgical departments in different hospitals. The distances between the laboratory and the hospitals

From: *Methods in Molecular Biology, vol. 188: Epithelial Cell Culture Protocols*
Edited by: C. Wise © Humana Press Inc., Totowa, NJ

have not appeared to be a limiting factor, since the survival time of both the biopsy and the cultured grafts is adequate for transportation (*see* **Note 3**). Moreover, the problems associated with transportation of the grafts can be solved by freezing the grafts. The availability of frozen cultured epithelium has also allowed different hospitals to utilize standard quality grafts produced on a large scale and, especially for those patients who required several transplantations, removed all problems of coordination between the cultivation and the surgical schedules. We have observed an average "take" of cultured autografts to be 95% and 50% in cultured allografts.

Although muscular fascia has been reported to be the ideal receiving bed, deep excision of the burned areas was avoided since, especially in young patients, the chances of subsequent retraction of the grafted area is increased. The main causes of graft failure are infection and hemorrhage. Bleeding is not a major problem when the grafts are applied on dermis. When grafts are made on excised granulating tissues, bleeding can be controlled by preparing the wound bed 24–48 h before graft application. Infection is less easily controlled. Cultured grafts appear to be more sensitive to bacterial infection than traditional split skin graft. Cadaver skin is a useful temporary covering, which can control infection and prepare an excellent receiving bed for cultured grafts (*9*), but sometimes it is difficult to use cadaver skin freely because of legal problems. Early coverage of burns with cultured allografts stored frozen in a skin bank could replace frozen cadaver skin (*10*).

Cultured allografts, either fresh or frozen, can have several clinical applications. We have evidence that deep partial skin thickness burns heal much faster when grafted with such cultures. In three full thickness skin lesions, grafting of allografts was followed by epidermal regeneration. However, DNA analysis of the regenerated epidermis did not show donor type cells. This suggests that lesions, which have full thickness skin defects, can be re-epithelialized by residual keratinocytes, whose growth and probably migration is strongly stimulated by the cultured allografts (*see* **Note 4**). Therefore, when we use such cultures, surgical excision of necrotic tissues is not performed too deeply, so as to keep the residual epithelial cells in the dermis.

2. Materials

1. Growth media: Dulbecco's modified Eagle's medium (DMEM) (Life Technologies) supplemented with 10% fetal calf serum (FCS) (Life Technologies), 1000 U/mL penicillin G (Sigma), 1 mg/mL kanamycin (Sigma), and 2.5 µg/mL amphotericin B (Sigma).
2. 10 µg/mL Mitomycin C (Sigma) in DMEM.
3. 3T3 Medium: DMEM supplemented with 5% FCS.
4. 3T3-J2 Cells.

5. Phosphate-buffered saline (PBS) (Life Technologies).
6. Sterilization solution: PBS supplemented with 1000 U/mL penicillin G, 1 mg/mL kanamycin, and 2.5 μg/mL amphotericin B.
7. 0.25% Trypsin, 0.02% EDTA (Life Technologies).
8. 1000 U/mL Dispase (GODO Shusei) in DMEM.
9. 400 U/mL Dispase in DMEM.
10. 50-μm Nylon mesh.
11. Epithelial cell culture medium: 3:1 mixture of DMEM and Ham's F12 supplemented with 5% FCS, 10^{-9} M cholera toxin, 5 μg/mL Hydrocortisone, 5 μg/mL transferrin, 10^{-9} M triiodothyronine, 5 μg/mL insulin, 100 U/mL penicillin, 0.25 μg/mL amphotericin B, 0.1mg/mL kanamycin, 10 ng/mL epidermal growth factor (EGF).
12. Freezing medium: DMEM supplemented with 10% glycerol as a cryoprotectant and 15% FCS.
13. Sterile collagen membrane (Meipac, Seika Company Ltd., Tokyo).
14. 4.5-mL Cryotubes (Nunc).
15. 0.1% Gentamicin ointment.
16. 3% Tetracycline ointment.
17. QIAamp Kit (Qiagen).
18. AmpliFLP PCR Kit (Perkin Elmer, cat. no. D1S80).

3. Method

3.1 Preparation of the Cultured Epithelium

1. Epithelial cell cultures should be established as previously described *(11)* (*see* **Fig. 1**).

3.1.1. Feeder Layers for Epithelial Cells

1. Treat 3T3-J2 with mitomycin C for 2 h at 37°C.
2. Rinse cultures with PBS to remove mitomycin C.
3. Plate out at 1×10^4 cells/cm^2.
4. Culture for 24 h in 3T3 Medium, before adding epithelial cells.

3.1.2. Epithelial Cells

1. Superfluous tissue obtained from patients during surgery can be used as a source of oral mucosa or skin segments.
2. Place the tissue in growth medium.
3. Clean the mucosa or skin and cut into small pieces.
4. To sterilize, immerse samples twice in sterilization solution, each for 30 min at 37°C.
5. Immerse twice in dispase, each time for 16 h at 4°C.
6. Treat the tissue with trypsin-EDTA solution for 30 min at room temperature.
7. To separate the different cell types, add 3T3 growth medium and stir for 30 min.
8. Filter the suspension through nylon mesh to remove satisfactory segments and retain the filtrate.
9. Make a suspension of purified epidermal and mucosal cells.

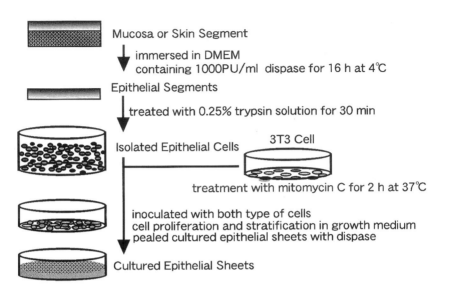

Fig. 1. Method of preparation of cultured mucosal epithelium.

10. Centrifuge twice for 5 min at 2500*g*.
11. Resuspend the cell pellet in DMEM.
12. Plate out epithelial cells at 1×10^4 cells/cm^2 onto the 3T3-J2 feeder layer.
13. To make the epithelial sheet, add epithelial cell culture medium and incubate at 5% CO_2 at 37°C.
14. Change the medium every 2 d.
15. Cultured epithelial sheets are graftable after 20 d in culture.
16. Efficiency of colony formation by the epithelial cells was determined by the speed at which cells reach confluence. Plate out epithelial cells (1×10^4 cells/10-cm dish) onto a feeder layer. Allow to proliferate for 5 d and then count the number of colonies (*see* **Notes 5** and **6**).

3.2. Preparation of Grafts

1. Use the cultured epithelium when it reaches confluence and exhibits pluristratification. This is usually 20 d after inoculation.
2. Wash with serum-free DMEM.
3. Incubate for 30 min in 400 U/mL dispase to detach the intact layer from the surface of the culture bottle.
4. Put the collagen membrane into the bottle and place it on top of the epithelium.
5. Remove the media.
6. The cultured epithelium will attach, although quite weakly, to the collagen membrane.
7. Carefully remove the collagen membrane and cultured epithelium together.

Table 1
The Participating Institutions
of the Aichi Bio-Skin Bank System

1. Department of Plastic and Reconstructive Surgery,
   Aichi Medical University

2. Burn care center,
   Social Insurance Chukyo Hospital

3. Department of Plastic and Reconstructive Surgery,
   Nagoya University School of Medicine

4. Department of Dermatology,
   Medical School Nagoya City University

5. Department of Plastic and Reconstructive Surgery,
   Fujita Health University School of Medicine

6. Department of Oral Surgery
   Nagoya University School of Medicine

3.3. Freezing and Thawing Technique

1. Freezing and thawing of cultured epithelium should be carried out in the manner based on the following technique *(12)* (*see* **Note 7**).
2. Peel cultured epithelial sheets off of the culture bottle with dispase II (*see* **Subheading 3.2.3.**) with the collagen membrane and store in a cryotube.
3. Equilibrate the cultured epithelial sheet with freezing medium for 30 min at 4°C.
4. Then place the cryotubes in a –20°C freezer for 1 h.
5. Transfer to a –80°C freezer overnight.
6. Store in a deep freezer (–145°C).
7. At the time of the grafting operation, place the cryotubes in water at 37°C to thaw rapidly for 1 min.
8. After thawing, place the cultured epithelial sheets in a sterile dish and wash in DMEM containing 10% FCS in the operation room.

3.4. Patients

1. One hundred and three patients admitted to the 6 surgery departments of 5 different hospitals located in the Aichi district were the subjects of this study (*see* **Table 1**). Informed consent was obtained in all cases from the patients or their relatives. The patients' ages ranged between 1 and 79 yr. Partial and full thickness skin defects covered between 10 and 95% of the body surface area.
2. In the case of autografting, within 1 wk of admission, each patient should have a full thickness specimen of skin or oral mucosa (1–4 cm^2) taken under local anesthesia.
3. Place the specimen in epithelial cell culture medium in a 50-mL centrifuge tube and transfer to the laboratory.

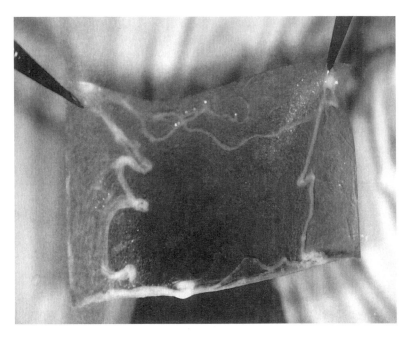

Fig. 2. Gross appearance of the cultured mucosal epithelium with the collagen membrane as a carrier.

3.5. Transplantation of Cultured Epithelium

1. Detach the cultured epithelium with dispase II (*see* **Subheading 3.3.**)
2. Wash in serum-free medium and place basal side up on sterile collagen membrane (**Fig. 2**).
3. Place the cultured epithelium sheets in a test tube containing serum-free DMEM and transport to the hospital or operating room.
4. Place the cultured epithelial grafts on the prepared sites (after skin debridement) with the basal cell layer directed against the wound bed.
5. Cover the prepared wound completely with grafts, making sure that there are no gaps or spaces.
6. Overlay the grafts with several layers mesh gauze, containing gentamicin and tetracycline ointment.
7. Change the dressings every 2 d.
8. Remove the gauze when the percentage of the wound covered by the epithelium has been determined and can be referred to as a clinically evident "take". This is usually between 6 and 14 d after the graft was made (*see* **Note 8**).
9. Since epithelial cells can grow from the edges of epithelium that have "taken", the percentage of full thickness skin lesions covered by the cultured epithelium can be calculated upon discharge from the hospital.

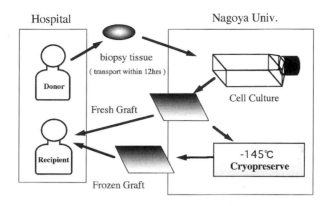

Fig. 3. The system of Bio-Skin Bank.

10. For the preparation of allografts, epithelial cells are grown from healthy donors, and all tests normally done for blood donors should be performed (*see* **Fig. 3**).
11. In most patients, autografts were made from their own healthy skin. Usually the healthy skin was taken as a split skin thickness piece and then grafted. To protect the areas from where the healthy skin had been taken, cultured allografts were placed on these donor sites.
12. In some patients, it is possible to use cultured grafts, if their own cultured epithelium has previously been cultured and frozen.
13. Frozen grafts should be kept at −145°C and shipped in dry ice to the hospital or operating room.
14. In the operating room, the tubes should be immersed for 10 min in a 37°C water bath and then opened.
15. Wash the grafts twice in sterile PBS and place on the site to be grafted.
16. To determine how long the allogenic cells live for, or was alive, extract DNA from a peripheral blood specimen (from the graft recipient) and from the skin biopsy (on the grafted site) *(13)* (*see* **Note 9**).
17. Extract the DNA using the QIAamp kit, according to the manufacturer's instructions.
18. Digest the purified DNA (3 µg) with *Hinf*I at 37°C for 2 h.
19. Carry out polymerase chain reaction (PCR), using the AmpiFLP kit according to the manufacturer's instructions.

4. Notes

1. **Fig. 4** shows the clinical results from the use of cultured autografts in 80 patients. The patients' ages ranged between 1 and 79 yr, the area of skin injury covered between 10 and 95% of the body surface. Grafts were applied on full and partial thickness skin wounds. In the burn wounds, the necrotic tissues were excised down to muscular fascia or fresh dermis in patients. In all other patients the recipient areas were excised down to vital dermal tissue.

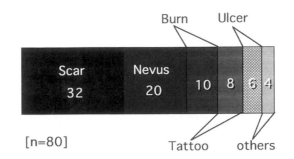

Fig. 4. Patients treated with autografts.

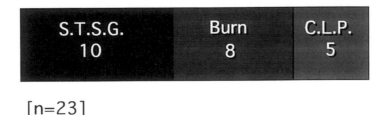

[n=23]

Fig. 5. Patients treated with allografts.

2. Twenty-three cases were treated by cultured allograft (**Fig. 5**). In most of the patients who received large split skin thickness mesh grafts, "fresh" or frozen cultured allografts were placed on the donor sites. These donor sites were completely re-epithelialized in all patients by 2–5 d after surgery. An interesting observation was made in patient 1: the donor site used as a source for split skin thickness grafts was partially covered with cultured allografts; this area healed in 5 d and subsequently showed no scarring, whereas the ungrafted area healed more slowly and later developed hypertrophic scars (**Fig. 6**). Also, 5 patients with cleft palate were treated by cultured mucosal allografts after usual palatoplasty.

3. Given the distance between the laboratory and some of the plastic surgery departments (up to 20 km), it was first necessary to establish a maximum time for transportation of biopsy and epithelium. It was observed that the best cell yield and colony-forming efficiency of isolated epithelial cells were obtained when the skin biopsies were kept at room temperature in culture medium containing 10% fetal bovine serum (FBS), and colony-forming efficiency did not change significantly within a 12-h test period (**Fig. 7**).

4. **Fig. 8** shows a case of a 30-yr-old woman who received fire burn to the left leg 3 wk ago. The conventional ointment care was applied, but partial thickness skin defect remained. The necrotic tissue was removed by a razor knife and previously prepared cultured epithelium was transplanted onto the recipient bed. Two

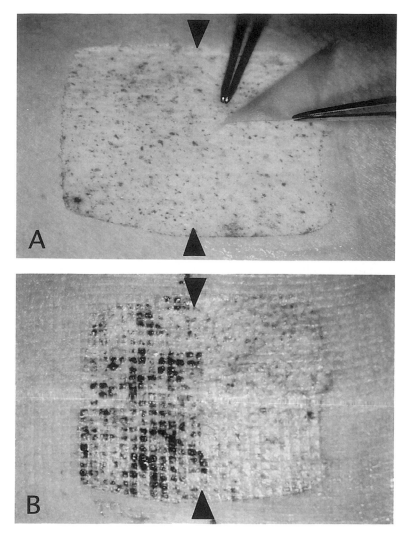

Fig. 6. (**A**) The cultured mucosal epithelium was placed on the donor site of split thickness skin graft. (**B**) Three days after allografting, the grafted area was epithelialized. However, the control side did not epithelialize; and hemorrhaging and exudate was noted.

weeks later, the grafted area was completely re-epithelialized, and the survival rate was 95%.
5. Epithelial cells from mucosa or skin started to from colonies within 3 d. The colony forming rate in mucosal epithelial cells was 7, and 5% in skin keratinocytes (**Fig. 9**).

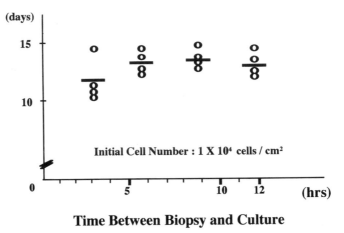

Fig. 7. Colony-forming efficiency of the time between biopsy and culture.

6. In 3 patients who received chemotherapy and radiotherapy for cancer treatment, we were unable to obtain confluent secondary cultures. This behavior was probably due to the declining growth potential of basal keratinocytes.

7. The viability of frozen grafts was monitored by light microscopy and by flow cytometry dissociated epithelial cells. The histology of vertical section of grafts before and after freezing was comparable and light microscopy showed very well-conserved epithelial cells in the frozen epithelium. From the analysis of flow cytometry, the cell viability after freezing stage was above 62% in any conditions. With the same cryoprotectant, cell viability of cultured epithelium stored at $-145°C$ was higher than at $-80°C$ (**Figs. 10** and **11**).

8. In patients more than 65-yr-old, the average take by the time the dressing was removed was 47%, whereas in all other patients the average take was 100% (**Fig. 12**).

9. In order to examine how long cultured allografts survive, a punch-biopsy of a supposedly full skin thickness burned area, whose epidermis has regenerated following application of cultured allografts, should be taken from the patients 1 mo after grafting. As a control, a peripheral blood sample is taken also, from the recipient. DNA is extracted, and the repetitive DNA sequences that are arranged in tandem repeats, termed variable number of tandem repeats (VNTR) should be analyzed. We analyze the alleles at the D1S80 locus, which contains VNTRs. If no difference is noted in the DNA bands, this indicates that, at least in the patients we examined, only autologous cells remain (**Fig. 13**). The sensitivity of this method is such that in mixing experiments, we have detected minor DNA populations at a level as low as 2%. Therefore, we do not believe that cultured allografts survive for very long, and their effect is to promote the proliferation of resident epidermal cells. In one case, a 50-yr-old man, who had a burn on his

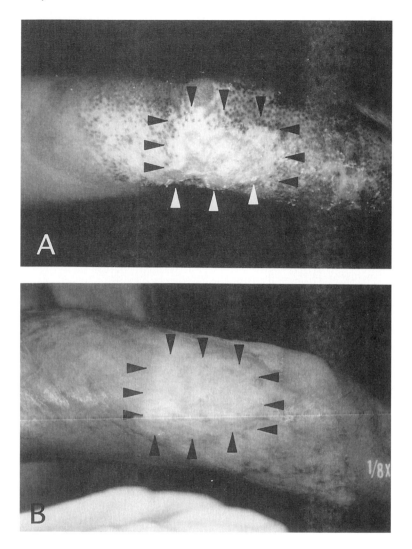

Fig. 8. A 30-yr-old female patient received fire burn (deep dermal burn, DDB) to the left leg 3 wk prior to treatment. (**A**) Before operation. (**B**) The grafted area was completely re-epithelialized after 2 wk.

arm, received 3 transplantations of frozen allografts, with no debridement to the burned area, and eventually, the ulcer healed completely (**Fig. 14**). We suggest that the best results are obtained when frozen allografts are transplanted immediately after the burn, to allow stimulation of residual keratinocytes and re-epithelialization.

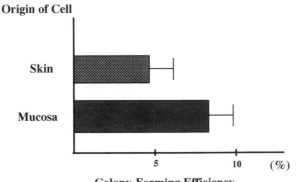

Fig. 9. Colony-forming efficiency of the skin and the mucosal cell.

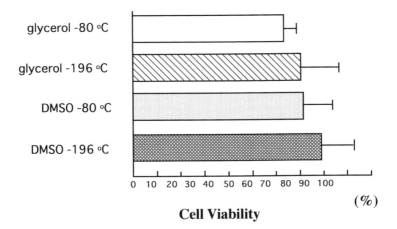

Fig. 10. Cell viability of cultured epithelium after 3 wk cryopreservation.

Acknowledgment

This study was supported by the Program for Promotion of Fundamental Studies in Health Sciences of the Organization for Drug ADR Relief, R & D Promotion and Product Review of Japan.

References

1. O'Connor, N. E., Mulliken, J. B., Banks-Schlegel, S., Kehinde, O., and Green, H., (1981) Grafting of burns with cultured epithelium prepared from autologous epidermal cells. *Lancet* **1,** 75–78.
2. Gallico, G. G., O'Connor, N. E., Compton, C. C., Kehinde, O., and Green, H. (1981) Permanent coverage of large burn wounds with autologous cultured human epithelium. *N. Engl. J. Med.* **311,** 448–451.

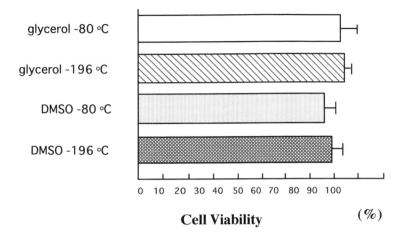

Fig. 11. Cell viability of cultured mucosal epithelium after 3 wk cryopreservation.

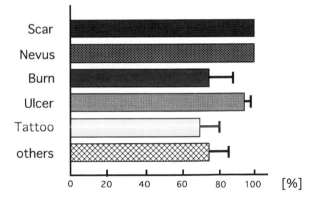

Fig. 12. Survival rate of autografts.

3. Gallico, G. G., O'Connor, N. E., Compton, C. C., Remensnyder, J. P., Kehinde, O., and Green, H. (1989) Cultured epithelial autografts for giant congenital naevi. *Plast. Reconstr. Surg.* **84,** 1–9.
4. Carter, D. M., Lin, A. N., Varghese, M. C., Caldwell, D., Pratt, L. A., Eisinger, M. (1987) Treatment of junctional epidermolysis bullosa with epidermal autografts. J. Am. Acad. Dermatol. **172, 246**–250.
5. Thivolet, J., Faure, M., Demidem, A., and Mauduit, G. (1996) Cultured human epidermal allografts are not rejected for a long period. *Arch. Dermatol. Res.* **278,** 252–254.
6. Phillips, T. J., Kehinde, O., Green, H., and Gilchrest, G. A. (1989) Treatment of skin ulcers with cultured epidermal allografts. *J. Am. Acad. Dermatol.* **21,** 191–199.

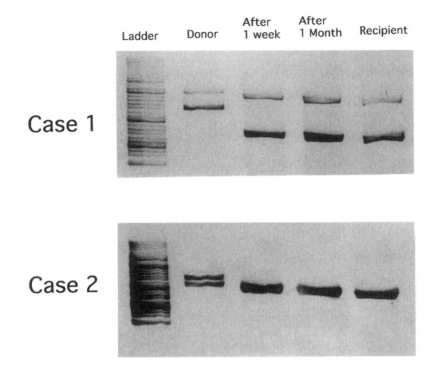

Fig. 13. VNTR analysis of 2 patients. No difference was noted in the DNA bands, indicating that only autologous cells remained.

7. Ueda, M. (1995) Formation of epithelial sheets by serially cultivated human mucosal cells and their applications as a graft material. *Nagoya J. Med. Sci.* **58,** 13–28.
8. Ueda, M., Sumi, Y., and Hata, K. (1999) Establishment of bio-skin bank: how we do it in our hospitals. *Ann. Plast. Surg.* **42,** 574–576..
9. Teepe, R. G. C., Ponec, R. W., and Hermans, R. P. (1986) Improved grafting method for treatment of burns with autologous cultured human epithelium. *Lancet* **1,** 385.
10. Langdon, R. C., Cuono, C. B., Birchall, N., Madri, J. A., Kuklinska, E., McGuire, J., and Moellman, G. E. (1988) Reconstruction of structure and cell function in human skin grafts derived from cryopreserved allogeneic dermis and autologous cultured keratinocytes. *J. Invest. Dermatol.* **81,** 478–485.
11. Rheinwald, J. G. and Green, H. (1975) Serial cultivation of strains of human epidermal keratinocytes: the formation of keratinizing colonies from single cell. *Cell* **6,** 331–344.

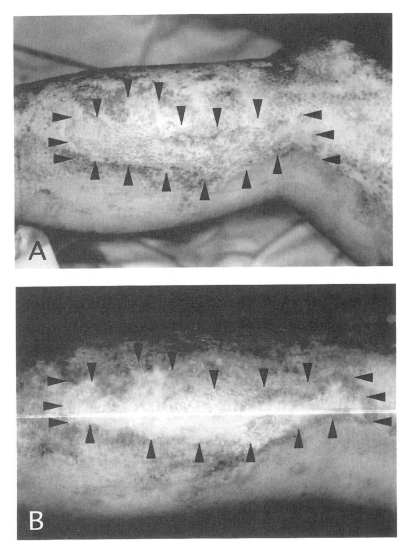

Fig. 14. A 50-yr-old man received burn in the arm. **(A)** Before operation. **(B)** The grafted area became flat skin, and the ulcer healed completely.

12. Hibino, Y., Hata, K., Horie, K., Torii, S., and Ueda, M. (1996) Structural changes and cell viability of cultured epithelium after freezing storage. *J. Craniomaxillofac. Surg.* **4,** 346–351.

13. Burt, A. M., Pallett, C. D., Sloane, J. P., et al. (1989) Survival of cultured allografts in patients with burns assessed with probe specific for Y chromosome. *BMJ* **298,** 915–917.

19

An Outgrowth Culture System of Normal Human Epithelium

An In Vitro Model to Study the Coordination of Cellular Migration and Proliferation

Tohru Masui

1. Introduction

In order to study the growth regulation of normal human epithelium, we have developed an outgrowth culture system *(1)*. Cinematographic observation has revealed that the cells migrate and proliferate in a coordinated manner. For example, an outgrowth will expand concentrically as a cell sheet, and the cell density will be consistent between different sized outgrowths (*see* **Fig. 1**). The increment in the radius of the outgrowth stays constant (about 1.5 mm/d) and is independent of the size of the explant or donor individuals. We can easily obtain 10^8 cells per specimen in 3 wk. Because of its constant growth pattern, the growth history of the cultures can be easily traced, and comparable cultures can be used for further analyses (*see* **Note 1**).

In conventional culture systems, the outgrowth serves as the source of epithelial cells. Therefore, cells from outgrowths are usually dissociated with trypsin and seeded in a controlled manner. This procedure has been thought to be important in quantitative studies of cultures. However, quantitative studies require a reproducible biological response and a way to determine the cell number. The outgrowth culture system satisfies these two requirements, and we have tried successfully to use the outgrowths in various experiments.

We have demonstrated that the outgrowth culture system is an attractive in vitro model for analyzing coordination mechanisms in growth of normal human epithelium in vivo (*see* **Note 2**).

From: *Methods in Molecular Biology, vol. 188: Epithelial Cell Culture Protocols*
Edited by: C. Wise © Humana Press Inc., Totowa, NJ

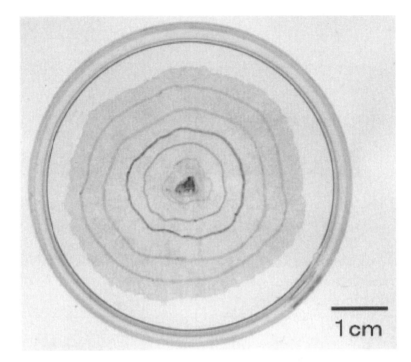

Fig. 1. Macroscopic appearance of outgrowth cultured in DMMC medium supplemented with 4% FBS. Concentric circles are the records of outgrowth expansion made
every 2 d.

2. Materials
2.1. Normal Human Tissue

Normal human ectocervical specimens can be obtained from uterine lei-
omyoma patients undergoing hysterectomy. Confirm the absence of atypia by
histological examination. Ethical issues should be satisfied before obtaining
tissue samples, according to the local regulations. Tissue should be used only
after the sample has been recorded photographically. Sterile conditions are not
necessary at this point.

2.2. Instruments and Plastics

1. Sterile scalpels with wide blades (Number 22).
2. Fine pointed scissors.
3. Forceps with wide tips, for the isolation of the epithelial layer.
4. Finely pointed steel needles, for scoring plastic.
5. Sterile 50-mL conical plastic tubes.
6. Petri dishes, 100 mm (Nunc).

2.3. Media

1. Washing medium: Dulbecco's modified Eagle's medium (DMEM) (Life Technologies) supplemented with 4 μg/mL fungizone (Life Technologies) and 1% fetal bovine serum (FBS).
2. Storage medium: if the tissue is to be kept over night at 4°C, then it is better to use Leibovitz's L-15 medium (Life Technologies) as the basal medium. The pH of L15 is independent of the air phase and therefore suitable for overnight storage.
3. Growth medium (DMMC): 1:1 DMEM:MCDB153HAA medium (*MCDB*) (*see* **Note 3**), supplemented with 1 μg/mL fungizone, 100 U/mL penicillin (Meiji Seika, Japan), and 50 μg/mL gentamicin (Sigma). MCDB medium is a special order (*2*) without phenol red, supplemented with growth factors, and containing 0.9 m*M* Ca^2.
4. Coating solution: HEPES-buffered saline containing 10 μg/mL of human fibronectin (Sigma), 30 μg/mL collagen type I (Nitta Gelatin, Japan), and 100 μg/mL bovine serum albumin (BSA) (Sigma).

3. Methods
3.1. Preparation of Culture Dishes

1. Score areas of about 1 mm^2 of the Petri dish surface with a fine needle. Usually 3 scratch marks per 100-mm dish is sufficient. The scratches provide attachment sites for the explants.
2. Coat dishes with coating solution for 1 h at room temperature.

3.2. Specimen Preparation

1. To remove the epithelium with a thin layer of stroma from the ectocervical area, hold the epithelium with forceps and slice away the thin sheet of epithelium and stroma with the scalpel.
2. Cut the sheet away from the ectocervical area using scissors.
3. Wash the tissue with washing medium 3 times.
4. Place the specimen in a 100-mm plastic dish with the epithelial surface up and cut it into about 1–3 mm^2 pieces.
5. Add 3 mL of growth medium to the dish, to prevent the tissue from drying out and floating.
6. Cut the specimen using a scalpel. The scalpel blade should be in a vertical position, and the cuts made by pushing down vertically onto the tissue. This cutting method results in minimal damage of the epithelial layer. Do not make horizontal cuts, because this damages the epithelial layer.

3.3. Outgrowth Culture

1. Place explants on the scored areas of the Petri dishes.
2. Leave to stand for 1 h to allow the explants to settle onto the dishes.
3. Add 3 mL of growth medium.

4. Place the dishes in an ordinary CO_2 incubator. Do this gently, so as not to disturb the attachment of the explants. If the explants do not attach at this stage, they will not attach or grow.
5. The next day, feed the cultures with 5 mL of growth medium.
6. Feed explants every 2 d.
7. After 5 d in culture, the amount of medium can be increased.
8. Since the cell densities of outgrowths are constant, cultures containing approximately the same number of cells can be easily selected. These can be used for a variety of further experiments. We have used them successfully to analyze the basic growth nature of the outgrowth culture (manuscript in preparation).

4. Notes

1. Since cell densities proved constant *(1)*, outgrowth area was used to express cell number. The outlines of outgrowths were marked on the bottom of the culture dishes every 2 d, and the areas were measured using an image analyzer. This method allowed us to follow the growth of each outgrowth *(1)*.
2. Coordination of migration and proliferation has been thought to be an essential element in epithelial growth. As has been described, at the site of a wound, epithelium starts to grow as a cell sheet *(3,4)*. In the outgrowth cultures, explants recognize the free space as a wound site and start to grow. Therefore, this system may provide a suitable model to study the initial phase of wound healing.
3. Obtaining good quality custom made MCDB media can be a problem. We are currently testing a new source of this, and if the production of the media proves to be reproducible, the Japanese Tissue Culture Association will support the company that produces it. Please contact the author if you experience problems in locating this reagent.

References

1. Masui, T. (1995) Establishment of an outgrowth culture system to study growth regulation of normal human epithelium. *In Vitro Cell. Dev. Biol. Anim.* **31,** 440–446.
2. Shipley, G. D. and Pittelkow, M. R. (1987) Control of growth and differentiation *in vitro* of human keratinocytes cultured in serum-free medium. *Arch. Dermatol.* **123,** 1541a–1544a.
3. Clark, R. A. F. (1985) Cutaneous tissue repair: basic biologic considerations. I. *J. Am. Acad. Dermatol.* **13,** 701–725.
4. Coomber, B. L. and Gotlieb, A. I. (1990) *In vitro* endothelial wound repair: interaction of cell migration and proliferation. *Arteriosclerosis* **10,** 215–222.

20

Application of Epithelial Cell Culture in Drug Transport in the Respiratory Tract

Jie Shen and Vincent H. L. Lee

1. Introduction

Drugs can be inhaled and absorbed throughout the conducting airway from the trachea down to the bronchioles and ultimately in the distal lung across the alveolar epithelium. The respiratory tract offers a large surface area, extensive vasculature, and significantly lower enzymatic activity to favor both local and systemic drug delivery. The respiratory tract is not only structurally but also functionally complex. This must be taken into account in selecting models to learn about the mechanisms as well as factors influencing drug deposition and absorption in the lung. These models fall in five categories: (*i*) in vivo animal lungs *(1–3)*; (*ii*) *in situ* perfused lungs *(4–6)*; (*iii*) in vitro isolated and perfused lungs or discs punched from strips of trachea *(7–9)*; (*iv*) in vitro isolated respiratory tract epithelial cells *(7,10)*; and (*v*) in vitro cultured epithelial cell monolayers *(11–15)*.

Epithelial cell culture of the respiratory tract not only allows studies of barrier properties and drug absorption in the lung, but it also eliminates the intrinsic complex anatomical arrangement of the lung and simplifies data interpretation. For the conducting airway, both tracheal and bronchial cell cultures of different animal species have been used to evaluate permeability of a wide variety of solutes and drugs as well as regulation of barrier properties of the airway epithelium *(12,13,16–19)*. A greater number of studies have reported development of distal alveolar epithelial cell culture and permeability data for various solutes and drugs across the cultured alveolar cell monolayers *(14,15,20–26)*.

Epithelial cell culture of the respiratory tract includes both primary cultures and transformed cells or carcinoma cell lines. While the later two provide a continuous sources of viable epithelial cells as a result of incessant proliferation,

From: *Methods in Molecular Biology, vol. 188: Epithelial Cell Culture Protocols*
Edited by: C. Wise © Humana Press Inc., Totowa, NJ

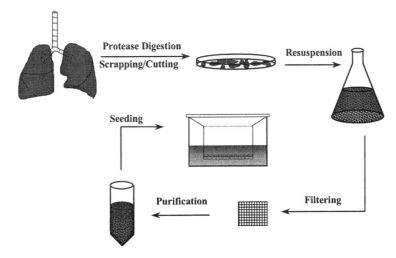

Fig. 1. Isolation and culturing of tracheal and alveolar epithelial cells for primary culture on permeable membrane support.

they often exhibit de-differentiated characteristics, and they lack development of tight junctions characteristic of the epithelial linings in vivo *(27,28)*. These drawbacks argue for primary cultured cell layers as a better alternative for drug transport studies. In this chapter, we will focus on methods of cultivating primary cultures of the respiratory epithelial cells for drug transport studies. **Fig. 1** schematically illustrates the principal steps involved in culturing tracheal and alveolar epithelial cells.

2. Materials

The following items are used for both epithelial cell cultures, unless otherwise stated.

1. Male New Zealand albino rabbits (*see* **Note 1**).
2. Sterile dissection kit.
3. 5000 U/mL Heparin (sodium injection, USP) (Elkins-Sinn) For alveolar epithelial cell culture.
4. Euthanasia injection solution: 6 g/mL sodium pentobarbital (Western Medical Supply).
5. Buffer A: 137.0 mM NaCl, 5.0 mM KCl, 0.7 mM Na$_2$HPO$_4$, 10.0 mM HEPES, and 5.5 mM glucose. For alveolar epithelial cell culture.
6. Buffer B: 137.0 mM NaCl, 5.0 mM KCl, 0.7 mM Na$_2$HPO$_4$, 10.0 mM HEPES, 5.5 mM glucose, and 3 mM EDTA. For alveolar epithelial cell culture.
7. Buffer C: 137.0 mM NaCl, 5.0 mM KCl, 0.7 mM Na$_2$HPO$_4$, 10.0 mM HEPES, 5.5 mM glucose, 1.2 mM MgSO$_4$, and 1.8 mM CaCl$_2$. For alveolar epithelial cell culture.

8. Porcine pancreatic elastase (Worthington Biochemical Corporation). For alveolar epithelial cell culture.
9. Lectin from *Bandeiraea simplicifolia* BS-1 (Sigma) for alveolar epithelial cell culture.
10. Deoxyribonuclease I (type IV, DNase I) (Sigma).
11. Protease E (type XIV) (Sigma).
12. Trypsin inhibitor (type II-S: soybean) (Sigma).
13. Human recombinant epidermal growth factor (EGF) (Sigma).
14. Hydrocortisone (Sigma).
15. Bovine serum albumin (BSA) (Sigma).
16. PC-1 medium: this is a defined medium containing predetermined amounts of insulin, transferrin, fatty acids, and other growth and attachment factors in a 1:1 DMEM:F12 (BioWhittaker). For tracheal epithelial cell culture.
17. Dulbecco's modified Eagle's medium nutrient mixture F-12 Ham (DMEM/F12) (Life Technologies) for alveolar epithelial cell culture.
18. Ca^{2+}-free minimum essential medium (S-MEM) (Life Technologies).
19. Ca^{2+}- and Mg^{2+}- free Hanks balanced salt solution (HBSS) (Life Technologies).
20. Certified fetal bovine serum (FBS) (Life Technologies).
21. Fungizone™ (Life Technologies).
22. Penicillin–streptomycin (Life Technologies).
23. L-glutamine (Life Technologies).
24. Gentamicin (Life Technologies).
25. ITS+ Premix: culture supplement containing insulin, transferrin, selenium, linoleic acid, and BSA (Collaborative Biomedical Products) for alveolar epithelial cell culture.
26. Recombinant human fibronectin (Collaborative Biomedical Products).
27. Type I rat tail collagen (Collaborative Biomedical Products).
28. Noncoated clear Transwells™ and Snapwells™ (Costar).
29. Bicarbonate Ringer's solution (BRS): 116.4 mM NaCl, 5.4 mM KCl, 1.8 mM CaCl$_2$, 0.81 mM MgSO$_4$, 0.78 mM NaH$_2$PO$_4$, 25 mM NaHCO$_3$, 15 mM HEPES, and 5 mM D-glucose.
30. 0.5% Triton X-100.
31. Epithelial voltohmmeter (EVOM™) and a pair of STX-2 electrodes (World Precision Instruments) (*see* **Note 5**).

3. Methods

3.1. Tracheal Epithelial Cell Culture

3.1.1. Isolating Tracheal Epithelial Cells

1. Upon euthanasia (1 mL solution/kg body weight), excise the rabbit trachea between the larynx and the bifurcation into the main stem bronchi (as shown in **Fig. 2**).
2. Place the excised trachea in ice-cold HBSS. Aseptically trim off the extraneous cartilage and connective tissue.
3. Cut excised trachea into 3 pieces of equal length, of approx 2 cm, open each longitudinally, and incubate in 0.2% protease E in S-MEM at 37°C for 90 min.

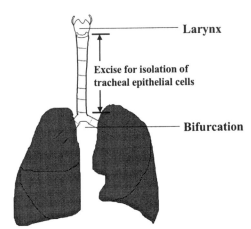

Fig. 2. Diagram of the trachea to be excised for isolation of tracheal epithelial cells.

4. Hold the pieces of trachea in place with a pair of forceps and gently scrape off the epithelial cell layer with a sterile scalpel blade.
5. Mix the cells in S-MEM containing 0.5 mg/mL DNase I solution and 10% FBS.
6. Centrifuge at 210g at room temperature for 10 min.
7. Aspirate the supernatant and reconstitute the cell pellet in S-MEM containing 10% FBS.
8. Repeat centrifugation and reconstitution once.
9. Filter cell suspension through a 40-µm cell strainer.
10. Centrifuge the filtrate and reconstitute the cell pellet in PC-1 medium supplemented with 100 U/mL penicillin, 100 µg/mL streptomycin, 50 µg/mL gentamicin, and 1 µg/mL fungizone.
11. Estimate cell viability and yield by the Trypan blue dye exclusion method (*see* **Note 2**).

3.1.2. Culturing Tracheal Epithelial Cells

1. Seed the isolated tracheal epithelial cell suspension onto a permeable membrane support in the Transwell device (*see* **Note 3**) at a density of 1.3 million cells/cm^2.
2. Add PC-1 medium to the basolateral side of the filter insert and bring the fluid level to the same as that on the apical side.
3. Maintain the cells in a humidified incubator with 95% air and 5% CO_2 at 37°C.
4. Twenty-four hours post initial seeding, remove the growth medium from both sides by aspiration.
5. Gently wash the adhered cells with fresh PC-1 medium pre-equilibrated at 37°C in 95% air/5% CO_2 (*see* **Note 4**).
6. Culture the cells in an air interface with their apical surfaces directly exposed to air. Add the growth medium to only the basolateral side of the filter insert to the same level as the apical side of the tracheal epithelial cells.
7. Change the growth medium daily.

3.1.3. Monitoring Tracheal Epithelial Cell Culture for Drug Transport Studies

1. Starting from d 3 onwards, monitor the transepithelial electrical resistance (TEER, expressed in $k\Omega$) and spontaneous potential difference (PD, expressed in mV) of the cell monolayers with EVOM (*see* **Note 5**).

3.2. Alveolar Epithelial Cell Culture

3.2.1. Isolating Alveolar Epithelial Cells

1. Inject the rabbit with heparin (1 mL/kg) to prevent blood clotting.
2. Five minutes later, inject the rabbit with the euthanasia solution (1 mL/kg).
3. Manually ventilate the lung via the trachea cannulated with a 60-mL syringe (use a tidal volume of about 35 mL).
4. Simultaneously, perfuse the lung vasculature with buffer B via the pulmonary vein.
5. Excise and lavage the lung 4 times each with alternating buffer A and buffer B.
6. Excise and lavage once with buffer C.
7. Excise and lavage once with 40 mL of S-MEM containing 2 U/mL porcine pancreatic elastase prewarmed to 37°C.
8. Allow the lung to completely deflate before each lavaging step.
9. Instill 40 mL of a 2 U/mL porcine pancreatic elastase solution through the trachea and incubate the lung at 37°C for 20 min.
10. Instill another 20 mL of 2 U/mL elastase solution through the trachea and incubate at 37°C for an additional 15 min.
11. Excise the trachea and the bronchi from the lung, and transfer the lung pieces to a S-MEM solution containing 1.67 mg/mL trypsin inhibitor and 25% FBS.
12. Mince the lung pieces and transfer to a sterilized Erlenmeyer flask (*see* **Note 6**).
13. Sequentially filter the lung tissue suspension through sterilized gauze, a 40-μm cell strainer, and a 15-μm nylon mesh.
14. Rinse all filters with fresh S-MEM solutions.
15. Centrifuge the cell suspension at 200*g* for 8 min at 4°C.
16. Reconstitute the cell pellets in buffer C containing 16 μg/mL BS-I lectin.
17. Incubate at room temperature for 30 min and subsequently filter through 40-μm cell strainers (*see* **Note 7**).
18. Centrifuge the filtered cell suspension and reconstitute the cell pellets in DMEM/F12 containing 10% FBS supplemented with 100 U/mL penicillin, 100 μg/mL streptomycin, 50 μg/mL gentamicin, and 1 μg/mL fungizone.
19. Estimate the cell viability and yield by the Trypan blue dye exclusion method (*see* **Note 2**).

3.2.2. Culturing Alveolar Epithelial Cells

1. Seed the isolated alveolar epithelial cell suspension onto a permeable membrane support in the Transwell device (*see* **Note 3**) at a density of 0.88 million cells/cm^2.
2. Add the DMEM/F12 medium to bathe the basolateral side of the filter insert.
3. Maintain the cells in a humidified incubator with 95% air and 5% CO_2 at 37°C.

4. Forty-eight hours post-seeding, remove the growth medium from both sides by aspiration.
5. Gently wash the adhered cells with serum-free DMEM/F12 medium supplemented with 1% ITS+, 10 ng/mL EGF, and 1 μ*M* hydrocortisone.
6. Add serum-free DMEM/F12 to both the apical and the basolateral sides of the filter insert.
7. Change the growth medium every other day.

3.2.3. Monitoring Drug Transport in the Alveolar Epithelial Cell Layers

1. Starting from day 3 onwards, monitor the transepithelial electrical resistance (TEER, kΩ) and spontaneous PD (mV) of the cell monolayers with EVOM (*see* **Note 8**).

3.3. Drug Transport Studies Using Cultured Epithelial Cell Layers

3.3.1. Uptake Experiment

1. Both alveolar and tracheal epithelial cells form polarized cell layers on the permeable membrane support when grown under conditions described above. Uptake measurement for various substrates can be carried out at either the apical or the basolateral membrane of the cultured cell monolayers (*see* **Note 9**). The Transwell™ filters are available in different sizes (6.5, 12, and 24.5 mm in diameter). The following description refers to the usage of cells grown on a 6.5-mm diameter filter device, unless otherwise indicated.
2. Equilibrate the cell layers in a BRS buffer for 1.5 h (*see* **Notes 10** and **11**) at a predetermined temperature, e.g., 4° or 37°C.
3. For apical uptake measurement, aspirate the incubation solution from both the apical and basolateral compartments of the cell layers.
4. Add 0.1 mL dosing solution containing the substrate to the apical compartment.
5. Then add 0.5 mL fresh BRS to the basolateral compartment to bring the basolateral fluid to the same level as the apical dosing fluid to avoid the creation of a hydrostatic pressure gradient.
6. For basolateral uptake measurement, aspirate the incubation solution from both the apical and basolateral compartments of the cell layers.
7. Add 0.1 mL fresh BRS to the apical compartment, and then add 0.5 mL dosing solution to the basolateral compartment.
8. Incubate the cells for a predetermined time at an appropriate temperature (*see* **Note 12**).
9. Terminate the incubation by aspirating both the dosing and sampling solutions in the opposite compartments.
10. Rinse the cell layers in ice-cold BRS 6 times.
11. Use a scalpel and a pair of forceps to excise the filter membrane with the cell layers attached from the Transwell.
12. Place the filter membrane with the cell layer in 0.5 mL 0.5% Triton X-100 for 3 h to lyse the cells.
13. Use 20 μL of the cell lysate for protein content determination (*see* **Note 13**) and use the rest for substrate quantification by a pertinent assay.

3.3.2. Transport Experiment

1. The primary cultured alveolar and tracheal epithelial cell layers mimic the epithelial lining of the airway and airspace in vivo. Therefore, transport experiments using the cultured cell layers are conducted to estimate the in vivo permeability of these mucosal linings to various solutes (*see* **Notes 14** and **15**).
2. Equilibrate the cell layers in a BRS buffer for 1.5 h at a predetermined temperature, e.g., 4° or 37°C.
3. For apical to basolateral transport, add 0.2 mL dosing solution to the apical compartment and 0.8 mL fresh BRS to the basolateral compartment.
4. For basolateral to apical transport, add 0.2 mL fresh BRS to the apical compartment first before adding 0.8 mL dosing solution to the basolateral compartment.
5. At predetermined times, pipet the solution in the sampling compartment up and down to create a stirring effect, and withdraw 0.1 mL solution from the apical side for the basolateral to apical transport study, or withdraw 0.2 mL solution from the basolateral side for the apical to basolateral transport study.
6. Replace the aliquot removed with the same volume of fresh BRS.
7. Measure the substrate amount in each sample using a pertinent assay.

3.3.3. Efflux Experiment

1. Cell layers cultured on a permeable membrane support allows substrate efflux from either side of the cell membrane to be measured (*see* **Note 16**).
2. Incubate the cell layers in a dosing solution in both apical and basolateral compartments with a suitable substrate concentration (which allows maximum loading of the substrate into the cells) for 1 h at 37°C.
3. Wash the filter with the cell layers attached in ice-cold BRS 6 times.
4. Transfer the filters to a new plate.
5. Add 0.2 mL fresh BRS buffer (37°C) to the apical and 0.8 mL to the basolateral compartment at time zero.
6. At predetermined time points, pipet the solution in the sampling compartment (either apical or basolateral) up and down to create a stirring effect. Withdraw 0.1 mL solution from the apical side for apical efflux study, or withdraw 0.2 mL solution from the basolateral side for basolateral efflux study.
7. Replace the aliquot removed with the same volume of fresh BRS (37°C).
8. At the end of the efflux experiment, excise the filter with the cell layers attached and place the filter in 0.5 mL 0.5% Triton X-100 to lyse the cells.
9. Measure the substrate amount in each sample as well as that remaining in the cells using a pertinent assay.

3.4. Data Analysis and Calculation

3.4.1. Uptake Experiment

1. Uptake is generally expressed in terms of total substrate amount accumulated intracellularly in unit time normalized by the cellular protein content, with units like pmol/min/mg protein or nmol/h/mg protein.

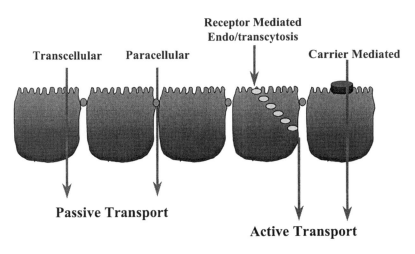

Fig. 3. Schematic presentation of solute transport pathways.

2. As shown in **Fig. 3**, transcellular transport can be either passive or active. Lipo-philic compounds can passively diffuse across the cell layers through the transcellular pathway, while hydrophilic compounds like mannitol may diffuse through the paracellular pathway. Transport could also take place in active pro-cesses through the membrane-associated transporter proteins or through recep-tor-mediated endo/transcytosis. To determine which pathway is undertaken by the substrate of interest, uptake should be measured at both 37°C, for total uptake, and 4°C, for the passive component of the uptake. The active component of the uptake is obtained by subtracting the passive component from total uptake. Active uptake processes are expected to demonstrate significant temperature depen-dency, with uptake much higher at 37°C than that at 4°C.

3. Uptake should also be measured over a range of substrate concentrations. For carrier- and receptor-mediated processes, uptake will demonstrate saturation as the substrate concentration increases in the dosing solution. Passive uptake pro-cesses, on the other hand, are independent of the substrate concentration and remain linear as the dosing concentration increases.

4. For uptake processes with an active component, uptake is described by **Eq. 1**:

$$\text{Uptake} = (V_{max} \times C)/(K_m + C) + K_d C \qquad \text{[Eq. 1]}$$

where V_{max} is the maximal uptake rate, K_m is the substrate concentration at half-maximal uptake, and C is the substrate concentration in the dosing solution. The nonsaturable passive coefficient, K_d, of the uptake rate can be determined by estimating the slope of linear substrate uptake at 4°C (*see* **Note 17**).

5. For carrier- and receptor-mediated uptake processes, inhibition studies should also be carried out. These studies allow delineation of substrate–ligand chemical structure requirement by the cellular uptake system and may shed some light on the nature of interaction between the substrate–ligand and the binding sites asso-

ciated with the cell membrane. This information would be of value in drug design. Inhibition may be competitive, noncompetitive, or uncompetitive, which can be determined by Dixon plots *(29)*. Competitive inhibitors, which are likely substrates for the cellular uptake systems themselves, can be rank ordered in terms of their relative affinities, reflected by the parameter K_i, for the uptake systems. K_i can be estimated by **Eq. 2**:

$$\text{Uptake}^{-1} = K_m[I]/V_{max} \times K_i \times C + (1 + K_m/C)/V_{max} \qquad \text{[Eq. 2]}$$

where [I] is the inhibitor concentration, and C is the substrate concentration. A lower K_i value for an inhibitor suggests a higher affinity towards the uptake system. Passive uptake processes, on the other hand, do not have a structural preference for any permeants and, therefore, cannot be specifically inhibited.

3.4.2. Transport Experiment

1. Transport is generally expressed in terms of unidirectional flux of a solute either in the apical to basolateral or the basolateral to apical directions through a unit cross section of a barrier in unit time, as described in **Eq. 3**:

$$J = M/(S \times t) \qquad \text{[Eq. 3]}$$

where J stands for flux, *M* is the drug amount, S is the surface area of the barrier, and t is the time allowed for transport to take place. Flux has units of pmol/(min $\times$ cm^2) or nmol/(h $\times$ m^2).

   Fig. 4 illustrates a typical time course of drug transport. The transport curve is convex to the time axis during the initial nonsteady state, becoming linear as it reaches steady state. When the linear line is extrapolated to the time axis, as shown in **Fig. 4**, the point of intersection is termed "lag time", which is the time required for a steady concentration gradient to be established across the epithelial cell layers. The lag time is governed by how fast the drug is transported, as well as the thickness of the cell layers. The slope of the linear portion of the curve equals the flux as defined in **Eq. 3** above.

3. A more commonly used parameter for characterization of transport is the permeability coefficient P_{app}, which can be estimated using **Eq. 4**:

$$P_{app} = M/(s \times t \times c) \qquad \text{[Eq. 4]}$$

where C is the initial dosing concentration. Since transcellular transport is usually proportional to the dosing concentration, P_{app} is a more accurate indicator for the intrinsic permeability of a substance across the cell layer than J. P_{app} has the unit of distance/time, usually in cm/h. (*see* **Notes 18** and **19**)

   From **Fig. 4**, P_{app} can be estimated by dividing the slope of the curve by the dosing concentration C.

3.4.3. Efflux Experiment

1. Efflux measurements can be taken at 4°C and 37°C to determine whether an active mechanism is involved.

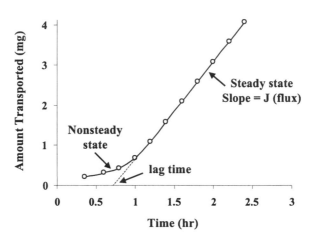

Fig. 4. Time course of drug transport.

2. If an active mechanism is involved, efflux can be measured in presence of competitive inhibitors in the extracellular space to determine whether trans-stimulation or trans-inhibition occurs. For bidirectional carriers, trans-stimulation of efflux may be observed when competitive inhibitors are present. On the contrary, for carriers that function mainly as efflux pumps, trans-inhibition of efflux in the presence of competitive inhibitors will be observed instead (*see* **Note 20**).

4. Notes

1. For alveolar epithelial cell culture, young (1.2 kg) and preferably pathogen-free rabbits (approx 1.2 kg) should be used to maximize the yield of alveolar epithelial cells free from contamination by cells of the immune system. For tracheal epithelial cell culture, on the other hand, larger animals may be used to ensure a large quantity of epithelial cells harvested from each animal. Moreover, during isolation of alveolar epithelial cells, the trachea is needed for ventilation and lavaging of the whole lung. Therefore, the same animal cannot be shared for isolation of both alveolar and tracheal epithelial cells. Tight monolayers of primary cultured human and rat alveolar epithelial cells maintained on permeable membrane support have also been developed as in vitro models for drug transport studies by other laboratories (*15,30*). For detailed information on how to isolate and culture rat or human alveolar epithelial cells, please refer to the corresponding publication (*15,30*).
2. Viability of isolated epithelial cells is crucial for cell differentiation and proliferation later on in culture. Usually isolated cells with less than 80% viability do not yield tight cell monolayers that are suitable for drug transport studies (unpublished observation).
3. The Transwell membrane inserts are precoated with collagen and fibronectin. The inserts are incubated with a DMEM/F12 solution containing 11.25 µg/mL BSA, 10 µg/mL recombinant human fibronectin, and 45 µg/mL type I rat

tail collagen for 2 h at 37°C. The coating solution is aspirated before the cells are seeded.

4. This washing step removes nonadherent cells that might be nonviable tracheal cells or contaminating cells such as red blood cells obtained during the cell isolation procedure.

5. Epithelial linings are known to consist of either monolayers or multilayers of cells joint by intercellular junctional complexes (tight junctions, intermediate junctions, and spot desmosomes). The presence of tight junctions prevents free lateral diffusion of ions and provides the cell layers with a measurable TEER. In the absence of tight junctions, solutes including drugs and ions could quickly diffuse between adjacent cells, and TEER values would not be significant. Epithelial cells are also known to actively transport ions, such as Na^+ and Cl^-, in a vectorial manner through the many ion channels and transporters present on the surface of their plasma membranes *(13,31)*. For example, the alveolar epithelium in vivo is known to actively absorb Na^+ in order to clear the alveolar space of fluid *(32)*. The electric current generated by net active ion transport allows a PD to develop across the epithelium. TEER and PD, therefore, have been used as two gauges to evaluate the viability of cultured cell layers and their suitability for drug uptake and transport studies. The EVOM and STX-2 electrodes are used to measure both TEER and PD. For tracheal cells grown at an air interface, medium pre-equilibrated to 37°C in 95% air/5% CO_2 needs to be added to both apical and basolateral sides, so that a pair of the STX-2 electrodes can be placed in the solution on both sides to measure TEER and PD across the cell layer. A peak PD value of around 70 mV is expected to develop on d 5, and a peak TEER value of around 1.2 k$\Omega \times$ cm^2 is expected to develop on d 7 *(13)*.

6. The cell suspension at this point should be swirled or pipetted up and down repeatedly to allow dissociation of alveolar epithelial cells from the underlying membrane.

7. The lectin from *Bandeiraea simplicifolia* binds to glycoproteins of both red blood cells and alveolar macrophages *(33)*. Incubation of the alveolar epithelial cell suspension with this lectin agglutinates these two contaminating cell types to form precipitates, thereby purifying the alveolar epithelial cells.

8. For alveolar epithelial cells in culture, a peak TEER value of 1.98 ± 0.02 k$\Omega \times$ cm^2, and a peak PD value of 34.5 ± 0.8 mV are expected to develop on d 6 *(14)*.

9. Uptake of solutes and/or drugs can be measured using the primary cell culture model described in this chapter. The advantage of these culture models is that both apical and basolateral membranes of the polarized cell layers are available for uptake measurement. Such an arrangement allows differentiated characterization of substrate uptake activities at the two membrane domains, which is important because polarized distribution of many transporter proteins has been observed in those epithelial cells *(34–36)*. Moreover, uptake experiments allow identification of the rate-limiting step in a multistep transcellular process.

10. For alveolar epithelial cell uptake and transport experiments, it is necessary to equilibrate the cells in BRS buffer containing 0.5% BSA to maintain a high TEER

value over long periods of time (up to 5 h). For tracheal cells, the presence of BSA in the BRS buffer does not seem to be necessary to maintain integrity of the tight cell monolayer.

11. For uptake and transport studies, it is crucial to use cell layers with optimal bioelectric parameters (*see* **Notes 5** and **8**), which are indicators for tight junction formation and active ion transport activities. Usage of "leaky" cell layers for uptake experiment will obscure the actual uptake site if the purpose of the experiment is to quantify apical membrane uptake versus basolateral membrane uptake. On the other hand, when leaky cell layers are used for transport studies, the paracellular route will constitute a larger contribution to the overall transport, thereby skewing the estimation of the in vivo permeability across the epithelium of interest.

12. It is important to select multiple short time frame (30 s, 1 min, 5 min, 10 min, etc.) for initial uptake experiments when the uptake rate is unknown. This step, known as the uptake time course measurement, allows determination of initial linear phase of uptake without the confounding influence of substrate efflux or metabolism. If initial samples are taken over an extended period of time, the measured uptake amount may reflect net accumulation as a balance between uptake and efflux activities rather than the result of a true uptake event. Once the time frame for initial linear uptake is determined, a sampling time equal to or shorter than that should be applied for subsequent uptake experiments.

13. It is inconvenient to measure the total cell number directly. Therefore, even though uptake amount is directly correlated with total cell number in the cultured cell layers, protein content of the epithelial cell layers is measured instead and used to normalize solute uptake.

14. Transport experiments can be carried out by dosing the drugs on either the apical side (to measure apical to basolateral transport) or the basolateral side of the cell layer (to measure basolateral to apical transport). A control experiment should be conducted using bare filters coated with collagen and fibronectin to assess whether the permeable membrane itself poses a significant diffusional barrier to solute transport. This is especially important for evaluating the permeability of lipophilic compounds.

15. In all transport experiments, mannitol ($C_6H_{14}O_6$) flux should also be measured to correct for paracellular permeability. Mannitol, a commonly used paracellular transport marker, travels strictly across cell layers through the paracellular route. Therefore, mannitol permeability can serve as a measure of cell layer integrity.

16. Similar to uptake measurements, efflux measurements can be particularly useful for characterizing the function of transporter proteins that assume a polarized distribution in epithelial cells, such as P-glycoprotein (P-gp) *(37)*.

17. The nonlinear least squares regression analysis program such as Prism™ may be used for fitting experimental data and calculating the three parameters (V_{max}, K_m, and K_d). V_{max} and K_m are also known as the Michaelis-Menten parameters, which describe the kinetics of uptake. V_{max} describes the capacity of the uptake process, whereas K_m depicts the affinity of the cellular uptake system towards a particular substrate.

18. For passive diffusion across the cell layers, either through transcellular or paracellular route, P_{app} is independent of changes in the dosing concentration. By contrast, for saturable processes such as carrier-mediated transcellular transport, P_{app} would decrease with increasing dosing concentration.

19. P_{app} for the paracellular marker mannitol has been estimated to be $(1.01 \pm 0.03) \times 10^{-7}$ cm/s across the primary cultured rabbit alveolar epithelial cell *(14)*, and $(1.2 \pm 0.3) \times 10^{-7}$ cm/s across the primary cultured rabbit tracheal epithelial cell *(13)*. If a similar sized hydrophilic compound exhibits a similar P_{app}, this compound might be traversing the epithelial cell layers passively through the paracellular route. On the other hand, if the compound of interest exhibits a much higher P_{app} than that of mannitol, there must be an active transport component contributing to this compound's translocation across the epithelial cell layers. This is because hydrophilic compounds cannot freely diffuse across epithelial cell membranes.

20. For bidirectional transporter proteins, the presence of competitive inhibitors outside the cells provides a driving force for substrate exchange to take place. Therefore, translocation of the inhibitor by the carrier into the cells would enhance the efflux of intracellularly accumulated substrate. This phenomenon has been reported previously *(38,39)*. On the other hand, for transporter proteins that specialize in efflux, such as P-gp and multidrug resistance protein (MRP), the extracellular competitive inhibitors might occupy the binding site on the carrier, thereby preventing it from gathering substrates from inside the cells to pump them out. This observation has lead to the approach of using competitive inhibitors to increase cellular accumulation of cytotoxic drugs when P-gp and MRP are over expressed on the cell membrane, as in the case of cancer treatment *(40)*

References

1. Folkesson, H. G., Westrom, B. R., Pierzynowski, S. G., Svendsen, J., and Karlsson, B. W. (1993) Lung to blood passage of albumin and a nonapeptide after intratracheal instillation in the young developing pig. *Acta Physiol. Scand.* **147,** 173–178.
2. Folkesson, H. G., Westrom, B. R., Dahlback, M., Lundin, S., and Karlsson, B. W. (1992) Passage of aerosolized BSA and the nona-peptide dDAVP via the respiratory tract in young and adult rats. *Exp. Lung Res.* **18,** 595–614.
3. Enna, S. J. and Schanker, L. S. (1972) Absorption of drugs from the rat lung. *Am. J. Physiol.* **223,** 1227–1231.
4. Ma, T., Fukuda, N., Song, Y., Matthay, M. A., and Verkman, A. S. (2000) Lung fluid transport in aquaporin-5 knockout mice. *J. Clin. Invest* **105,** 93–100.
5. Saumon, G., Soler, P., and Martet, G. (1995) Effect of polycations on barrier and transport properties of alveolar epithelium in situ. *Am. J. Physiol.* **269,** L185–L194.
6. Rannels, D. E., Pegg, A. E., Clark, R. S., and Addison, J. L. (1985) Interaction of paraquat and amine uptake by rat lungs perfused *in situ*. *Am. J. Physiol.* **249,** E506–E513.

7. Charon, J. P., McCormick, J., Mahta, A., and Kemp, P. J. (1994) Characterization of sodium-dependent glucose transport in sheep tracheal epithelium. *Am. J. Physiol.* **267,** L390–L397.

8. Saldias, F. J., Comellas, A., Guerrero, C., Ridge, K. M., Rutschman, D. H., and Sznajder, J. I. (1998) Time course of active and passive liquid and solute movement in the isolated perfused rat lung model. *J. Appl. Physiol.* **85,** 1572–1577.

9. French, M. C. and Wishart, G. N. (1985) Isolated perfused rabbit lung as a model to study the absorption of organic aerosols. *J. Pharmacol. Methods* **13,** 241–248.

10. Murata, M., Tamai, I., Sai, Y., Nagata, O., Kato, H., and Tsuji, A. (1999) Carrier-mediated lung distribution of HSR-903, a new quinolone antibacterial agent. *J. Pharmacol. Exp. Ther.* **289,** 79–84.

11. Kim, K. J., Matsukawa, Y., Lee, V. H.L., and Crandall, E. D. (1995) Characteristics of albumin absorption across rat alveolar epithelial cell monolayers. *FASEB J.* **9,** A569.

12. Yamashita, F., Kim, K. J., and Lee, V. H. (1998) Dipeptide uptake and transport characteristics in rabbit tracheal epithelial cell layers cultured at an air interface. *Pharm. Res.* **15,** 979–983.

13. Mathias, N. R., Kim, K. J., Robinson, T. W., and Lee, V. H.L. (1997) Development and characterization of rabbit tracheal epithelial cell monolayer models for drug transport studies. *Pharm. Res.* **12,** 1499–1505.

14. Shen, J., Elbert, K. J., Yamashita, F., Lehr, C.-M., Kim, K.-J., and Lee, V. H.L. (1999) Organic cation transport in rabbit alveolar epithelial cell monolayers. *Pharm. Res.* **16,** 1279–1286.

15. Elbert, K. J., Schäfer, U. F., Schäfers, H.-J., Kim, K. J., Lee, V. H.L., and Lehr, C.-M. (1999) Monolayers of human alveolar epithelial cells in primary culture for pulmonary absorption and transport studies. *Pharm. Res.* **16,** 601–608.

16. Mathias, N. R., Kim, K. J., and Lee, V. H. (1996) Targeted drug delivery to the respiratory tract: solute permeability of air-interface cultured rabbit tracheal epithelial cell monolayers. *J. Drug Target.* **4,** 79–86.

17. Yamashita, F., Kim, K. J., and Lee, V. H. (1997) Gly-L-Phe transport and metabolism across primary cultured rabbit tracheal epithelial cell monolayers. *Pharm. Res.* **14,** 238–240.

18. Yu, X. Y., Undem, B. J., and Spannhake, E. W. (1996) Protective effect of substance P on permeability of airway epithelial cells in culture. *Am. J. Physiol.* **271,** L889–L895.

19. Devalia, J. L., Godfrey, R. W., Sapsford, R. J., Severs, N. J., Jeffery, P. K., and Davies, R. J. (1994) No effect of histamine on human bronchial epithelial cell permeability and tight junctional integrity *in vitro. Eur. Respir. J.* **7,** 1958–1965.

20. Morimoto, K., Yamahara, H., Lee, V. H.L., and Kim, K. J. (1993) Dipeptide transport across rat alveolar epithelial cell monolayers. *Pharm. Res.* **10,** 1668–1674.

21. Saha, P., Kim, K. J., and Lee, V. H.L. (1994) Influence of lipophilicity on β-blocker transport across rat alveolar epithelial cell monolayers. *J. Control. Rel.* **32,** 191–200.

22. Morimoto, K., Yamahara, H., Lee, V. H.L., and Kim, K. J. (1994) Transport of thyrotropin-releasing hormone across rat alveolar epithelial cell monolayers. *Life Sci.* **54,** 2083–2092.

23. Matsukawa, Y., Yamahara, H., Yamashita, F., Lee, V. H., Crandall, E. D., and Kim, K. J. (2000) Rates of protein transport across rat alveolar epithelial cell monolayers. *J. Drug Target* **7,** 335–342.
24. Matsukawa, Y., Lee, V. H., Crandall, E. D., and Kim, K. J. (1997) Size-dependent dextran transport across rat alveolar epithelial cell monolayers. *J. Pharm. Sci.* **86,** 305–309.
25. Matsukawa, Y., Yamahara, H., Lee, V. H., Crandall, E. D., and Kim, K. J. (1996) Horseradish peroxidase transport across rat alveolar epithelial cell monolayers. *Pharm. Res.* **13,** 1331–1335.
26. Forbes, B., Wilson, C. G., and Gumbleton, M. (1999) Temporal dependence of ectopeptidase expression in alveolar epithelial cell culture: implications for study of peptide absorption. *Int. J. Pharm.* **180,** 225–234.
27. Gruenert, D. C., Finkbeiner, W. E., and Widdicombe, J. H. (1995) Culture and transformation of human airway epithelial cells. *Am. J. Physiol.* **268,** L347–L360.
28. Foster, K. A., Oster, C. G., Mayer, M. M., Avery, M. L., and Audus, K. L. (1998) Characterization of the A549 cell line as a type II pulmonary epithelial cell model for drug metabolism. *Exp. Cell Res.* **243,** 359–366.
29. Segel, I. H. (1976) Enzymes, p. 208–319. In *Biochemical calculations.* New York.
30. Cheek, J. M., Kim, K. J., and Crandall, E. D. (1989) Tight monolayer of rat alveolar epithelial cells: bioelectric properties and active sodium transport. *Am. J. Physiol.* **256,** C668–C693.
31. Kim, K. J., Cheek, J. M., and Crandall, E. D. (1991) Contribution of active Na^+ and Cl^- fluxes to net ion transport by alveolar epithelium. *Respir. Physiol.* **85,** 245–256.
32. Goodman, B., Kim, K.-J., and Crandall, E. D. (1987) Evidence for active sodium transport across alveolar epithelium of isolated rat lung. *J. Appl. Physiol.* **62,** 703–710.
33. Simon, R. H., McCoy, J. P., Chu, A. E., Dehart, P. D., and Goldstein, I. J. (1986) Binding of *Griffonia simplicifolia*I lectin to rat pulmonary alveolar macrophages and its use in purifying type II alveolar epithelial cells. *Biochim. Biophys. Acta* **885,** 34–42.
34. Lubman, R. L., Chao, D. C., and Crandall, E. D. (1995) Basolateral localization of Na^+-HCO_3^- cotransporter activity in alveolar epithelial cells. *Respir. Physiol* **100,** 15–24.
35. Oelberg, D. G., Xu, F., and Shabarek, F. (1994) Sodium-coupled transport of glucose by plasma membranes of type II pneumocytes. *Biochim. Biophys. Acta* **1194,** 92–98.
36. Gaillard, D., Ruocco, S., Lallemand, A., Dalemans, W., Hinnrasky, J., and Puchelle, E. (1994) Immunohistochemical localization of cystic fibrosis transmembrane conductance regulator in human fetal airway and digestive mucosa. *Pediatr. Res.* **36,** 137–143.
37. Lechapt-Zalcman, E., Hurbain, I., Lacave, R., et al. (1997) MDR1-Pgp 170 expression in human bronchus. *Eur.Respir. J.* **10,** 1837–1843.
38. Temple, C. S., Stewart, A. K., Meredith, D., et al. (1998) Peptide mimics as substrates for the intestinal peptide transporter. *J. Biol. Chem.* **273,** 20–22.

39. Takeuchi, A., Masuda, S., Saito, H., Hashimoto, Y., and Inui, K. (2000) Trans-stimulation effects of folic acid derivatives on methotrexate transport by rat renal organic anion transporter, OAT-K1. *J. Pharmacol. Exp. Ther.* **293,** 1034–1039.

40. Larrivee, B. and Averill, D. A. (2000) Modulation of adriamycin cytotoxicity and transport in drug-sensitive and multidrug-resistant Chinese hamster ovary cells by hyperthermia and cyclosporin A. *Cancer Chemother. Pharmacol.* **45,** 219–230.

21

Applications of Epithelial Cell Culture in Studies of Drug Transport

Staffan Tavelin, Johan Gråsjö, Jan Taipalensuu, Göran Ocklind, and Per Artursson

1. Introduction

The popularity of epithelial cell lines in studies of drug transport processes can probably be explained by the ease with which new information is derived from these rather simple in vitro models. Drug transport studies in epithelial cell monolayers grown on permeable supports are easy to perform under controlled conditions, resulting in the generation of a wealth of information. This information can generally be relatively easily translated into fundamental principles, since the homogenous epithelial cell cultures lack the complexity and variability found in more complex whole tissue models. In fact, much of our more recent knowledge about active and passive drug transport mechanisms has been obtained from studies in various epithelial cell cultures (*1*). The good correlation between passive drug transport through various epithelial cell monolayers and that seen across the human intestine in vivo now makes it possible to use the cell cultures for studies on structure-absorption relationships (examples are found in **refs.** *2–4*). Indeed, both cell culture and transport experiments across epithelial cell monolayers have been automated, and these models are now used as a screening tool in drug discovery programs in many drug companies for the prediction of intestinal drug permeability.

In this chapter, we present the basic protocols used in our laboratory in studies of passive and active drug transport across epithelial cell monolayers grown on permeable supports. Protocols for the characterization and quality control of the cell monolayers are presented initially, since the reproducible performance of the cell cultures are a requirement for reliable quantitative drug transport studies. In the final part, the most commonly used mathematical expressions

From: *Methods in Molecular Biology, vol. 188: Epithelial Cell Culture Protocols*
Edited by: C. Wise © Humana Press Inc., Totowa, NJ

for the calculation of epithelial drug transport are presented. Our protocols have been developed for the popular human intestinal epithelial cell line Caco-2. However, they should be readily adaptable to other monolayer-forming epithelial cell lines.

2. Materials
2.1. Cells

The most commonly used cell line for studies of drug transport is Caco-2, which originates from a human colonic adenocarcinoma *(5)*. There are several reasons for its popularity. First, despite its cancerous origin, its behavior is similar to its normal in vivo counterpart *(6)*. Second, it is of human origin. Third, the oral route is the most important drug administration route and the degree of intestinal absorption of a drug may determine the clinical success or failure of a drug candidate *(7)*. Fourth, the first correlation between drug permeability in vitro, and drug absorption in the human was based on studies in this cell line *(2)*. Caco-2 cells can be obtained from several sources, including the American Type Culture Collection (ATCC) (http://www.atcc.org/) or from the European Collection of Cell Cultures (ECACC) (http://www.ecacc.org/). Caco-2 cells exhibit morphological and functional similarities to intestinal (absorptive) enterocytes *(8,9)*. The cells form tight junctions and express many brush border enzymes, some CYP450 isoenzymes, and some phase II enzymes such as glutathione-S-transferases, sulfotransferase, and glucuronidase. These enzymes are all relevant in studies of presystemic (drug) metabolism *(10–12)*. More recently, a method has been developed to induce functional expression of CYP450-3A4 in Caco-2 cells *(13)*. Many active transport systems that are normally found in small intestinal enterocytes have been characterized in this cell line. These include transport systems for sugars, amino acids, peptides and vitamins *(14–21)*. The influence of efflux systems, such as P-glycoprotein (P-gp) and multidrug resistance-associated proteins (MRPs), on intestinal drug transport has been extensively studied in this cell line *(22–25)*. The unusually high degree of differentiation, together with the fact that these cells differentiate spontaneously in normal serum-containing cell culture medium, has resulted in Caco-2 becoming one of the most popular cell lines for studies of epithelial integrity and transport. Cell lines may have different characteristics depending on the interval of passage number at which the cells are studied. It is, therefore, important to define a limited number of passages that are used for the experiments. Caco-2 cells obtained from ATCC and ECACC are usually at passage number 20–40, while in our laboratory, we use Caco-2 cells at passage 90–105. We have thoroughly characterized the Caco-2 cells and found that the integrity, for example, is constant within this interval of passages. Caco-2 cells

Table 1
Selected Examples of Monolayer-Forming
Epithelial Cell Lines Used in Drug Transport Studies

Cell line	Origin	Main characteristics	References
Caco-2	Human colonic adenocarcinoma	Villus enterocyte-like, differentiates spontaneously.	*(11,31)*
T84	Human colonic adenocarcinoma	Crypt cell-like.	*(32,33)*
HT29-clones	Human colonic	Goblet cell-like, forms mucus layer. Crypt cell-like, leaky.	*(34–36)* *(37,38)*
IEC cell lines	Rat fetal intestinal epithelium		
2/4/A1	Rat fetal intestinal epithelium	Crypt cell-like, leaky, temperature-sensitive differentiation.	*(3,39)*
LLC PK$_1$	Pig kidney epithelium	Low expression of efflux systems, expression systems for transport proteins.	*(33,40–43)*
MDCK	Dog kidney epithelium	Low expression of efflux systems, expression systems for transport proteins.	*(4,30,44)*

require 21 d to differentiate using the well-established culture protocol presented here *(26)*. Recently, culture protocols that speed up the differentiation process to a varying degree (usually to less than 1 wk) have been published *(27,28)*, and at least one of these protocols is commercially available (http://www.bd.com/labware) and has been evaluated *(29)*. However, only limited information regarding the performance of these faster culture protocols is available. Therefore, a thorough characterization of Caco-2 cell cultures grown according to the accelerated protocols will be required in order to investigate the reproducibility of these protocols.

The time-demanding culture protocol of the Caco-2 cell line has stimulated the evaluation of alternative epithelial cell lines (*see* **Table 1**). Some of these cell lines have single properties that resemble more closely the human intestinal epithelium than does Caco-2. For instance, 2/4/A1 cells form leaky monolayers that better mimic the passive drug permeability in the small intestine *(3)*. Other cell lines (such as MDCK and LLC PK$_1$) are popular because of the low endogenous expression of transporters, which makes them suitable as expression systems, for example, for selected ABC transporters *(30)*.

2.2. Equipment and Consumables

In addition to the general equipment required for growing and maintaining cell cultures, the following equipment and materials are required. Optional pieces of equipment that are required for characterization of the cell monolayers grown on permeable supports and other tasks are given in conjunction to the method descriptions.

1. Permeable cell culture supports: there are several types of permeable cell culture supports commercially available from different suppliers (*see* **Table 2**). The cell culture supports are available in different sizes (for example, 6.5, 12, 24, and 98 mm diameter). The porous membranes on which the cells are grown are usually made from polycarbonate, cellulose, or materials with similar characteristics. We prefer to use polycarbonate filters, since Caco-2 cells attach readily to these supports without the need for an extracellular matrix such as collagen (*see* below). In addition, the hydrophilic polycarbonate supports do not restrict the diffusion of water and most drugs. Permeable supports are available with different pore diameters from 0.1–3.0 µm. Many inserts may be obtained with different pore densities. A low pore density is suitable for transillumination microscopy because of the lower opacity, and a high pore density is suitable for drug transport studies. Most permeable supports are shipped in multiwell culture plates. Additional multiwell plates without permeable supports must be obtained for the transport experiments. We generally use cell culture supports with a diameter of 12 mm and a pore diameter of 0.4 µm. For simplicity, in all the following protocols, all volumes and time intervals are optimized for these supports. A schematic representation of epithelial cells grown on permeable supports is shown in **Fig. 1**.
2. Incubator, water bath, and plate warmer set to 37°C: it is important to control the temperature during the transport experiment since the integrity of the cell monolayers, and hence the rate of drug transport, depends on temperature. Therefore, all our experiments with epithelial cell monolayers grown on permeable supports are performed in an incubator at 37°C, and all buffers are preheated in a water bath. In order to avoid rapid cooling of the cell monolayers during sampling, we place the tissue culture plate with the inserts on a thermostatically controlled plate warmer. We use a custom-built plate warmer, especially designed for cell culture plates, but there are commercially available warmers that may be used for this purpose, such as the Kitazato microscopic stage warmer (http://www.kitazatosupply.com/e-index.html). Plate warmers must be checked for local variations in temperature before use.
3. Plate shaker: a plate shaker is placed in the incubator to allow for stirring of the inserts. Stirring of the inserts at for example 100–500 rpm on a conventional plate shaker seems to give more reproducible results and does not affect the integ-

Table 2
Selected Cell Culture Supports
Suitable for Microscopy or Drug Transport Studies

Company/Name	Material[a]	Comment[b]	Web address
Becton Dickinson			http://www.bd.com/labware/
BD Falcon™	PWT	Microscopy	library/cellculture.html
	FP	Drug transport	
BD Biocoat™	FP, PET	Pre-coated with extracellular matrices (collagen I or IV, laminin, fibronectin or matrigel)	
Corning Costar®			http://www.scienceproducts.
Transwell	PC	Drug transport	corning.com/
Transwell-Clear	PC	Microscopy	
Transwell-COL	PC	Pre-coated with bovine collagen I and III	
Snapwell	PC	Detachable filter, suitable for mounting in specific diffusion chamber, for example for electrophysiolgical characterization	
Millipore			http://www.millipore.com/
Millicell	CM	Microscopy	analytical/products.nsf/docs/
	HA	Microscopy	millicell
	PCF	Drug transport studies	
NUNC®			http://nunc.nalgenun.com/
Anopore® membrane	n/a	Microscopy	products/catalog/cellculture/ gr1-18.html
Polycarbonate membrane	PC	Drug transport studies	

[a]PET (polyethylene terephthalate), FP (hydrophilic fluoropolymer), PC and PCF (polycarbonate), (polystyrene), HA (mixed cellulose esters), n/a (no information available).

[b]More information regarding recommended use of the specific supports may be obtained from the suppliers' web addresses.

rity of Caco-2 cell monolayers (more vigorous stirring may affect the integrity of less adherent cell monolayers) (*45*). Stirring also reduces the thickness of what is known as the "aqueous boundary layer" (ABL), which is adjacent to the epithelial cell surface (*45*). If the ABL significantly contributes to the overall resistance of

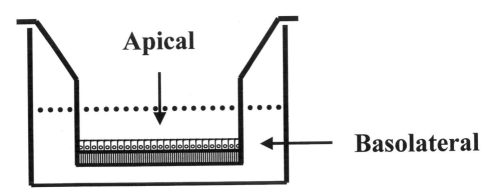

Fig. 1. A schematic representation of an epithelial cell monolayer grown on a permeable support. The apical and basolateral chambers are indicated. The dotted line represents the surfaces of the experimental medium in the two chambers.

the system, it is likely that the cellular permeability is underestimated. This phenomenon is primarily observed when the transport of rapidly absorbed drugs is studied. In our laboratory, the inserts are agitated on a calibrated enzyme-linked immunosorbent assay (ELISA) plate shaker (IKA® Shüttler MTS4).
4. Endohm® tissue resistance measurement chamber connected to an Evohm resistance meter (World Precision Instruments). Other transepithelial electrical resistance (TER) measurement systems are available (Millicell ERS from Millipore).
5. Fine-pointed scalpel blades.

2.3. Chemicals and Buffers

All culture media and supplements listed below may be purchased from a general supplier, such as Life Technologies. All media and buffers must be prepared under aseptic conditions.

1. Culture Medium: usually culture media of identical compositions can be used to maintain and expand the cell cultures in the flasks as well as to culture the cells on the permeable supports. However, to reduce the risk for contamination, separate media bottles are used for the two types of culture. The standard culture media composition used for culturing Caco-2 cells in flasks or on permeable supports is described in **Table 3**.

In our laboratory, the antibiotics are added only to cells grown on permeable supports. Exclusion of the antibiotics from the maintenance cultures allows for rapid detection of contaminated cultures. In addition, we also screen our cell cultures for mycoplasma contamination every second month.

In order to avoid batch-to-batch variations in FCS, we evaluate several batches of FCS for cell proliferation, time-dependent development of TER, and mannitol permeability. We then purchase a 1-yr supply of the most suitable batch. A less

Table 3
Standard Culture Medium Composition

Ingredient	Volume	Storage	Cat. no.[a]
Dubecco's modified Eagle's medium (DMEM) (high glucose 4.5 g/L without Na-pyruvate)	500 mL	4°C	41965-039
Nonessential amino acids (MEM)	5 mL	4°C	11140-035
Fetal calf serum (FCS)	50 mL	−20°C	—[b]
Streptomycin–penicillin solution	5 mL	−20°C	15140-114

[a] The catalogue numbers refer to materials from Life Technologies, unless otherwise stated, but these materials may be obtained from other suppliers.

[b] The most suitable batch of FCS should be chosen among batches from more than one supplier (*see* below).

Table 4
Trypsin-EDTA Solution Composition

Ingredient	Volume	Storage	Cat. no. [a]
PBS	40 mL	room temperature	14190-094
Trypsin (10×)	5 mL	−20°C	25090-028
2% EDTA (sodium salt) solution	5 mL	room temperature	2820549; ICN Biomedicals

[a] The catalogue numbers refer to materials from Life Technologies, unless otherwise stated, but these materials may be obtained from other suppliers.

validated alternative may be to use a better defined medium, for example one that is serum-free *(46)*.

The culture medium must be used within 1 mo if stored at 4°C.

2. Serum-free media (SFM): DMEM without additives.
3. Phosphate-buffered saline (PBS): Ca^{2+}- and Mg^{2+}-free, sterile, and without phenol red (Life Technologies, cat. no. 14190-094). PBS in opened bottles should be used within 1 mo if stored at 4°C.
4. Trypsin-EDTA solution (*see* **Table 4**).

   Caco-2 cells attach strongly to the plastic surface. Therefore, we use a more concentrated trypsin-EDTA solution (0.25%, w/v) than that recommended for many other cell lines. Other cell lines may be less adherent. For these cell lines the trypsin concentration may be reduced to 0.025% (w/v). The trypsin-EDTA solution is stable for 1 mo at 4°C.
5. Hank's balanced salt solution (HBSS): the most commonly used medium in drug transport experiments is HBSS. A buffer system must be added to HBSS in order to maintain the desired pH.

Table 5
Composition of HBSS[a]

Ingredient	Amount	Storage	Supplier	Cat. no.
Hanks' balanced salts premixture without phenol red		4°C	Life Technologies	11201-019
Sodium bicarbonate (Na_2HCO_3)	0.35 g	Room temperature	Life Technologies	066-01810
HEPES	5.96 g (25 mM)	Room temperature	Sigma	H-9136

[a]Add the HBSS premixture, Na_2HCO_3 and HEPES to a 1000-mL volumetric flask.
Add 500 mL of ultrapure water (for example MilliQ).
Allow the ingredients to dissolve completely under stirring with a magnetic stirring bar.
Add ultrapure water to almost 1000 mL (to allow for pH adjustment).
Adjust the pH to 7.4 by adding aliquots of NaOH (1 M).
Add ultrapure water up to 1000 mL.
Sterile-filter through bottle-top filters (0.22 µm; Nunc) to sterile bottles. The filtration step minimizes the risk of contamination and prolongs the shelf life of the medium.

Hepes (4-[2-hydroxyethyl]-1-piperazineethanesulfonic acid) and Mes (2-[N-morpholino]ethane-sulfonic acid) are the most frequently used buffers for the maintenance of physiological (pH = 7.4) and slightly acidic (pH = 6.0–6.5) pH values, respectively.

For the preparation of 1000 mL HBSS, pH 7.4, *see* **Table 5**.

For the preparation of HBSS, pH 6.0, 1000 mL, replace HEPES with 10 mM Mes (1.95 g) (Sigma M-8652). HBSS is stable for 1 mo at room temperature if protected from light.

6. Matrigel (Sigma or Becton Dickinson) or EHS (Promega).
7. Trypan blue.
8. 3% Paraformaldehyde in PBS.
9. 0.1% Triton X-100 in PBS.
10. Rhodamine-phalloidin (Molecular Probes): 1:150 in PBS.
11. 50% Glycerol in PBS.
12. 0.2% Triton X-100 in PBS.
13. Z0-1 Antibody (Zymed, cat. no. 61-7300).
14. Fluorescein isothiocyanate (FITC) anti-rabbit IgG (Amersham, N1034).
15. Microscope slides and coverslips.
16. RNeasy Minikit (Qiagen).
17. Lysis buffer for protein extraction: 50 mM Tris-HCl, pH 7.4, 10 mM EDTA, 1% sodium dodecyl sulfate (SDS). Supplemented with a complete mini-proteinase inhibitor cocktail (Roche Diagnostics).
18. Bicinchoninic acid (BCA) Assay (Pierce).

2.4. Drugs

It is preferable to use the more easily dissolved salt form of a drug. Many registered drugs can be obtained from Sigma. Other registered or experimental drugs can often be obtained from the respective drug companies. The drug must be chemically pure. Impurities may damage the cells, resulting in erroneous transport experiments. Impurities or degraded drug may also interfere with the analysis of transported drug. If the drug to be studied is available with a radioactive label, preferably stably labeled with ^{14}C, it may facilitate and speed the analysis considerably. If a labeled drug has a high specific radioactivity, it can be detected in very small amounts. Problems associated with the use of radiolabeled drugs are that they may contain radioactive impurities (for example ^{3}H-water) that will interfere with the analysis and that their potential degradation during the experiment may be overlooked. Labeled drugs are expensive, and only a few are commercially available. Due to the limitations associated with radiolabeled drugs, most investigators prefer to use unlabeled drugs in their studies.

1. ^{14}C-mannitol (NEN Life Sciences) 50 Ci/mol, 0.1 mCi/mL.

3. Methods
3.1. Culturing of Epithelial Cells on Permeable Supports
3.1.1. Seeding Density

In various laboratories $0.5–5 \times 10^5$ Caco-2 cells/cm^2 are seeded onto the permeable supports. In our laboratory, 4.4×10^5 Caco-2 cells/cm^2 are seeded onto the supports. For other cell lines, the optimal cell density has to be determined. This is done by measuring the development of TER or, preferably, ^{14}C-mannitol permeability over time and by microscopic examination. A low seeding density may require a longer culture period prior to obtaining confluent monolayers than a high seeding density. Sensitive cell lines may de-differentiate or detach from the support during this period. On the other hand, too high a seeding density may result in multilayer-formation for some cell lines, which is undesirable for drug transport studies.

3.1.2. Seeding Cells on Permeable Supports

This is a protocol that we use for seeding Caco-2 cells on permeable cell culture supports (Transwell Costar, 0.4 µm pore size, 12 mm in diameter). This protocol may also be used for other epithelial cell lines. Caco-2 cells attach readily to uncoated supports, but other cell lines may require a matrix-coated support for proper cell attachment. A schematic representation of an epithelial cell monolayer grown on a permeable support is shown in **Fig. 1**. If matrix-coated inserts are used (*see* **Subheading 3.1.3.**), the coating is performed in advance, and the wetting step is excluded.

1. To wet the supports, add 0.1 mL of medium to the apical (top) side of the supports and 1.5 mL to the basolateral (bottom) side. Place the inserts in the 37°C incubator for 30 min (or until the cell suspension is ready).
2. Harvest the Caco-2 cells by trypsinization. To do this, first remove the culture medium.
3. Wash the cells once with cold PBS.
4. Add 5 mL (to a 75-cm^2 flask) trypsin-EDTA.
5. Rock the flask gently and then pour off most of the trypsin-EDTA, so that there is just enough left to cover the surface.
6. Leave the flask at 37°C for the minimum amount of time needed to detach the cells.
7. Add FCS containing culture medium to the detached cell suspension to inactivate the trypsin (*see* **Note 1**). Adding 10 mL medium to a culture flask with 75 cm^2 growth surface is sufficient.
8. Count the cells (*see* **Note 2**).
9. Pellet the cells by centrifugation at 200–400g (1100–1500 rpm in a rotor with a radius of 16 cm) for 5 min and discard the trypsin-containing medium.
10. Resuspend the pellet carefully in fresh culture medium to a cell concentration of 1×10^6 cells/mL.
11. Add 0.5 mL (0.5×10^6 cells) of the cell suspension to the apical side of the permeable support (*see* **Note 3**).
12. Place the supports in the CO_2 incubator for 5 h. Remove the apical medium and replace with 0.6 mL fresh medium (*see* **Note 4**).
13. Change the medium (*see* **Note 5**) every second day for 21 d to obtain well-differentiated monolayers suitable for drug transport experiments (*see* **Note 6**).

3.1.3. Coating of Permeable Supports with Matrigel

The attachment of epithelial cell lines to the permeable support can be improved by coating the support with an extracellular matrix. Matrix proteins commonly used are various types of collagens and a matrix mixture obtained from Engelbreth-Holm-Swarm sarcoma and marketed as matrigel and as EHS. Apart from improved attachment, improved morphology and differentiation of the cells may be obtained.

Below follows the protocol to coat permeable supports (12 mm in diameter) with 15 µg/cm^2 matrigel.

1. Aliquot matrigel from the stock solution into sterile vials in amounts sufficient for one batch of cell monolayers. Use precooled pipets and work on ice. Keep aliquots frozen and avoid repeated freeze-thawing of the matrix.
2. Thaw an aliquot of matrigel on ice. Note that too rapid thawing may cause precipitation of matrix components. Keep precooled SFM on ice. Use precooled pipets.

3. For each support, use 16.95 µg matrigel diluted in cold SFM to a final volume of 250 µL.
4. Multiply the volumes in step 3 by the total number of inserts. Add 10% to account for losses during pipetting.
5. Add matrigel to SFM and mix thoroughly. Keep the mixture on ice.
6. Add 250 µL of matrigel mixture to each insert.
7. Leave the inserts at 37°C for 2 h to allow the matrigel to attach to the surface. If the coated inserts are not used immediately, they may be stored at 4°C for 24 h. Do not allow the inserts to dry out.
8. The coated inserts are now ready to use. Remove the remaining coating solution immediately prior to seeding the cells onto the coated inserts.

3.2. Characterization of Epithelial Cell Monolayers

If there is little or no knowledge about the cell line available, a thorough examination of the monolayer integrity, including TER and mannitol permeability, changes over time, and microscopic examination of the monolayers should be performed. In addition, the specific features to be studied should be characterized with regard to expression, localization, and function (*see* **Subheading 3.2.5.**). In order to maintain reproducible results of the transport experiments, the investigator should always perform a routine characterization of each batch of cell monolayers. Prior to each transport experiment, a routine examination of the monolayers may be carried out by measuring TER (*see* **Subheading 3.2.1.**) or ^{14}C-mannitol permeability (*see* **Subheading 3.2.2.**) on selected monolayers.

3.2.1. Assessment of TER of Caco-2 Cell Monolayers

TER measurements of cell monolayers grown on permeable supports give information about the resistance to ion flux across the monolayer. Since the ion flux across the cell membranes is small compared with that through the tight junctions of the paracellular spaces, TER reflects the integrity of the tight junctions between the cells. It should be noted that the equipment used here is suitable only for routine characterization of TER. For quantitative electrophysiological characterization, we use home-built equipment described elsewhere (*47*).

TER depends on temperature. At room temperature, the TER value of a cell monolayer is higher than it is at 37°C. For instance, in our experience, the TER of a Caco-2 cell monolayer may increase by approx 200 $\Omega \times cm^2$ if the temperature drops from 37°C to room temperature (22°C) during a transport experiment. Lack of proper temperature control is probably a major factor responsible for the variable TER values reported for Caco-2 cell monolayers in the literature (*48*). Therefore, it is important to carefully control the temperature in order to obtain reliable TER values. TER is usually measured at 37°C.

The TER of Caco-2 cell monolayers should increase with time in culture, reaching a maximum after 10–14 d. In our laboratory we commonly obtain

TER values of 200–250 $\Omega \times cm^2$ for Caco-2 cell monolayers at passage 90–105. TER values ranging from 62 to 1290 $\Omega \times cm^2$ have been reported for Caco-2 cells *(48)*. Apart from improper control of temperature, these differences may be related to use of different clones or passage numbers of Caco-2 cells *(48)*. For instance, in our laboratory, we obtain TER values of around 350 $\Omega \times cm^2$ for Caco-2 cells at passage 30–40. The use of different pieces of equipment may also contribute to the wide span of TER values that have been reported *(48)*.

1. Add 2.4 mL HBSS to the Endohm chamber and put the chamber into an incubator set to 37°C. Allow the chamber to reach 37°C.
2. Remove the cell culture medium from the permeable supports and place the supports in empty wells. Add HBSS preheated to 37°C to the apical side (0.5 mL) and to the basolateral side (1.5 mL).
3. Allow monolayers to equilibrate for 15–30 min at 37°C before TER measurements (*see* **Note 7**).
4. Remove the apical HBSS and transfer the supports to the Endohm chamber. Add 0.25 mL preheated HBSS to the apical side. Place the lid (containing the apical electrodes) onto the support. Make sure that no air bubbles are trapped in the chamber.
5. Wait 30 s to 1 min before measuring (*see* **Note 8**).
6. Repeat steps 1–5 with an empty insert to obtain background values.
7. Calculate TER by multiplying the resistance value (after subtraction of the background) from the reader by the surface area of the monolayer (cm^2) to obtain TER (*see* **Note 9**) expressed as $\Omega \times cm^2$.
8. Discard the monolayer (*see* **Note 10**).

3.2.2. Transport of Mannitol Across Caco-2 Cell Monolayers

An alternative and more relevant method to assess monolayer integrity is to study the transport of a hydrophilic marker molecule (such as a model drug) that is passively transported across the monolayer. Passive transport across an epithelial cell monolayer can either occur through the cell (transcellular) or through the tight junctions (paracellular) (**Fig. 2**). Since hydrophilic molecules are not distributed into the lipophilic cell membranes to any large extent, their transport across the monolayer is restricted to the paracellular route. The transport rate of a hydrophilic marker molecule should decrease over time in culture reaching a minimum in confluent cell monolayers with fully developed tight junctions. The most common hydrophilic marker molecule used to characterize paracellular transport across cell monolayers is ^{14}C-labeled mannitol. 21- to 35-d-old Caco-2 cell monolayers grown in our laboratory have a permeability to mannitol of approximately 1 to 2×10^{-7} cm/s (*see* **Subheading 3.4.**).

Transport studies require rigorous temperature control as TER measurements do. All media should therefore be preheated in a water bath. In addition, the cell monolayers should be kept in a humid atmosphere at 37°C. The latter

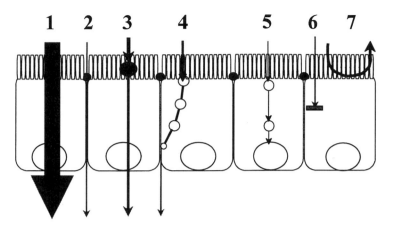

Fig. 2. Schematic representations of the different transport routes and barriers for drugs in an epithelial cell monolayer. Transcellular (**1**), paracellular (**2**), carrier-mediated (**3**) (note that the carrier may be situated in the apical or the basolateral membrane), trancytosis (**4**), endocytosis (**5**), intestinal metabolism (**6**), and efflux (**7**) (note that the efflux protein may be situated in the apical or the basolateral membrane).

can be accomplished by placing the inserts in a thermostated chamber set to 37°C, into which water trays are placed. The water will saturate the air in the chamber, minimizing evaporation from the inserts during the experiment. In order to avoid rapid cooling during sampling, we place the tissue culture plate on a thermostatically controlled plate warmer.

1. Prepare the ^{14}C-mannitol solution by pipetting approx 1×10^6 counts per minute (cpm)/permeable support into a 50-mL polypropylene test tube.
2. Add an appropriate amount of preheated HBSS to the tube and mix thoroughly.
3. Remove the cell culture medium from 3 to 4 permeable supports and place them in empty wells. Add HBSS preheated to 37°C to the apical side (0.5 mL) and to the basolateral side (1.5 mL). Pre-incubate the monolayers for 15–30 min (*see* **Note 7**).
4. Remove the HBSS and transfer the inserts to new wells.
5. Add 0.4 mL of ^{14}C-mannitol solution to the apical side of the monolayers and 1.2 mL preheated HBSS to the basolateral side. Sample 10–50 μL from the apical chamber at t = 0 for determination of the initial radioactivity of each support (*see* **Note 11**).
6. Place the inserts into a 37°C incubator on a plate shaker set to 100–500 rpm (*see* **Note 12**).
7. Sample 600 μL from the basolateral chamber every 20 or 30 min for 120–360 min (*see* **Note 13**). Replace each sample with fresh preheated HBSS.
8. Immediately after the final sampling, take 10–50 μL from the apical chamber to determine the final apical concentration (*see* **Note 11**).
9. Determine the radioactivity of the samples in a liquid scintillation counter.
10. Calculate the permeability coefficient of mannitol across the cell monolayers (*see* **Subheading 3.4.**).

3.2.3. Assessment of Membrane Integrity Using Rhodamine–Phalloidin

Visualization is an important additional tool to assess the cell morphology and monolayer integrity. It can be used to verify the monolayer homogeneity and tightness of the cultured epithelium. Unfortunately, direct visualization by light microscopy is not possible with normal permeable supports such as Transwell, due to the high pore density that scatters the illuminating light. Special inserts with lower pore density (for example Transwell Clear and Falcon Cyclopore cell culture inserts) must be used. However, these permeable supports are not suitable for transport studies, since the low pore density limits the transfer of compounds to the basolateral side of the cells.

Fluorescence microscopy is a more powerful tool for examining the integrity and changes in barrier properties at a cellular level. General fluorescent markers, such as nuclear stains and actin-binding agents (such as rhodamine-labeled phalloidin) can be used to assess the continuous and gross morphology of various monolayer-forming epithelial cell lines.

Actin staining with rhodamine-labeled phalloidin has been used as an indirect method to study the integrity of tight junctions, since actin distribution often (but not always) correlates with changes in tight-junction properties *(50)*.

1. Remove the cell culture medium from the permeable supports and place them in empty wells.
2. Wash the cells by adding HBSS to the apical side (0.5 mL) and to the basolateral side (1.5 mL).
3. Remove the HBSS from the permeable supports and fix the cells by adding 250 µL 3% paraformaldehyde/PBS to the apical side of each monolayer for 2 min at room temperature.
4. Remove the paraformaldehyde solution and wash 2×10 min in 500 µL PBS.
5. Remove the PBS and wash the cells in 500 µL 0.1% Triton X-100 in PBS on an ELISA plate shaker at 60 rpm for 1 min.
6. Repeat the washing step for 10 min.
7. Remove the Triton X-100 in PBS and incubate with 250 µL rhodamine–phalloidin 1:150 in PBS for 30 min.
8. Remove the rhodamine–phalloidin solution and wash in 500 µL PBS for 60 s.
9. Repeat the washing step for 2×10 min.
10. Wash the cells once in 50% glycerol in PBS, and carefully cut out the monolayer and supporting filter membrane from the cell culture insert with a fine-pointed scalpel.
11. Mount on a microscope slide in 50% glycerol in PBS under a cover glass.
12. Examine the monolayer in a fluorescence microscope.
13. Preferably, the examination should be carried out immediately after the staining procedure. If this is not possible, the monolayers may be kept for up to 24 h at 4°C in the dark.

3.2.4. Assessment of Membrane Integrity Using ZO-1 Antibody

Antibodies raised against the tight-junction protein ZO-1 provide a more specific tool to study the tight junctions of an epithelial cell monolayer. ZO-1 antibodies are available as a rabbit polyclonal antibody (Zymed, cat. no. 61-7300) and a mouse monoclonal antibody (Zymed, cat. no. 33-9100)

This protocol can also be used to stain for other tight junction associated proteins such as occludin. Occludin antibodies are available as a polyclonal antibody (Zymed, cat. no. 71-1500) and a mouse monoclonal antibody (Zymed, cat. no. 33-1500).

1. Perform **Subheading 3.2.3., steps 1–6.**
2. Remove the Triton X-100 in PBS. Incubate with 150 µL anti-ZO-1 1:1000 in 0.2% Triton X-100 in PBS for 30 min.
3. Remove the antibody solution and wash in 500 µL PBS for 60 s.
4. Repeat the washing step for 2 × 10 min.
5. Incubate with 150 µL FITC anti-rabbit Ig, diluted 1:100 in PBS in the dark for 30 min.
6. Remove the antibody solution.
7. Wash in PBS for 30 s.
8. Wash in PBS 2 × 10 min.
9. Wash the cells once in 50% glycerol in PBS solution and carefully cut out the monolayer and supporting filter membrane from the cell culture insert with a fine-pointed scalpel.
10. Mount on a microscope slide in 50% glycerol in PBS under a cover glass.
11. Examine the monolayer in a fluorescence microscope.
12. Preferably, the examination should be carried out immediately after the staining procedure. If this is not possible, the monolayers may be kept for up to 24 h at 4°C in the dark.

3.2.5. Extraction of RNA and Protein from Epithelial Cells Grown on Permeable Supports

During the initial characterization of an epithelial cell line, it may be desirable to study the expression of selected markers in the filter-grown cell monolayers. Since the extraction of RNA and proteins from filter-grown cells may be somewhat tricky, we present a protocol for this extraction below. The extract may then be used for assessment by conventional molecular biological techniques such as reverse-transcription polymerase chain reaction (RT-PCR) and Western blot.

1. Wash the cell monolayers (*see* **Note 14**) in HBSS and cut them out from the cell culture insert using a fine-pointed scalpel.
2. Place the filters in a microcentrifuge vial (*see* **Notes 15** and **16**), freeze immediately in liquid N_2, and store at –80°C until needed.

3. Total RNA from Caco-2 cell filters can be successfully isolated (*see* **Notes 17** and **18**) using the RNeasy minikit, whereas proteins are extracted as described below.
4. For protein extraction, apply 600 µL lysis buffer for protein extraction to the microcentrifuge vial containing the Caco-2 cell filters.
5. Ensure that the filters are completely submerged in the lysis buffer, and mix thoroughly in order to flush the filters with lysis buffer.
6. Centrifuge briefly, to deposit the extract in the vial.
7. Homogenize and shear the extract for 15 s, using a tissue homogenizer (*see* **Note 19**).
8. Transfer the extract to a new vial and measure the protein concentration (*see* **Note 20**).
9. Store the extract at –80°C pending Western blot analysis.

3.3. Drug Transport Studies

Transport processes across absorptive epithelia are mediated through one or several of the following routes: passive transcellular, paracellular, active transcellular (transporter-mediated), or transcytosis (**Fig. 2**).

In this section, we present a method for studying passive transport. In addition, we present a standard protocol for the studies of active transport. There are some important issues to consider prior to carrying out drug transport experiments:

1. pH. In our laboratory, we perform the transport experiments at pH 7.4 in both the apical and the basolateral chambers, unless we want to study the influence of a proton gradient (*see* **Subheading 3.3.2.**). An alternative may be to perform the transport experiments at an apical pH of 6.0–6.5 (which corresponds to the small intestinal microclimate in vivo) and a basolateral pH of 7.4.
2. The solubility of the drug. Many drugs are poorly soluble in physiological buffers, such as HBSS. For drug transport experiments in Caco-2 cells, a 0.1–1 mM solution of a rapidly transported drug, and a 5–10 mM solution of a slowly transported drug, should preferably be used to allow for easy detection of the transported amount by conventional high-pressure liquid chromatography (HPLC) (with UV-detection). It may be necessary to dissolve a hydrophobic drug in a co-solvent prior to dilution in the buffer. The following concentrations of co-solvents can be used without affecting the integrity of Caco-2 cell monolayers: 0.1% (v/v) dimethyl sulfoxide (DMSO) or 1% (v/v) ethanol.
3. Adsorption onto the plastic surface. Solubility problems are generally not an issue when radiolabeled drugs are used, since they can be used in very low molar concentrations (in less than micromolar). However, it is recommended that at least 0.1 mM of the corresponding unlabeled drug is added to the radioactive drug solution in order to avoid nonspecific adsorption onto the plastic surface. The excess of unlabeled drug is added to saturate the nonspecific adsorption sites of the plastic surfaces. Adsorption may be detected by calculating the mass balance of the drug after the transport experiment.

4. The time interval between sampling. The transport experiment must be designed so that the experiment is completed well before the drug concentration in the receiver chamber has reached the equilibrium concentration of the system or before almost all the amount of drug has been removed by the samplings. The difference between donor and receiver concentration should not fall below 10% of the initial difference between donor and receiver concentrations. With a thorough error analysis and a careful consideration about the error tolerance of the experiment, these limits can be extended. The time it takes to reach these critical values depends on the transport rate (permeability coefficient) of the drugs, but can be regulated by the amount of sample and the sampling frequency. Since the transport rates of different drugs in Caco-2 can differ by a factor of more than 10,000, the interval between sampling will vary from a few minutes for rapidly transported drugs (such as lipophilic drugs) to 1 h for slowly transported drugs (such as hydrophilic peptides). Educated guesses of the optimal time interval are based on the physicochemical properties of the drug (such as its lipophilicity or the number of hydrogen bonding atoms) or on preliminary experiments. An estimate of, for example, the lipophilicity of the drug can be obtained by computer calculations (for example at: http://www.daylight.com/).

5. Methods of analysis. Transport experiments have traditionally been carried out under sink conditions. This has been done in order to allow the investigator to apply slightly simpler mathematics in the analysis. The definition of sink conditions is that the concentration in the receiver chamber must never exceed 10% of the concentration in the donor chamber. The use of sink condition analysis, therefore, further restricts the choice of time interval and/or sampling volumes in the design of the drug transport experiment. In the theoretical section below, we present mathematical treatments both of the traditional approach that requires sink conditions (*see* **Subheadings 3.4.2.** and **3.4.3.**) and of the novel and more general approach, which is not restricted to sink conditions (*see* **Subheadings 3.4.4.–3.4.8.**).

6. The toxicity of the drug. There are several commercial kits available for studying the toxicity of a compound (for example, measurements of intracellular dehydrogenase activity with the MTT-assay [3-(4,5-dimethylthiazol-2-yl)-2,5,-diphenyl tetrazolium bromide] [Sigma] or membrane permeability by following lactic dehydrogenase [LDH] leakage [Boehringer Mannheim] from the cells). In our laboratory, we routinely use the ^{14}C-mannitol transport experiment as a tool to assess the effect of drugs or pharmaceutical additives on epithelial integrity. This is because we have found that changes in ^{14}C-mannitol permeability are a more sensitive indicator of initial drug toxicity than general toxicity tests such as the MTT and LDH assays. An integrity test may be carried out by comparing the flux of mannitol across the monolayers in the presence and the absence of a drug or additive. We have observed that if the mannitol flux is higher in the presence of the added compound than it is in the control monolayers, it is likely that the compound expresses a dose-dependent toxicity to the cells or that the compound affects in some other way the barrier properties of the cell monolayer. If a compound is toxic to the cells, the investigator should try to reduce the concentration of the compound until the mannitol permeability is comparable to its value in the control monolayers.

3.3.1. Passive Drug Transport

Passive transport is driven by the concentration gradient in the monolayer, i.e., the concentration difference between the donor chamber and the receiver chamber. It typically displays nonsaturable kinetics, cannot be inhibited by structural analogues, and does not require metabolic energy. The following experiments are routinely performed in our laboratory to investigate whether the transport is passive: (*i*) determination of the permeability coefficient of the drug in the apical to basolateral direction and the basolateral to apical direction. The permeability coefficient should be independent of transport direction; and (*ii*) determination of the permeability coefficient of the drug over a concentration interval (for example 10^{-6}–10^{-3} mmol/L). The permeability coefficient should be independent of concentration.

Below, we present a protocol for the determination of Caco-2 permeability to a drug that is absorbed by passive transport.

1. Prepare the drug solution by dissolving (*see* **Note 21**) desired amount of the drug in HBSS. Make sure that the drug is completely dissolved. Sterile filter the solution through a 0.22-μm filter fitted to a plastic syringe into a test tube (*see* **Note 22**). If a radiolabeled drug is used, pipet the required amount of drug into a test tube and allow the solvent to evaporate (*see* **Note 23**) prior to adding the unlabeled filtered drug. Preheat the solution in a water bath at 37°C.
2. Preheat the required amount of HBSS to 37°C.
3. Remove the cell culture medium from 3–6 permeable supports and place them in empty wells. Add HBSS preheated to 37°C to the apical side (0.5 mL) and to the basolateral side (1.5 mL). Pre-incubate the monolayers for 15–30 min (*see* **Note 7**).
4. Transfer the inserts to new wells. Add 0.4 mL of drug solution to the apical chambers and 1.2 mL HBSS to the basolateral chambers. Sample 10–50 μL from the apical chamber at t = 0 for determination of the initial donor concentration of each permeable support (*see* **Note 11**).
5. Place the inserts in the incubator (37°C) on the plate shaker set to 100–500 rpm (*see* **Note 12**).
6. Sample 200–800 μL (*see* **Note 24**) from the basolateral chambers after 3–60 min (*see* **Note 25**). Replace each sampled volume with fresh preheated HBSS.
7. Repeat step 6 at least 4 times to achieve statistically reliable results (*see* **Note 13**).
8. Immediately after the final sampling, take 10–50 μL from the apical chamber to determine the final donor concentration of each permeable support (*see* **Note 11**).
9. Determine the concentrations of the samples by HPLC or determine the radioactivity of the samples in a liquid scintillation counter.
10. Calculate the permeability coefficient of the drug across the cell monolayers (*see* **Subheading 3.4.**).

The cumulative fraction transported (*see* **Subheading 3.4.2.**) of a passively transported drug across Caco-2 cell monolayers should increase linearly with

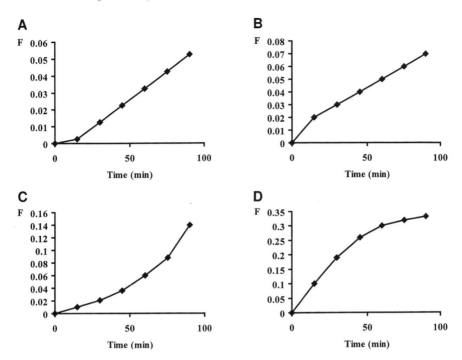

Fig. 3. Schematic representation of different deviations from linearity for "cumulative fraction transported" (F) in drug transport experiments in epithelial cell monolayers (*see* text for details).

time as long as the experiment is performed under sink conditions. However, deviations from this situation may sometimes be observed (**Fig. 3**). Here we list 4 situations that may be observed where the transport is non-linear, and we give plausible explanations of the observed phenomena: (*i*) less drug is transported during the first sampling interval. This may be caused by poor temperature control at the beginning of the experiment, or by the fact that partitioning of the drug into the cell monolayer is the rate-limiting step (**Fig. 3A**); (*ii*) more drug is transported during the first sampling interval. This is sometimes observed when the transport of radiolabeled drugs is studied. The reason may be that radiolabeled low molecular weight impurities (such as ^{3}H-water) are present in the drug solution and are transported at a higher rate than the drug. Another reason may be that the cell monolayer is affected by a too harsh application of the drug solution (**Fig. 3B**); (*iii*) the transport rate increases with time. The reason for this phenomenon is decreased integrity of the cell monolayer over time, caused, for example, by the drug being toxic to the cells, or the reason may be decreased viability of the cell monolayer during the transport experiment due to contamination. Poor temperature control, resulting in an increase in temperature over time, may also lead to this observation (**Fig. 3C**); and (*iv*) the transport rate decreases with time. The most likely explanation of this phenomenon is that the sink condition is significantly exceeded, resulting in a more shallow concentration gradient between the donor and receiver chamber. However, as described in the theoretical section (*see* **Subheading 3.4.4.–3.4.8.**), this problem can be overcome by using a more general equation for the calculation of permeability that does not require sink conditions (**Fig. 3D**).

3.3.2. Active Transport

In contrast to passive transport, active transport occurs in the absence of an external driving force (concentration gradient). Active transport processes are mediated by transporter proteins located in the apical and/or in the basolateral cell membranes. An active transport process displays saturation kinetics, is substrate-specific, functions against a concentration gradient, and is energy-dependent. Characterization of an active transport process in epithelial cell monolayers is complicated due to several factors, including: (*i*) the process may involve more than one transporter situated in either or both of the apical and basolateral membranes. In addition, passive transcellular or paracellular diffusion always occurs simultaneously with the active process; (*ii*) the determination of the cytosolic concentration of drug may be experimentally demanding; and (*iii*) specific inhibitors of transporter-mediated transport processes are not always available. Well-differentiated epithelial cell monolayers such as Caco-2 are, therefore, mainly used to study the "apparent" contribution of transport proteins to the transport of various compounds. This may still be useful, since the presence of several transporters and efflux systems allows their identification, and since studies in differentiated epithelial cell monolayers may reflect the in vivo situation, provided that the epithelial cell line expresses the transporter(s) of interest at a physiologically relevant level. However, once an apparent transport mechanism has been identified, it should preferably be followed up in an epithelial expression system with low inherent expression of transporters or efflux systems, such as LLC PK$_1$ or MDCK cells (*see* **Table 1**).

The functional characterization of active transport can be carried out by several methods. Here we present some of the more straightforward experiments:

1. Determination of the permeability coefficient of the drug in the apical to basolateral direction and in the basolateral to apical direction. The permeability coefficient should depend on transport direction.
2. Determination of the permeability coefficient of the drug over a concentration interval (such as 10^{-6}–10^{-3} mM). The permeability coefficient should be saturable, i.e., the transport rate should depend on concentration.
3. Determination of the permeability coefficient of the drug in the presence of and absence of inhibitors to transport proteins. Known substrates for the transport

protein or structural analogues to the drug of interest can be used as competitive inhibitors.

4. Determination of the permeability coefficient of the drug at low temperature (4°C). The low temperature should inhibit significantly any active energy-dependent transport processes.

5. pH-dependence. Some transporters are proton-coupled and require a slightly acid pH for activity. For instance, to study the function of PepT1, a proton-coupled peptide transporter, an acid pH of around 6.0 must be used apically to obtain significant co-transport.

Apart from the experiments above, additional experiments can be performed such as inhibition of Na^+/K^+-ATPase by replacing sodium with choline and by the addition of oubain. Another experiment that decreases active transport is the inhibition of the cellular metabolism by adding sodium azide and 2-deoxyglucose. However, these methods are not always suitable, since for example the inhibition of Na^+/K^+-ATPase may, in our experience, give a rather small inhibition of the transport, and the metabolic inhibition has a time-dependent effect on the monolayer integrity.

A good availability of specific inhibitors and substrates would significantly facilitate the studies of active transport in epithelial cell monolayers. Unfortunately, it is relatively unusual that an inhibitor is specific to one transport protein. Rather, as an increasing number of members of various transporter and efflux protein families are being discovered, several inhibitors that previously were considered to be specific have been found to interact with several family members (51). The picture is becoming even more complex in the case of the well-studied efflux protein P-glycoprotein (P-gp), since there is also a substrate overlap between P-gp and the drug-metabolizing enzyme cytochrome P-450 3A4 (and 3A5) (52). Since this research field is currently undergoing rapid development, which will be further accelerated by the recent publications of the human genome (53,54), we do not find it meaningful to give recommendations about more or less specific inhibitors and substrates for the various transport and efflux systems. Instead, we direct the reader to the most recent literature treating the transport system of interest. However, we note that traditional substrates and inhibitors, such as glycylsarcosine for the peptide transporter PepT1 and verapamil for the efflux protein P-gp (and other efflux proteins), are generally available in radiolabeled form, which facilitates the analysis of inhibition experiments.

Below, we present a protocol that we use for the initial investigation of active transport in Caco-2 cell monolayers. We recommend that the radiolabeled drug is added at a low but defined concentration (such as 1 μM) in order not to saturate the transporter (note that it is important to check the adsorption to the plastic surfaces when such low concentrations are used).

1. Perform all the steps in **Subheading 3.3.1.**
2. Perform all the steps in **Subheading 3.3.1.**, but add the drug to the basolateral chamber instead.
3. Withdraw the samples (50–100 µL) from the apical receiving chamber and replace the sampled volume in the apical chamber with fresh HBSS at regular time intervals.
4. Calculate the permeability coefficient of the drug across the cell monolayers (*see* **Subheading 3.4.**).
5. If a clear difference between the flux rates in the two directions is observed, repeat the experiment, but add unlabeled drug (at concentrations between, for example, 10^{-6}–10^{-3} M) to investigate if the difference in flux rate is concentration-dependent (*see* **Note 26**).
6. If an inhibitor is available for the transporter of interest, it should be added both to the apical and to the basolateral chamber to keep the inhibitor concentration at a constant level during the experiment (*see* **Note 27**).
7. If no clear difference is observed, the transport may be passive, or alternatively, the expression and/or function of the transporter may not be optimal under the experimental conditions. In this case, it may be wise to study if the transporter depends on, for example, the presence of a proton gradient. A proton gradient is accomplished by using HBSS, pH 6.0, on the apical side and HBSS, pH 7.4, on the basolateral side.

3.4. Calculations

Studies of passive drug permeability in Caco-2 cells are currently performed in a large number of academic and commercial laboratories on a daily basis. As outlined above (*see* **Subheading 3.3.**), the experiments are generally performed under sink conditions in order to avoid bias by back-diffusion of significant amounts of compound from the receiver chamber. As we shall see, the requirement for sink conditions is not absolute, and it is possible to obtain reliable permeability coefficients also under non-sink conditions by applying a more general mathematical expression *(55)*. This more general approach has the advantage of being less dependent on the design of the experiment, but perhaps the disadvantage of being less appealing, since a more complex mathematical expression is used.

3.4.1. Physical Background and Derivation of Fundamental Equations

The passive drug permeability experiments described in **Subheading 3.3.1.** involve the study of the barrier properties of epithelial cell monolayer with respect to different drugs. In our case, the barrier separates a donor solution from a receiver solution.

The diffusive flow of substance in a medium, such as an epithelial barrier, depends on the concentration gradient of the substance and the diffusion coefficient of the substance in the medium. The concentration profile and the concentration gradient in the barrier will depend on its morphology and chemical composition. Epithelial barriers have a rather complicated morphology and are not chemically homogeneous. To obtain a qualitative picture of the features controlling the barrier properties and what the measures reflect we, however, consider the barrier as a chemically homogeneous slab. The experimentally determined barrier measures shall thus be seen as slab-shaped and homogeneous barrier equivalents.

With these simplifications, the relation between the flow and the concentration profile in the barrier is expressed by Fick's first law *(56)*:

$$J = D \times [dC(x)]/dx \qquad \text{[Eq. 1]}$$

where J is the flow in the direction from the donor side of the barrier, x is the distance from the donor compartment, and $C(x)$ is the concentration in the barrier at the coordinate x in the barrier.

If we denote the receiver concentration by C_R and the donor concentration by C_D, the concentration in the barrier will equal $K \times C_D$ at the donor side and $K \times C_R$ at the receiver side, where K is the distribution coefficient between the medium in the barrier and the aqueous donor and receiver solutions. The gradient (dC/dx) then equals $K \times (C_R-C_D)/h$, where h is the thickness of the barrier. Further, the flow must equal the rate of appearance of substance on the receiver side, divided by the cross-sectional area of the barrier (A). Thus:

$$J = \frac{dM_R}{dt} \times \frac{1}{A} = -D \times \frac{dC}{dx} = -K \times D \times \frac{C_R - C_D}{h} \Rightarrow$$
$$\frac{dM_R(t)}{dt} = \frac{K \times D}{h} \times A \times (C_D - C_R) \qquad \text{[Eq. 2]}$$

where M_R is the amount of substance in receiver chamber. The quantity $K \times D/h$ is conventionally called permeability coefficient (P) and reflects the rate by with a substance passes the barrier (**Fig. 4**). Since both K and D depend on the chemical properties of the substance and the barrier, the permeability coefficient will, in addition to the thickness of the barrier, also be dependent on the chemical properties of the substance and the barrier.

In most types of drug transport experiments, and specifically in the type of transport experiment treated here, C_D, C_R, and M_R will change with time. Emphasizing this time dependence and introducing the permeability coefficient, **Eq. 2** can be written:

$$\frac{dM_R(t)}{dt} = P \times A \times [C_D(t) - C_R(t)] \qquad \text{[Eq. 3]}$$

which is a differential equation with the variables $C_D(t)$, $C_R(t)$ and $M_R(t)$.

Depending on the experimental conditions, different treatment of **Eq. 3** can be applied in the analysis to determine the permeability coefficient (*see* below).

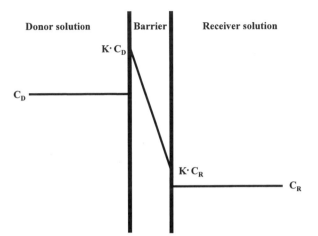

Fig. 4. Schematic representation of the concentration profile in the donor solution–barrier–receiver solution system. The jumps in the interfaces between the barrier and the aqueous phases are due to the distribution coefficient between the barrier and the aqueous phase. The constancy of the concentration profiles in the donor and receiver solutions, respectively, are due to the stirring of the solutions.

3.4.2. Analysis Approximating the Receiver Concentration as Zero (Sink Conditions)

When the transport rate is low, neither the donor nor the receiver concentration will change significantly with time. Both the donor and receiver concentrations can, under these circumstances, be approximated as being constant on the right side of **Eq. 3**. This is the conventional and the simplest possible treatment of **Eq. 3**. In the analysis, the concentration levels are set to the initial concentrations. The receiver concentration is thus set to zero.

Since the receiver concentration is regarded as zero, the term sink conditions is generally used for these types of experiments. Conventionally, a maximum receiver concentration less than 10% of the donor concentration is accepted, if the experiment is to be regarded as a sink condition experiment.

With these approximations, **Eq. 3** becomes:

$$\frac{dM_R(t)}{dt} = P \times A \times C_{D0} \Rightarrow \frac{dM_R(t)}{dt} \times \frac{1}{A \times C_{D0}} = P \qquad \text{[Eq. 4]}$$

Integrating gives (*57*):

$$\frac{M_R(t)}{C_{D0}} = P \times A \times t + const \qquad \text{[Eq. 5]}$$

Since M_R is initially zero (at time zero), the constant term also is zero and vanishes.

The analysis is easily improved by considering the change of C_D. The donor concentration $[C_D(t_i)]$ can be calculated at each sample occasion (i) from the donor concentration at the previous occasion $[C_D(t_{i-1})]$ and the amount that has entered the receiver chamber during that time interval.

$$C_D(t) = C_D(t_{i-1}) - \frac{[C_R(t) - f \times C_R(t_{i-1})] \times V_R}{V_D} \qquad \text{[Eq. 6]}$$

where V_R is the receiver chamber volume, V_D is the donor chamber volume, $f = 1 - V_S/V_R$ is the sample replacement dilution factor, and V_S is the sample volume. For each time interval between two samplings, C_D is regarded as constant with a value equal to the average of the C_D determined of the beginning and of the end of the interval. Integration of **Eq. 4** then gives:

$$\frac{1}{A} \times \sum_{k=1}^{i} \frac{M_{Rk}}{[C_D(t_{k-1}) + C_D(t_k)]/2} = \frac{1}{A} \times \sum_{k=1}^{i} \frac{[C_R(t_k) - f \times C_R(t_{k-1})] \times V_R}{[C_D(t_{k-1}) + C_D(t_k)]/2} = P \times t_i \qquad \text{[Eq. 7]}$$

where t_i is the time point for the sampling occasion i, t_k is the time point for the sampling occasion k, M_{Rk} is the amount that has passed the barrier during interval k sample occasion i and $C_R(t_k)$ is the measured concentration at sample occasion k. P is then determined from the slope obtained from the linear curve-fit of **Eq. 7**. Linear curve-fit routines are provided in Excel with the functions Slope and Intercept (**Figs. 5** and **6**).

The left and middle part of **Eq. 7** can be regarded as the "weighted normalized cumulative amount of transported drug". The amount transported in each interval has been weighted with the inverse average driving force (donor concentrations) for the intervals, respectively. The normalization is carried out by dividing by the epithelial cross-sectional area of the cell monolayer. For simplicity, the not totally correct term "cumulative fraction transported" is commonly used in the literature, and also used in this chapter for the somewhat inconvenient expression "weighted normalized cumulative amount of transported drug".

3.4.3. Determination of Permeability Coefficients Using Sink Conditions Analysis

1. Determine the receiver concentrations at different time points according to **Subheading 3.3.1.**
2. Calculate C_D according to **Eq. 6**.
3. Check that the ratio C_R/C_D is less than 0.1 at each sampling point used in the analysis (sink conditions).
4. Calculate the cumulative fraction transported according to the middle part of **Eq. 7** for each sample occasion.
5. Determine P by linear curve-fit of **Eq. 7** to values of cumulative fraction absorbed.

	A	B	C	D	E	F	G	H	I
1	A (cm²)		t (s)	Cr exp (uM)	Cr rel	cumulative fraction transported (cm)	theor	diff^2 Cr	Cd (uM)
2					=D2/I2	=0	=P*C2+B$13	=(G2-F2)^2	=Cd0
3	Vd (cm³)				=D3/I3	=(D3-D2*f)/(I3+I2)*2*Vr/A+F2	=P*C3+B$13	=(G3-F3)^2	=I2-(D3-D2*f)*Vr/Vd
4	Vr (cm³)				=D4/I4	=(D4-D3*f)/(I4+I3)*2*Vr/A+F3	=P*C4+B$13	=(G4-F4)^2	=I3-(D4-D3*f)*Vr/Vd
5	Vs (cm³)				=D5/I5	=(D5-D4*f)/(I5+I4)*2*Vr/A+F4	=P*C5+B$13	=(G5-F5)^2	=I4-(D5-D4*f)*Vr/Vd
6	f	=1-Vs/Vr			=D6/I6	=(D6-D5*f)/(I6+I5)*2*Vr/A+F5	=P*C6+B$13	=(G6-F6)^2	=I5-(D6-D5*f)*Vr/Vd
7					=D7/I7	=(D7-D6*f)/(I7+I6)*2*Vr/A+F6	=P*C7+B$13	=(G7-F7)^2	=I6-(D7-D6*f)*Vr/Vd
8	Cd0 (uM)				=D8/I8	=(D8-D7*f)/(I8+I7)*2*Vr/A+F7	=P*C8+B$13	=(G8-F8)^2	=I7-(D8-D7*f)*Vr/Vd
9									
10									
11									
12	P (cm/s)	=SLOPE(F2:F8,C2:C8)							
13	intercept	=INTERCEPT(F2:F8,C2:C8)							
14	SSE	=SUM(H2:H8)							
15									
16									
17									
18									

Fig. 5. An example of an Excel spreadsheet with formulas for permeability coefficient determination from six determined receiver concentrations under sink condition. Values for cross sectional area (A), donor and receiver solution volumes (Vd, Vr), the sample volume (Vs), and initial donor concentration (Cd0) must be inserted in the B column on the rows as indicated by the A column. The experimentally determined concentrations and corresponding sample time points shall be inserted in the D and C columns, respectively. The determined permeability coefficient (P) is reported in cell B12. Since the formulas in cell B6, and the F, G, and I columns refer to the names of the variables and not to the cell designation of the cells in the B column, the referred cells in that column must be given the names of the variables. Therefore, cell B1 must be given the name A, cell B3 the name Vd, cell B4 the name Vr, cell B5 the name Vs, cell B6 the name f, cell B8 the name Cd0, and cell B12 the name P.

The E column contains values of the ratio between the receiver and donor concentrations at each sampling occasion and shall be used to check that sink condition is not exceeded. The F column contains values of the cumulative fraction of transported drug calculated from the experimentally determined receiver concentration (D column). The G column contains values of the theoretical cumulative fraction of transported drug according to the linear curve fit. The H column contains values of the squared difference between experimentally and theoretically determined cumulative fraction of transported drug. The SSE is reported in cell B14. The I column contains values of the donor concentration calculated from the experimentally determined receiver concentration (D column).

3.4.4. Analysis Regarding the Continuous Change of the Concentrations (Non-Sink Conditions)

To solve the differential **Eq. 3** considering the continuous change of the donor and receiver concentrations, the equation must be expressed in a single variable. In this case, it is practical to express the equation in $C_R(t)$. $M_R(t)$ and $C_D(t)$ are, therefore, to be expressed in $C_R(t)$.

	A	B	C	D	E	F	G	H	I
1	A (cm²)	1.131	t (s)	Cr exp (uM)	Cr rel	cumulative fraction transported (cm)	theor	diff^2 Cr	Cd (uM)
2			0	0.0	0.000	0.0000	0.0026	6.945E-06	496.600
3	Vd (cm³)	0.400	600	22.1	0.051	0.0506	0.0470	1.263E-05	430.300
4	Vr (cm³)	1.200	1200	26.7	0.070	0.0914	0.0914	1.308E-09	383.350
5	Vs (cm³)	0.6	1800	28.6	0.085	0.1363	0.1359	1.975E-07	337.600
6	f	0.500	2400	27.2	0.091	0.1793	0.1803	9.104E-07	298.900
7			3000	25.3	0.096	0.2234	0.2247	1.532E-06	263.800
8	Cd0 (uM)	496.600	3600	23.5	0.102	0.2699	0.2691	7.481E-07	231.250
9									
10					0.3000				
11					0.2500				
12	P (cm/s)	7.401E-05			0.2000		♦ cumulative fraction		
13	intercept	0.003			0.1500		transported (cm)		
14	SSE	2.297E-05			0.1000		— — — theor		
15					0.0500				
16					0.0000				
17					0	1000	2000	3000	4000
18									

Fig. 6. The figure shows the same Excel spreadsheet as in **Fig. 5**, after the experimental data has been inserted and the permeability coefficient has been determined. The experimental data is the same as in **Fig. 8**. The experimentally and theoretically determined cumulative fraction of transported drug vs the time has been plotted in a graph that has been added to the spreadsheet. The graph can be an aid to get an idea about the deviations between experimental and theoretical data and the linearity of the cumulative fraction transported.

The amount of drug on the donor side equals the difference between the total amount in the system (M_{tot}) and the amount in the receiver chamber. $C_D(t)$ is then obtained by simply dividing the donor side amount with the donor solution volume (V_D), i.e.:

$$C_D(t) = \frac{M_{tot} - C_R(t) \times V_R}{V_D} \qquad [\text{Eq. 8}]$$

further:

$$\frac{dM_R(t)}{dt} = \frac{dC_R(t)}{dt} \times V_R \qquad [\text{Eq. 9}]$$

Eqs. **3**, **8**, and **9** then give:

$$\frac{dC_R(t)}{dt} = \frac{P \times A}{V_R} \times \left(\frac{M_{tot}}{V_D} - C_R(t) \times \frac{V_R + V_D}{V_D} \right) \qquad [\text{Eq. 10}]$$

which has the solution (55,58):

$$C_R(t) = \left(\frac{M_{tot}}{V_D + V_R} \right) + \left(C_{R0} - \frac{M_{tot}}{V_D + V_R} \right) \times e^{-P \times A \times \left(\frac{1}{V_R} + \frac{1}{V_D} \right) \times t} \qquad [\text{Eq. 11}]$$

where the initial condition $C_R(0) = C_{R0}$ has been considered.

	A	B	C	D	E	F	G
1	A (cm²)			t (s)	Cr exp (uM)	Cr theor (uM)	diff^2 Cr	Mtot (nmol)
2						=Cr0	=(D2-E2)^2	
3	Vd (cm³)					=G3/(Vr+Vd)+(Cr0-G3/(Vr+Vd))*EXP(-A*P*(1/Vd+1/Vr)*C3)	=(D3-E3)^2	=Cr0*Vr+Cd0*Vd
4	Vr (cm³)					=G4/(Vr+Vd)+(E3*f-G4/(Vr+Vd))*EXP(-A*P*(1/Vd+1/Vr)*(C4-C3))	=(D4-E4)^2	=G3-Vs*E3
5	Vs (cm³)					=G5/(Vr+Vd)+(E4*f-G5/(Vr+Vd))*EXP(-A*P*(1/Vd+1/Vr)*(C5-C4))	=(D5-E5)^2	=G4-Vs*E4
6	f	=1-Vs/Vr				=G6/(Vr+Vd)+(E5*f-G6/(Vr+Vd))*EXP(-A*P*(1/Vd+1/Vr)*(C6-C5))	=(D6-E6)^2	=G5-Vs*E5
7						=G7/(Vr+Vd)+(E6*f-G7/(Vr+Vd))*EXP(-A*P*(1/Vd+1/Vr)*(C7-C6))	=(D7-E7)^2	=G6-Vs*E6
8	Cd0 (uM)					=G8/(Vr+Vd)+(E7*f-G8/(Vr+Vd))*EXP(-A*P*(1/Vd+1/Vr)*(C8-C7))	=(D8-E8)^2	=G7-Vs*E7
9	Cr0 (uM)							
10								
11								
12	P (cm/s)							
13								
14	SSE	=SUM(F2:F8)						
15								
16								
17								
18								

Fig. 7. An example of an Excel spreadsheet with formulas for permeability coefficient determination from six determined receiver concentrations under non-sink condition. Values for cross sectional area (A), donor and receiver solution volumes (Vd, Vr), the sample volume (Vs), and initial donor and receiver concentrations (Cd0, Cr0) must be inserted in the B column on the rows as indicated by the A column. The experimentally determined concentrations and corresponding sample time points shall be inserted in the D and C columns, respectively.

The initial guess of permeability coefficient (P) shall be inserted in cell B12. The curve fit routine will change this value and report the finally determined P in the same cell.

Since the formulas in cell B6 and the F, G, and I columns refer to the names of the variables and not the cell designation of the cells in the B column, the referred cells in that column must be given the names of the variables. Therefore cell B 1 must be given the name A, cell B3 the name Vd, cell B4 the name Vr, cell B5 the name Vs, cell B6 the name f, cell B8 the name Cd0, cell B9 the name Cr0, and cell B12 the name P.

The E column contains values of the theoretical determined receiver concentrations at each sampling occasion. The F column contains values of the squared difference between experimentally and theoretically determined receiver concentration. The SSE is reported in cell B14. The G column contains values of the total amount of substance in the chamber system calculated from the experimentally determined receiver concentration (D column).

For the curve fit procedure Solver, cell B14 shall be indicated as the target cell that is to be minimized, and cell B 12 shall be indicated as the cell that shall be changed in order to minimize cell B14. The constraint $P >= 0$ should be added, in order reduce the risk of finding a false solution.

Eq. 11 describes the concentration development with time in the receiver chamber for an undisturbed system. Since substance is removed and the receiver concentration is instantaneously diluted on every sampling occasion, **Eq. 11** does not strictly hold.

Nevertheless, the equation holds within each sample interval. With the knowledge of initial receiver concentrations and total amount of drug for each interval, the final receiver concentrations of each interval can be determined. The time in this case is to be counted from the beginning of each interval rather than from the onset of the experiment.

The initial receiver concentration for each interval is calculated according to:

$$C_{R0,i} = C_{R,i-1}(t_{end,i-1}) \cdot f = C_{R,i-1}(t_{end,i-1}) \times (V_R - V_S)/V_R \qquad \text{[Eq. 12]}$$

where $C_{R0,i}$ is the initial receiver concentration of interval i, $C_{R,i-1}(t_{end,i-1})$ is the receiver concentration at the end of the previous interval, and $t_{end,i-1}$ is the elapsed time from the beginning of the previous interval to the end of that interval.

The total amount of drug for each interval is calculated from:

$$M_{tot,i} = M_{tot,i-1} - M_{samp,i-1} = M_{tot,i-1} - C_{R,i-1}(t_{end,i-1}) \times V_S \qquad \text{[Eq. 13]}$$

where $M_{tot,i}$ is the amount of drug in the system during interval i, $M_{samp,i-1}$ is the amount of drug in sample, and $M_{tot,i-1}$ is the amount of drug in the system during the previous interval.

For the first interval, the initial receiver concentration of the experiment is used for C_{R0} (which in general is zero), and total amount of drug used in the experiment for M_{tot} (which for zero C_{R0} equals $C_{D0} \cdot V_D$).

The theoretical final concentration values of the intervals are used in a non-linear curve-fit to the experimental concentrations to determine P. The curve-fitting is carried out by minimizing the sum of squared residuals (SSE), where:

$$SSE = \Sigma[C_{R,i,obs} - C_{R,i}(t_{end,i})]^2 \qquad \text{[Eq. 14]}$$

in which $C_{R,i,obs}$ is the observed receiver concentration at the end of interval i, and $C_{R,i}(t_{end,i})$ is the corresponding concentration calculated according to **Eq. 11** *(59)*. The Solver tool provided in Excel can be used to minimize SSE (**Figs. 7** and **8**).

3.4.5. Remarks About the Nonlinear Curve-Fitting

The theoretical C_R values will, according to **Eq. 11**, be dependent of the value of P. Thus, with different P, different theoretical concentration characteristics are generated. In the curve-fitting, the theoretical concentration characteristics that best corresponds to the experimental values, in the meaning of least SSE, is termed the fitted curve, and the corresponding P is termed the curve-fit determined permeability coefficient.

To make the search for this best value of P in the Solver tool; specify the target function (SSE) that is to be minimized and the variable (P) that is allowed to change in order to minimize SSE (**Fig. 9**).

The method also requires an initial guess of the P value. This is easily obtained in an intermediate step, where the experiment is analyzed as if sink

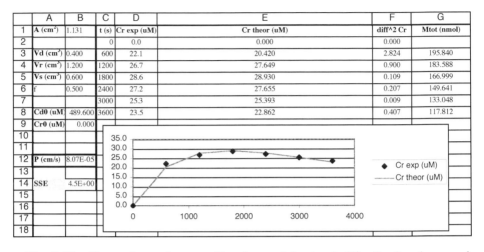

	A	B	C	D	E	F	G
1	A (cm²)	1.131	t (s)	Cr exp (uM)	Cr theor (uM)	diff^2 Cr	Mtot (nmol)
2			0	0.0	0.000	0.000	
3	Vd (cm³)	0.400	600	22.1	20.420	2.824	195.840
4	Vr (cm³)	1.200	1200	26.7	27.649	0.900	183.588
5	Vs (cm³)	0.600	1800	28.6	28.930	0.109	166.999
6	f	0.500	2400	27.2	27.655	0.207	149.641
7			3000	25.3	25.393	0.009	133.048
8	Cd0 (uM)	489.600	3600	23.5	22.862	0.407	117.812
9	Cr0 (uM)	0.000					
10							
11							
12	P (cm/s)	8.07E-05					
13							
14	SSE	4.5E+00					
15							
16							
17							
18							

Fig. 8. The figure shows the same Excel spreadsheet as in **Fig. 8**, after the experimental data has been inserted and the permeability has been determined. The experimental data is the same as in **Fig. 6**. The experimentally and theoretically determined receiver concentration vs the time has been plotted in a graph that has been added to the spreadsheet. The graph can be an aid to get an idea about the deviations between experimental and theoretical data.

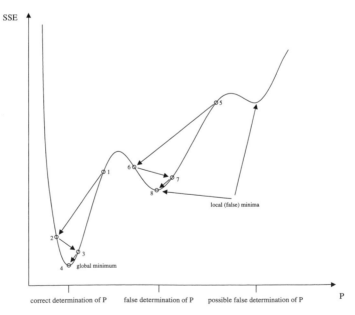

Fig. 9. A schematic plot of the *SSE* vs *P* characteristics. Points 1 to 4 show the search path from the initial *P* guess (point 1) to the correct *P* determination at the global minimum (point 4). Points 5 to 8 show the search path from another initial *P* guess (point 5), where the search has been trapped in a local (false) minimum.

conditions are appropriate. If more than one experiment is done with the same drug, the same initial guess can be used for all experiments with that drug.

There is, in principle, one risk with the use of numerical curve-fitting routines. The SSE function can have several false (local) minima in addition to the global minimum, and the routine could therefore find a false minimum rather than the global (**Fig. 9**). A visual inspection of the correspondence between the theoretical and experimental data in a graph should be sufficient to decide if the P that has been found corresponds to the global minimum or not. If a false minimum is found, the curve-fit must be repeated with a new initial guess of P. Under such circumstances, the curve-fitting is to be more of an art than a science, and there are several strategies as to how to proceed. Thus, it is cumbersome to propagate for one single method. As a suggestion, however, the initial guess for the next trial can be changed one or two orders of magnitude up or down from the previous initial guess *(59)*. However, in our experience, the problem of false minima hardly ever appears in the curve-fitting of **Eq. 11**.

3.4.6. Determination of Permeability Coefficient Using Non-Sink Conditions Analysis

1. Determine the receiver concentrations at different time points according to **Subheading 3.3.1.**
2. Find an initial approximation for P by making an intermediate sink condition determination of P for the studied drug.
3. Determine P by nonlinear curve-fitting of **Eq. 11** to experimentally determined values. Interval-specific values for initial concentration and total amount are used in the equation.

3.4.7. Recalculations of the Receiver Concentration for the Nonlinear Curve-Fit Determination of the Permeability Coefficient

1. Use the initial amount and the initial receiver concentration (in general zero) to determine the final receiver concentration for the first sample interval according to **Eq. 11**.
2. Determine the initial receiver concentration and the total amount for the next sample interval according to **Eqs. 12** and **13**.
3. Determine the final receiver concentration for that sample interval according to **Eq. 11**. Count the time from the beginning of the interval. Go to point 2 for the next interval.
4. Repeat points 2 and 3 until the last sample interval has been treated.
5. Use the final concentration values of the intervals obtained in point 3 for the nonlinear curve-fit determination of P.

3.4.8. Treatment of Initial Imperfections

As mentioned in **Subheading 3.3.1.**, imperfections in the experiment during a time interval in the beginning of the experiment may appear. These imperfections may cause deviations of the transport rate in that interval that does not correspond to the actual cell monolayer permeability. If this occurs, all measurements made in that interval should be excluded from the permeability determination. In the sink condition analysis, this is simply treated by doing the linear curve-fit to the remainder of the experimental values.

In the non-sink condition analysis, some recalculations must be made:

1. The initial receiver and donor concentrations become the receiver and donor concentrations just after the first sampling after the excluded interval, respectively. The initial receiver concentration (C_{R0new}) thus becomes:

$$(C_{R0new}) = C_R (t_{exc+1}) \times f \qquad \text{[Eq. 15]}$$

   where t_{exc+1} is the first sample time point after the excluded interval.
2. The initial donor concentration (C_{D0new}) must be calculated from the donor concentration at the onset of the experiment (C_{D0}), which is adjusted for the amount that has been transported to the receiver chamber, i.e.:

$$(C_{D0new}) = C_{D0} - \frac{C_R(t_{exc+1}) \times V_R + \sum_{i=1}^{N_{exc}} C_R(t_i) \times V_S}{V_D} \qquad \text{[Eq. 16]}$$

   where N_{exc} is the number of samples in the excluded interval, and the summation is carried out over all samples in the excluded interval.
3. Finally, the time must be counted from t_{exc+1}.

3.4.9. Comparison Between the Two Methods of Analysis

The non-sink condition analysis is more general and imposes less restriction on the experimental conditions than the analysis assuming sink conditions. For high permeability drugs, sink condition analysis requires short experimental times or frequent sampling. This could be undesirable if the aim is to study the system under a longer time, or if the sampling procedure disturbs the experiment. It is also more probable for non-sink condition analysis than for sink condition analysis, that the guesses of the optimal time interval (*see* **Subheading 3.3.**) is appropriate, and that the redesign of the experiment regarding sample intervals becomes unnecessary.

The non-sink analysis is based on the exact solution of the differential **Eq. 3**, while the sink condition approach is based on approximations (**Fig. 10**). Therefore, even for experiments that are run under sink conditions, non-sink condition analysis gives permeability coefficients in better accordance with the true permeability coefficients of the epithelial cell monolayer. The difference between the determination of the permeability coefficients according to the two methods is demonstrated by comparing the results in **Figs. 6** and **8**. In this example, there is about 10% underestimation of the permeability coeffi-

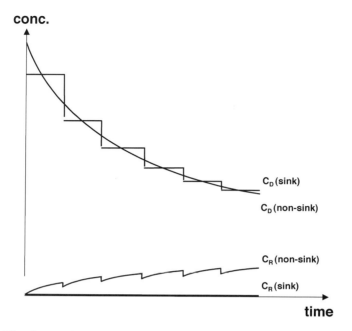

Fig. 10. The figure shows, schematically, how the receiver and donor concentrations are regarded in the sink condition and non-sink condition analysis, respectively. The saw-tooth shaped non-sink receiver curve is due to the instantaneous dilution in the sampling procedure, when the sampled volume is replaced by the same amount pure experimental medium. The diffusive driving force is the difference between the donor and receiver concentrations. In the sink condition analysis, the driving force is systematically overestimated, which leads to the permeability coefficient becoming systematically underestimated.

cient using the sink condition analysis as compared to using the non-sink condition analysis.

As mentioned above, the sink condition analysis can be used to generate a starting approximation for the nonlinear curve-fit applied in the non-sink condition analysis. It also has a strong advantage in the discovery of initial experimental imperfections (*see* **Subheadings 3.3.1.** and **3.4.8.**), which will show up as nonlinearities in the sink condition interval of the experiment. It is, therefore, recommended that both types of analysis are used complementarily, but that the final value of the permeability coefficients are determined using the non-sink condition analysis.

In spite of the generality of the non-sink condition analysis, it also may put restrictions on the experimental conditions (*see* **Subheading 3.3.**). If the receiver concentration rises so rapidly, that many or all sample concentrations lies too close to the equilibrium value, the non-sink condition analysis will fail or give very insecure values. It is necessary in these cases to shorten the experiment and sample more frequently.

3.4.10. A Remark About Statistics

In each experiment, the errors in the determination of receiver concentrations will, when curve-fitting to these values, propagate into the determination of the permeability coefficient. If the variances of the individual samples are known or can be estimated, it is possible to estimate the standard deviation of each determined permeability coefficient. This is seldom reported in scientific articles, and the reason for not doing this is that the biological variance is assumed to be much higher than the variance of a single determination. This is, in most cases, probably a correct assumption, but should be checked for every case. Since this is a standard method, it can be found in any textbook in the field of curve-fitting *(59)*.

4. Notes

1. The serum will inactivate the trypsin. This is a necessary step since the trypsin will otherwise remain active in the following steps of the procedure and may eventually kill the cells.
2. The counting of the cells is most conveniently carried out using a hemocytometer mounted in a light microscope. We use Trypan blue to detect damaged cells. No more than 5% of the cells should be stained.
3. When the cell suspension is added to the permeable support, great care must be taken so that no cells accidentally end up in the basolateral chamber. This may lead to the formation of a monolayer, also on the opposite (downward) facing of the supporting filter.
4. This step removes nonadherent cells and reduces the risk for multilayer formation.
5. The medium change is most conveniently carried out by aspirating the old medium using a vacuum tubing attached to a narrow pipet (for example, a 1-mL pipet). First, remove the basolateral and then the apical medium to reduce the risk of drying the cells. When the fresh medium is added, add the apical medium first and then the basolateral medium.
6. After 21 d, many essential functional properties of the Caco-2 cell monolayers are stabilized, and, in our experience, the monolayers are suitable for drug transport studies for an additional 14 d.
7. This equilibration step is necessary to give time for the cells to adapt to the medium change.
8. We have noticed that the TER of the cell monolayers drops with time in the chamber. This may be caused by leakage of ions from the electrodes, which in turn affects the cells. Therefore, we measure TER after a short but defined time interval.
9. The resistance of a monolayer depends on the surface area. A larger surface area will result in a higher ion flux and thus a lower resistance. Therefore, TER is

calculated by multiplying the resistance with the surface area to give the cell monolayer specific TER.

10. Due to possible toxic effects caused by ion leakage (Ag^+) from the electrodes, the monolayers used for TER measurements must not be used for other experiments.

11. Sampling from the donor solution at $t = 0$ and at the end of the experiment, allows for the calculation of the mass balance, which will detect possible loss of drug due to, for example, adsorption to the plastic surface.

12. Stirring the inserts at a moderate rate will reduce the effects of the aquous boundary layer adjacent to the cell monolayers (this is particularly important for studies of rapidly transported drugs).

13. The number of sampling occasions during a drug transport experiment affects the accuracy of the determination. Sampling occasions (4–6) are required for accurate determination of the permeability coefficient of the drug. Many sampling occasions also give information about possible lag times and other deviations from linearity. However, in some cases, a single time-point sampling (for example after 60 min) may be sufficient *(49)*.

14. Permeable supports containing Caco-2 cells from a TER measurement or a transport assay can be further processed for analysis of transcript and protein expression. For each of these applications, it is sufficient to save cell monolayers from three permeable supports (12 mm ϕ).

15. Use 2.0-mL cryogenic vials with straight walls, to ensure access for the tissue homogenizer tool (for example, Heidolph DIAX 900 tissue homogenizer equipped with a 6-G tool).

16. Alternatively, the cells can be lysed by applying the appropriate extraction buffer directly onto the cell monolayer, without removing the support from the cell culture insert, and subsequently transferring the extract to a vial for storage. This procedure is equally efficient in extracting RNAs and proteins from the cells, but considerably more laborious due to the high viscosity of the resulting cell lysate.

17. In order to minimize the risk of affecting the RNA population by subjecting the cells to a lengthy procedure, we save filters for RNA isolation immediately after a TER measurement. We do not save filters that have been used for drug transport experiments, since the RNA population may have been altered during the relatively long time that is required for such experiments.

18. Add 400 µL of the lysis buffer (provided by the manufacturer) to a microcentrifuge vial containing filters with Caco-2 cells and ensure that the filters are thoroughly submerged in the buffer. Homogenize and shear the extract for 15 s, using a tissue homogenizer, and process the extract according to the manufacturer's instructions. For sensitive assays such as quantitative RT-PCR, an on-column DNase treatment step, according to the manufacturer's instructions (Qiagen), is recommended. Expected yield is approximately 30 µg of total RNA.

19. Alternatively, this can also be accomplished by repeatedly passing the extract through a 21-G needle until the viscosity of the extract is reduced.

20. This procedure results in approx 1 µg of protein per µL of extract, as determined by the BCA assay using bovine serum albumin (BSA) as a standard.

21. As described in **Subheading 3.3.**, the solubility of the drug in the experimental medium may be insufficient to allow for transport of detectable amounts of the drug. In this case, the drug may be predissolved in a co-solvent such as ethanol prior to dilution in the experimental medium (to a final concentration of 1% ethanol [v/v]) or DMSO (to a final concentration of 0.1% DMSO [v/v]).

22. Note that some drugs adhere to plastic surfaces.

23. The evaporation step removes radioactively labeled solvents (such as ^{3}H-water and ethanol) that are often present in the drug solutions. It may sometimes be necessary to repeat the evaporation step in order to completely remove the labeled solvent.

24. The sample volume may be varied to optimize the experimental conditions. For instance, for rapidly transported drugs, it may be necessary to remove large samples to maintain the concentration gradient between the donor and the receiver chamber. Large samples also allow for repeated analysis, for example, by HPLC.

25. The time interval may be varied to optimize the experimental conditions. For instance, for rapidly transported drugs, samples must be taken at short time intervals to maintain the concentration gradient. For slowly transported drugs, samples must be taken at long time intervals to allow for detectable concentrations to reach the receiver chamber.

26. Care must be taken not to use toxic concentrations. Many compounds are more toxic to the cells when added to the basolateral side than when added to the apical side.

27. Note that the inhibitor may be toxic to the cells. The investigator should always perform a separate experiment to assess the effect of the inhibitor on the integrity of the cell monolayers (for example ^{14}C-mannitol). The optimal concentration of inhibitor may be found in the literature.

Acknowledgments

We thank Dr. Lucia Lazorova for excellent proof reading of this chapter and valuable hints. This work was supported The Swedish Medical Research Council and The Wallenberg Foundation.

References

1. Artursson, P. and Borchardt, R. T. (1997) Intestinal drug absorption and metabolism in cell cultures: Caco-2 and beyond. *Pharm. Res.* **14,** 1655–1658.

2. Artursson, P. and Karlsson, J. (1991) Correlation between oral drug absorption in humans and apparent drug permeability coefficients in human intestinal epithelial (Caco-2) cells. *Biochem. Biophys. Res. Commun.* **175,** 880–885.

3. Tavelin, S., Milovic, V., Ocklind, G., Olsson, S., and Artursson, P. (1999) A conditionally immortalized epithelial cell line for studies of intestinal drug transport. *J. Pharmacol. Exp. Ther.* **290,** 1212–1221.

4. Irvine, J. D., Takahashi, L., Lockhart, K., et al. (1999) MDCK (Madin-Darby canine kidney) cells: a tool for membrane permeability screening. *J. Pharm. Sci.* **88,** 28–33.

5. Fogh, J. Fogh, J. M., and Orfeo, T. (1977) One hundred and twenty-seven cultured human tumor cell lines producing tumors in nude mice. *J. Natl. Cancer Inst.* **59,** 221–226.

6. Pageot, L. P., Perreault, N., Basora, N., Francoeur, C., Magny, P., and Beaulieu, J. F. (2000) Human cell models to study small intestinal functions: recapitulation of the crypt-villus axis. *Microsc. Res. Tech.* **49,** 394–406.

7. Prentis, R. A., Lis, Y., and Walker, S. R. (1988) Pharmaceutical innovation by the seven UK-owned pharmaceutical companies (1964–1985). *Br. J Clin. Pharmacol.* **25,** 387–396.

8. Pinto, M., Robine-Leon, S., Appay, M., et al. (1983) Enterocyte-like differentiation and polarization of the human colon carcinoma cell line Caco-2 in culture. *Biol. Cell* **47,** 323–330.

9. Grasset, E., Pinto, M., Dussaulx, E., Zweibaum, A., and Desjeux, J. F., (1984) Epithelial properties of human colonic carcinoma cell line Caco-2: electrical parameters. *Am. J. Physiol.* **247,** C260–C267.

10. Boulenc, X., Bourrie, M., Fabre, I., et al. (1992) Regulation of cytochrome P450IA1 gene expression in a human intestinal cell line, Caco-2. *J. Pharmacol. Exp. Ther.* **263,** 1471–1478.

11. Hidalgo, I. J., Raub, T. J., and Borchardt, R. T. (1989) Characterization of the human colon carcinoma cell line (Caco-2) as a model system for intestinal epithelial permeability. *Gastroenterology* **96,** 736–749.

12. Howell, S., Kenny, A. J., and Turner, A. J. (1992) A survey of membrane peptidases in two human colonic cell lines, Caco-2 and HT-29. *Biochem. J.* **284,** 595–601.

13. Schmiedlin-Ren, P., Thummel, K. E., Fisher, J. M., Paine, M. F., Lown, K. S., and Watkins, P. B. (1997) Expression of enzymatically active CYP3A4 by Caco-2 cells grown on extracellular matrix-coated permeable supports in the presence of 1alpha,25-dihydroxyvitamin D3. *Mol. Pharmacol.* **51,** 741–754.

14. Mesonero, J., Matosin, M., Cambier, D., Rodriguez-Yoldi, M. J., and Brot-Laroche, E. (1995) Sugar-dependent expression of the fructose transporter GLUT5 in Caco-2 cells. *Biochem. J.* **312,** 757–762.

15. Hu, M. and Borchardt, R. T. (1992) Transport of a large neutral amino acid in a human intestinal epithelial cell line (Caco-2): uptake and efflux of phenylalanine. *Biochim. Biophys. Acta* **29,** 233–244.

16. Tamura, K., Lee, C. P., Smith, P. L., and Borchardt, R. T. (1996) Effect of charge on oligopeptide transporter-mediated permeation of cyclic dipeptides across Caco-2 cell monolayers. *Pharm. Res.* **13,** 1752–1754.

17. Said, H. M., Ortiz, A., Kumar, C. K., Chatterjee, N., Dudeja, P. K., and Rubin, S. (1999) Transport of thiamine in human intestine: mechanism and regulation in intestinal epithelial cell model Caco-2. *Am. J. Physiol.* **277,** C645–C651.

18. Kuo, S. M. (1998) Transepithelial transport and accumulation of flavone in human intestinal Caco-2 cells. *Life Sci.* **63,** 2323–2331.

19. Ma, T. Y., Dyer. D. L., and Said, H. M. (1994) Human intestinal cell line Caco-2: a useful model for studying cellular and molecular regulation of biotin uptake. *Biochim. Biophys. Acta* **1189,** 81–88.

20. Said, H. M. and Ma, T. Y. (1994) Mechanism of riboflavine uptake by Caco-2 human intestinal epithelial cells. *Am. J. Physiol.* **266,** G15–G21.

21. Ng, K. Y. and Borchardt, R. T. (1993) Biotin transport in a human intestinal epithelial cell line (Caco-2). *Life Sci.* **53,** 1121–1127.

22. Hunter, J., Hirst ,B. H., and Simmons, N. L. (1993) Drug absorption limited by P-glycoprotein-mediated secretory drug transport in human intestinal epithelial Caco-2 cell layers. *Pharm. Res.* **10,** 743–749.

23. Hochman, J. H., Chiba, M., Nishime, J., Yamazaki, M., and Lin, J. H. (2000) Influence of P-glycoprotein on the transport and metabolism of indinavir in Caco-2 cells expressing cytochrome P-450 3A4. *J. Pharmacol. Exp. Ther.* **292,** 310–318.

24. Hirohashi, T., Suzuki, H., Chu, X. Y., Tamai, I., Tsuji, A., and Sugiyama, Y. (2000) Function and expression of multidrug resistance-associated protein family in human colon adenocarcinoma cells (Caco-2). *J. Pharmacol. Exp. Ther.* **292,** 265–270.

25. Fujita, T., Yamada, H., Fukuzumi, M., Nishimaki, A., Yamamoto, A., and Muranishi, S. (1997) Calcein is excreted from the intestinal mucosal cell membrane by the active transport system. *Life Sci.* **60,** 307–313.

26. Artursson, P., Palm, K., and Luthman, K. (1996) Caco-2 monolayers in experimental and theoretical predictions of drug transport. *Adv. Drug Deliv. Rev.* **22,** 67–84.

27. Lentz, K. A., Hayashi, J., Lucisano, L. J., and Polli, J. E. (2000) Development of a more rapid, reduced serum culture system for Caco-2 monolayers and application to the biopharmaceutics classification system. *Int. J. Pharm.* **200,** 41–51.

28. Liang, E., Chessic, K., and Yazdanian, M. (2000) Evaluation of an accelerated Caco-2 cell permeability model. *J. Pharm. Sci.* **89,** 336–345.

29. Chong, S., Dando, S. A., and Morrison, R. A. (1997) Evaluation of Biocoat intestinal epithelium differentiation environment (3-day cultured Caco-2 cells) as an absorption screening model with improved productivity. *Pharm. Res.* **14,** 1835–1847.

30. Borst, P., Evers, R., Kool, M., and Wijnholds, J. (1999) The multidrug resistance protein family. *Biochim. Biophys. Acta* **1461,** 347–357.

31. Artursson, P. (1990) Epithelial transport of drugs in cell culture. I. A model for studying the passive diffusion of drugs over intestinal absorptive (Caco-2) cells. *J. Pharm. Sci.* **79,** 476–482.

32. Madara, J. L., Stafford, J., Dharmsathaphorn, K., and Carlson, S. (1987) Structural analysis of a human intestinal epithelial cell line. *Gastroenterology* **92,** 1133–1145.

33. Thwaites, D. T., Hirst, B. H., and Simmons, N. L. (1993) Passive transepithelial absorption of thyrotropin-releasing hormone (TRH) via a paracellular route in cultured intestinal and renal epithelial cell lines. *Pharm. Res.* **10,** 674–681.

34. Wils, P., Warnery, A., Phung-Ba, V., and Scherman, D. (1994) Differentiated intestinal epithelial cell lines as *in vitro* models for predicting the intestinal absorption of drugs. *Cell. Biol. Toxicol.* **10,** 393–397.

35. Wikman, A., Karlsson, J., Carlstedt, I., and Artursson, P. (1993) A drug absorption model based on the mucus layer producing human intestinal goblet cell line HT29–H. *Pharm. Res.* **10,** 843–852.

36. Collett, A., Sims, E., Walker, D., et al. (1996) Comparison of HT29-18-C1 and Caco-2 cell lines as models for studying intestinal paracellular drug absorption. *Pharm. Res.* **13,** 216–221.

37. Quaroni, A. and Isselbacher, K. J. (1981) Cytotoxic effects and metabolism of benzo[a]pyrene and 7,12-dimethylbenz[a]anthracene in duodenal and ileal epithelial cell cultures. *J Natl Cancer Inst.* **67,** 1353–1362.

38. Duizer, E., Penninks, A. H., Stenhuis, W. H., and Groten, J. P. (1997) Comparison of permeability characteristics of the human colonic Caco-2 and rat small intestinal IEC-18 cell lines. *J. Control. Release* **49,** 39–49.

39. Paul, E. C. A., Hochman, J., and Quaroni, A.(1993) Conditionally immortalized intestinal epithelial cells. Novel approach for study of differentiated enterocytes. *Am. J. Physiol.* **265,** C266–C278.

40. Miller, J. H. and Heath, L. N. (1989) Growth, enzyme activity, sugar transport, and hormone supplement responses in cells cloned from a pig kidney cell line LLC-PK1. *J. Cell. Physiol.* **139,** 538–549.

41. Tanigawara, Y., Okamura, N., Hirai, M., et al. (1992) Transport of digoxin by human P-glycoprotein expressed in a porcine kidney epithelial cell line (LLC-PK1). *J. Pharmacol. Exp. Ther.* **263,** 840–845.

42. Evers, R., Zaman, G. J., van Deemter, L., et al. (1996) Basolateral localization and export activity of the human multidrug resistance-associated protein in polarized pig kidney cells. *J. Clin. Invest.* **97,** 1211–1218.

43. Terada, T., Saito, H., Mukai, M., and Inui, K. (1997) Characterization of stably transfected kidney epithelial cell line expressing rat H+/peptide cotransporter PEPT1: localization of PEPT1 and transport of beta-lactam antibiotics. *J. Pharmacol. Exp. Ther.* **281,** 1415–1421.

44. Cho, M. J., Thompson, D. P., Cramer, C. T., Vidmar, T. J., and Scieszka, J. F. (1989) The Madin Darby canine kidney (MDCK) epithelial cell monolayer as a model cellular transport barrier *Pharm. Res.* **6,** 71–77.

45. Karlsson, J. and Artursson, P. (1992) A new diffusion chamber system for the determination of drug permeability coefficients across the human intestinal epithelium that are independent of the unstirred water layer. *Biochim. Biophys. Acta* **1111,** 204–210.

46. Jumarie, C. and Malo, C. (1991) Caco-2 cells cultured in serum-free medium as a model for the study of enterocytic differentiation *in vitro. J. Cell. Physiol.* **149,** 24–33.

47. Wikman Larhed, A. and Artursson, P. (1995) Co-cultures of human intestinal goblet (HT29-H) and absorbtive (Caco-2) cells for studies on epithelial transport and integrity. *Eur. J. Pharm. Sci.* **3,** 171–183.

48. Delie, F. and Rubas, W. (1997) A human colonic cell line sharing similarities with enterocytes as a model to examine oral absorption: advantages and limitations of the Caco-2 model. *Crit. Rev. Ther. Drug Carrier Syst.* **14,** 221–286.

49. Lazorova, L., Gråsjö, J., Artursson, P., et al. (1998) Quantification and imaging of mannitol transport through Caco-2 cell monolayers using a positron-emitting tracer. *Pharm. Res.* **15,** 1141–1144.

50. Lindmark, T., Nikkilä, T. and Artursson, P. (1995) Mechanisms of absorption enhancement by medium chain fatty acids in intestinal epithelial Caco-2 cell monolayers. *J. Pharmacol. Exp. Ther.* **275,** 958–964.

51. de Bruin, M., Miyake, K., Litman, T., Robey, R. and Bates, S. E. (1999) Reversal of resistance by GF120918 in cell lines expressing the ABC half-transporter, MXR. *Cancer Lett.* **146,** 117–126.

52. Benet, L. Z., Izumi, T., Zhang, Y., Silverman, J. A. and Wacher, V. J. (1999) Intestinal MDR transport proteins and P-450 enzymes as barriers to oral drug delivery. *J. Control. Release* **62,** 25–31.

53. International Human Genome Sequencing Consortium (2001) Initial sequencing and analysis of the human genome. *Nature* **409,** 860–921.

54. Venter, J., Adams, M., Myers, E., et al. (2001) The sequence of the human genome. *Science* **291,** 1304–1351.

55. Palm, K., Luthman, K., Ros, J., Gråsjö, J., and Artursson, P. (1999) Effect of molecular charge on intestinal epithelial drug transport: pH-dependent transport of cationic drugs. *J. Pharmacol. Exp. Ther.* **291,** 435–43.

56. Dawson, D. (1991) Chapter 1. Principles of membrane transport, p. 1–45. In *Handbook of physiology, section 6: the gastrointestinal system.* (Rauner B, ed.). American Physiological Society; Bethesda.

57. Karlsson, J. and Artursson, P. (1991) A method for determination of cellular permeability coefficient and aqueous boundary layer thickness in monolayers of intestinal epithelial (Caco-2) cells grown in permeable filter chambers. *Int. J. Pharm.* **71,** 55–64.

58. Spiegel, M. (1968) *Mathematical handbook of formulas and tables.* McGraw-Hill Book Company, New York.

59. Bevington, P. and Robinson, D. (1992) *Data reduction and error analysis for the physical sciences. 2nd ed.* McGraw-Hill, New York.

22

X-Ray Microanalysis of Epithelial Cells in Culture

Godfried M. Roomans

1. Introduction

X-ray microanalysis is a technique of elemental analysis that is carried out in an electron microscope. The technique is based on the generation of characteristic X-rays in atoms of the specimen by the incident beam electrons. These X-rays are characteristic for the element from which they originate, and hence contain information on which elements are present in the specimen (and how much of each). In addition to characteristic X-rays, the beam electrons generate background or continuum X-rays that do not carry information on the elemental composition of the sample, but the amount of background radiation is related to the total mass of the analyzed volume in the specimen and is used in quantitative analysis *(1,2)* (**Fig. 1**). The lowest concentration of an element that can be detected is in the order of a few mM/kg, and the smallest amount is in the order of 10^{-18} g. The spatial resolution of the analysis depends on the thickness of the specimen. The best spatial resolution is obtained in (thin) sections, where as a rule of thumb, the diameter of the analyzed volume is about half the section thickness. If bulk specimens are analyzed, as is done in the scanning electron microscope, the spatial resolution depends on the accelerating voltage and the composition of the specimen. A typical value for analysis of freeze-dried biological material at an accelerating voltage of 20 kV is about 10 μm *(1)*.

X-ray microanalysis of cultured epithelial cells can be a useful technique to elucidate (patho)physiological mechanisms of ion transport. The advantages of the use of cell cultures in general are well-known: the cell culture system is simpler, since it usually consists of only one cell type, systemic effects can be avoided, and especially in the case of human cells, in vivo experiments are often not possible because of practical or ethical constrictions. Preparation of cell cultures for X-ray microanalysis is often simpler than the preparation of

From: *Methods in Molecular Biology, vol. 188: Epithelial Cell Culture Protocols*
Edited by: C. Wise © Humana Press Inc., Totowa, NJ

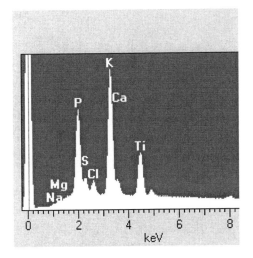

Fig. 1. Energy-dispersive X-ray spectrum from a cultured bronchial epithelial cells showing peaks for endogenous elements, as well as for Ti from the titanium grid on which the cells were grown. The peak at 0 keV is an artificially generated peak used to calibrate the energy scale.

tissue, because dissection artifacts can be avoided. The main advantage of X-ray microanalysis over other techniques used for investigating ion transport (e.g., radioactive tracers, fluorescent probes) is that with X-ray microanalysis all elements of interest can be measured simultaneously.

Cell lines, primary cell cultures, and isolated epithelial cells have been used *(3–7)*. Examples of epithelial cells studied include sweat gland cell lines *(8)* and cell lines from colon cancer *(9,10)*, prostate cancer *(11,12)*, and breast cancer *(13)*, keratinocyte cell lines *(14)*, primary cultures from sweat glands *(15)*, respiratory epithelium *(16)*, tracheal glands *(17,18)*, uterine epithelium *(19)*, and isolated nasal epithelial cells *(20)*.

Since X-ray microanalysis of epithelial cells in culture is usually carried out to investigate problems of ion transport, conventional fixation techniques for electron microscopy cannot be used, and it is necessary to use cryotechniques. X-ray microanalytical studies on epithelial cells can be carried out in different ways (**Fig. 2**). Cells can be grown on a substrate, frozen, and cryosectioned; the sections are then analyzed in the same way as cryosections from tissue. Cells can be grown on a solid substrate (either permeable or impermeable), frozen, freeze-dried, and analyzed in the scanning electron microscope (SEM) at relatively low accelerating voltage *(10,13,21–23)* (**Fig. 3**). Cells can also be grown on ultrathin plastic films on electron microscopy grids, frozen, freeze-dried, and analyzed in the scanning transmission electron microscope (STEM) at relatively high accelerating voltage *(9,14,15,24,25)* (**Fig. 4**).

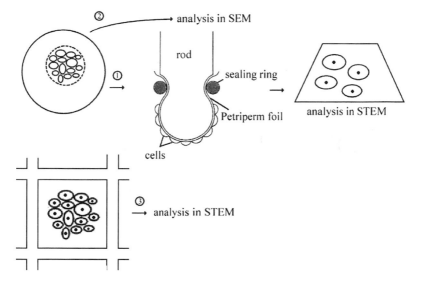

Fig. 2. Schematic of methods for preparation of cultured epithelial cells for X-ray microanalysis. Cells cultured on a solid substrate may be punched out, mounted on a rod, and cryosectioned in a cryoultramicrotome; the sections can be analyzed in the STEM *(1)*. They can also be rinsed to remove the culture medium, frozen, freeze-dried, and analyzed in the SEM *(2)*. Finally, they can be grown on a thin plastic film on a grid, rinsed to remove the culture medium, frozen, freeze-dried, and analyzed in the STEM.

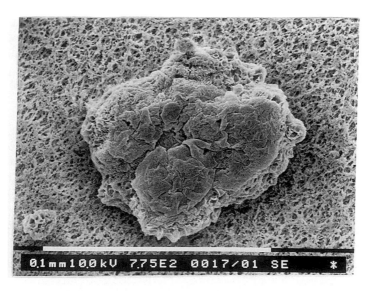

Fig. 3. Scanning electron micrograph of a HT29 colon cancer cell grown on a Millipore filter for analysis in the SEM.

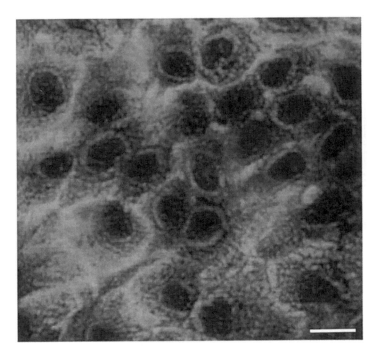

Fig. 4. Digitized scanning transmission electron micrograph of keratinocytes cultured on a thin Formvar film on a titanium grid for analysis in STEM. Bar = 5 μm.

Analysis of thin sections of cultured cells, and analysis of whole cells on a solid substrate or on a thin plastic film on a grid are techniques that each have their advantages and disadvantages.

X-ray microanalysis of thin cryosections of cultured cells allows analysis at the subcellular level to be carried out, i.e., one can analyze different cell organelles and different regions of the cytoplasm (or the nucleus) separately. This is not possible with the other methods. The washing step, which may introduce artifacts (*see* **Note 3**) is avoided. Quantitative analysis is theoretically straightforward. However, the method is technically difficult and requires specialized equipment (cryoultramicrotome), a skilled operator, and considerable effort, in effect, limiting the number of cells that can be analyzed within a reasonable period of time. Analysis requires a (scanning) transmission electron microscope.

X-ray microanalysis of cells cultured on a solid substrate is a technically easy method. The specimens are sturdy, easy to handle, and easy to analyze. The disadvantages are the necessity of the washing step and problems with quantitative analysis, because it is often impossible to avoid overpenetration of the specimen by the electron beam (*see* **Note 5**). In general, only the thickest part of the cell can be analyzed, no analysis at the subcellular level is possible.

Sensitivity of analysis at low accelerating voltage is lower than at high accelerating voltage. Analysis requires a SEM.

X-ray microanalysis of cells cultured on thin films on grids in the STEM is more sensitive, and quantitative analysis is more straightforward. It may be possible to analyze areas with cytoplasm only, and compare these with the area containing both nucleus and cytoplasm. The specimens are, however, more fragile, and when the film breaks during handling of the grid, the grid cannot be analyzed, and part of an experiment may be spoiled. Analysis requires a (scanning) transmission electron microscope. The contribution of the titanium or gold grid to the spectrum may be a problem, especially in quantitative analysis.

The final choice will be dependent on the type of cells, the problem investigated, and the availability of equipment. If analysis at the subcellular level is necessary, or if the cells do not withstand the rinsing procedure, analysis of sections may be the only option. In other cases, analysis of cells cultured on thin films is to be preferred, because of the problems in quantitative analysis connected with overpenetration of the beam. Nevertheless, analysis on a solid substrate may yield results of equivalent biological significance in many projects.

2. Materials

2.1. X-Ray Microanalysis of Cryosections of Cultured Cells

1. Cell culture media. Minimal essential medium (MEM), Dulbecco's modified Eagle's medium (DMEM), Ham's F-12 medium, or RPMI 1640 medium (Life Technologies), that may or may not be supplemented with up to 10% fetal bovine serum (FBS) (Life Technologies), and should be supplemented with 100 U/mL penicillin (Sigma) and 100 mg/mL streptomycin (Sigma). Instructions about which media are appropriate for a particular cell type are generally given by the provider of the cells (e.g., the American Type Culture Collection, commercial providers, or the laboratory in which the cell line was generated).
2. Incubator for cell culture.
3. Sterile hood for cell culture manipulation.
4. Inverted light microscope.
5. Centrifuge.
6. Petriperm dishes (Heraeus Instruments).
7. 3 mg/mL Collagen S type I from calf skin (Roche) for coating culture dishes (*see* **Subheading 3.1.1.**).
8. 1 mg/mL Fibronectin from human plasma (Sigma) for coating culture dishes (*see* **Subheading 3.1.1.**).
9. 1 mg/mL Bovine serum albumin (BSA) (Sigma) for coating culture dishes (*see* **Subheading 3.1.1.**).
10. Plexiglass rod (made locally).
11. Liquid propane or ethane cooled by liquid nitrogen.
12. Cryoultramicrotome (*see* **Subheading 2.5.** for suppliers).

13. Pioloform (polyvinyl butyral) film (SPI Supplies).
14. Thermanox (ICN Biochemicals).
15. n-Heptane.
16. 2% Agar (melting point 27–30°C)
17. 20% Gelatin.
18. Formvar film (Merck).
19. Electron microscope (scanning or scanning transmission) (*see* **Subheading 2.5.** for suppliers).
20. Electron microscopy grids.
21. Freeze-drier.

2.2. X-Ray Microanalysis of Cells Cultured on a Solid Substrate

1. Tissue culture plastic: flasks, pipets (Nalge-Nunc International).
2. Trypsin-EDTA: 2.5 g trypsin, 1.86 g EDTA per liter phosphate-buffered saline (PBS).
3. Cellulose nitrate (Schleicher & Schuell) or cellulose nitrate–cellulose acetate filters (Millipore), pore size about 0.2 µm.
4. Cell culture medium (*see* **Subheading 2.1., step 1**).
5. Ringer's solution: 140 mM NaCl, 5 mM KCl, 5 mM HEPES, 1 mM MgCl$_2$, 1.5 mM CaCl$_2$, and 5 mM D-glucose.
6. 300 mM mannitol (in distilled water).
7. 150 mM ammonium acetate (in distilled water).

2.3. X-Ray Microanalysis of Cells Cultured on a Thin Film on a Grid

1. Titanium grids.
2. 70% Ethanol.
3. Glass slides: 76 × 26 mm, ISO NORM 8037 (Menzel).
4. 0.5% (w/v) Formvar dissolved in 1,2-dichloroethane.
5. Glass dish.
6. 12-mm Round glass coverslips.
7. Carbon coater (Balzers, cat. no. CED020).
8. UV light (2 Osram HNS 15W OFR lamps).
9. 0.3% Pioloform.
10. 15-mm Circular Thermanox coverslips.

2.4. X-Ray Microanalysis of Isolated Human Nasal Epithelial Cells

1. 0.6-mm Sterile cytology brushes (can be bought at local pharmacies as dental brushes).
2. Cell culture medium (*see* **Subheading 2.1., step 1**).
3. Cell-Tak (Becton Dickinson).

2.5. Suppliers

2.5.1. Electron Microscopes

1. Hitachi Science Systems, 1040 Ichige, Hitachinaka, Ibaraki Pref 312-0033, Japan.
2. JEOL, 1–2 Musashino 3-chome, Akishima, Tokyo 196-8558, Japan.

3. LEO, Clifton Road, Cambridge CB1 3QH, U.K.
4. Philips Electron Optics (now FEI Company), P.O. Box 218, 5600 MD Eindhoven, The Netherlands.

2.5.2. Energy-Dispersive X-ray Microanalysis Systems

1. EDAX, Inc., 91 Mckee Drive, Mahwah, NJ 07430, U.S.A.
2. NORAN Instruments, Inc., 2551 W. Beltline Highway, Middleton, WI 53562-2697, U.S.A.
3. Oxford Instruments Microanalysis Group, Halifax Road, High Wycombe HP12 3SE, U.K.

2.5.3. Cryoultramicrotomes

1. Leica Microsystems AG, Ernst-Leitz-Strasse 17-37, 35578 Wetzlar, Germany.
2. RMC, Boeckeler Instrument, Inc., 4650 South Butterfield Drive, Tucson, AZ 85714, U.S.A.

2.5.4. Carbon Evaporators

1. Balzers, FL9496 Balzers, Liechtenstein.

3. Methods

3.1. X-Ray Microanalysis of Cryosections of Cultured Cells

Cryopreparation and X-ray microanalysis of cultured cells largely follows the procedures for cryopreparation and analysis of tissue. Many variants of these methods have been described in the literature, and a comprehensive treatment is outside the scope of this chapter. In the following, emphasis is placed on those steps in the procedure that are specific for cultured (epithelial) cells.

3.1.1. Coating of Culture Dishes or Other Substrates

1. The coating solution consists of 1 mL of a sterile 3 mg/mL collagen S solution, 1 mL of a sterile 1 mg/mL fibronectin solution, 10 mL of a sterile 1 mg/mL BSA solution, and 88 mL of the cell culture medium used for the particular cell type.
2. Place 1 mL of the coating solution per 25 cm^2 of area to be coated in a culture dish and leave it for about 2 h; remove the remaining solution by aspiration. The dishes can be used immediately or stored at $-20°C$ for later use.
3. Other substrates (culture flasks, coverslips) can be coated similarly.

3.1.2. Preparation of Cells Cultured in Culture Dishes

1. Culture cells in coated Petriperm dishes. Place 0.1 mL of a cell suspension containing approx 10^6 cells/mL in the dish and let the cells attach for maximum 2 h at 37°C. Add 2 mL of the appropriate medium and place the culture dishes in an incubator with appropriate gas supply (e.g., 5% CO_2/95% air) at 37°C. Change medium every 48 h. Check cell growth by light microscopy.

2. After the cells have reached confluence, punch out (with a metal punch) a round area with a diameter of 10 mm from the cell culture.
3. If the experiment involves incubation of the cells in experimental solutions, this should be done at this stage.
4. The punched foil with the cells should now be stretched over the round-shaped end of a 2-mm-thick plexiglass rod and cryofixed by rapid immersion into liquid propane or ethane cooled by liquid nitrogen.
5. Mount the specimen in a cryoultramicrotome (26–28).

3.1.3. Preparation of Cells Cultured on Thin Films or Coverslips

1. Culture cells on a thin polyvinyl butyral (Pioloform) film or on a Thermanox coverslip.
2. If nessessary, coat these as described above (see **Subheading 3.1.1.**).
3. After the cells have reached confluence and after the experiment has been carried out, rapidly freeze the Pioloform film with the cells on in liquid propane or ethane cooled by liquid nitrogen.
4. Glue the frozen specimen to the specimen holder of the cryoultramicrotome using n-heptane as a cryoglue (4,25).

3.1.4. Preparation of Cell Pellets

1. If pelleted cells are to be used, the cells should, after being cultured in a flask or Petri dish, be trypsinized as follows. Remove the culture medium, add 2 mL trypsin-EDTA per 25 cm^2 of culture area, and let this solution briefly cover the cells. Decant the trypsin-EDTA and incubate the flask for 10 min at 37°C. Resuspend the cells in the previously used culture medium (containing serum). To obtain a pellet, the cells should be centrifuged for 1 min at 800g.
2. Coherence of the cells in the pellet may be improved by adding a very small amount (about the same volume as the pellet) of molten agar or gelatin to the pellet, resuspending the pellet, and centrifuging again. Alternatively, cells can be resuspended in a small volume (20–40 µL) of 300 mM mannitol, and placed frozen in a small container made by moulding aluminum foil around the tip of a micropipet.
3. The amount of agar, gelatin, or mannitol should be very small, otherwise the final specimen will contain too few cells per unit volume.
4. Freeze the cells rapidly in liquid propane or ethane cooled by liquid nitrogen, or against a liquid nitrogen cooled metal block in a commercial rapid freezing apparatus.
5. Mount the specimen in a cryoultramicrotome.
6. It has to be taken into consideration that at least in some cell types, the ion content of the cell is affected by centrifugation (29). It is recommended to carry out centrifugation of suspended cells for X-ray microanalysis at low speeds, because this would be the best way of retaining the elemental concentrations at their in vivo levels (30).

3.1.5. Cryoultramicrotomy

1. Cut cryosections of the specimen (mounted as described in the previous subsections, *see* **Subheadings 3.1.2.–3.1.4.**) of approximately 100 nm thick, using glass or diamond knives at a temperature below −100°C.
2. Transfer the sections to electron microscopy grids covered with a thin plastic film such as Formvar (*see* **Subheading 3.3.**).
3. Press the sections onto the grids with a brass rod or weight.
4. Freeze-dry the sections for several hours, and transfer to the electron microscope.
5. Carry out analysis in STEM at high accelerating voltage. Carry out quantitative analysis using the continuum method for thin sections (*see* **Note 1**).

3.2. X-Ray Microanalysis of Cells Cultured on a Solid Substrate

1. Cells are cultured in a medium appropriate for the particular cell type in plastic flasks in an incubator.
2. Harvest subconfluent cells with trypsin-EDTA as described above (*see* **Subheading 3.1.4., step 1**) and seed the cells directly on sterile cellulose nitrate or cellulose nitrate–cellulose acetate filters or another suitable substrate (*see* **Note 2**).
3. Place the filters in a Petri dish.
4. After the cells have attached to the filters, which takes about 3 h, add 3 to 4 mL complete culture medium and allow the cells to grow for 2 to 3 d before the experiment.
5. Check the cells using an inverted light microscope for growth and possible presence of infection each time the medium is changed.
6. If the experiment consists of exposing the cells to physiological stimuli, this can be done in medium or in a physiological buffer (Ringer's solution), for the appropriate time.
7. Terminate the incubation by washing the filters, respectively, with one of the following washing fluids: (*i*) distilled water, (*ii*) 150 m*M* ammonium acetate, or (*iii*) 300 m*M* mannitol for 15–20 s only to remove the NaCl-rich experimental solution. The washing fluid should have a temperature of about 4°C (*see* **Note 3**).
8. To wash the filters, the fluid is placed in a beaker on a magnetic stirrer, and the filter is dipped in the fluid and held with forceps.
9. Take out the filter and remove excess fluid by blotting with a filter paper. Freeze the cells immediately in liquid propane cooled by liquid nitrogen (*see* **Note 4**).
10. Freeze-dry the cells overnight.
11. Coat the dried filters with a conductive carbon layer to avoid charging in the electron microscope.
12. Store the filters in a vacuum container or over a drying agent if they are not analyzed immediately.
13. Mount the filters on a specimen holder (carbon is suitable) and analyze the cells on the filter in a SEM. An accelerating voltage of 10–20 kV is appropriate (*see* **Note 5**). Acquisition times between 50 and 100 s are required. Only one spectrum should be acquired from each cell (*see* **Note 6**).

14. Quantitative analysis can be performed by using the ratio (P/B) of the characteristic intensity (peak, P) to the background intensity (B) in the same energy range as the peak and comparing this P/B ratio with that obtained by analysis of a standard *(2)*.

15. Alternatively, standardless analysis can be carried out if the microscope is equipped with a thin-window detector, which allows the detection of light elements (C, N, and O) (*see* **Notes 1** and **7**).

3.3. X-Ray Microanalysis of Cells Cultured on a Thin Film on a Grid

Cells are cultured in a medium appropriate for the particular cell type in plastic flasks in an incubator.

3.3.1. Preparation of Titanium Grids with a Formvar Film

Prepare 75 mesh titanium grids (*see* **Note 8**) with a Formvar film using the following procedure.

1. Clean the grids in 70% ethanol.
2. Clean a glass slide by immersing it in ethanol.
3. Remove it instantly and dry with lens tissue.
4. Dip the slide into a solution of 0.5% Formvar dissolved in 1,2-dichloro ethane and withdraw carefully. The thickness is dependent on the speed of withdrawal; faster withdrawal gives thicker films. Thicker films can also be produced by increasing the Formvar concentration.
5. Leave the slide to dry in a vertical position.
6. Score around the slide on all four sides with a razor blade. This defines the limits of the film to be dislodged from the slide.
7. Fill a deep glass dish with distilled water and place a light so that it reflects on the water surface.
8. Clean the water surface by moving a clean glass rod over the surface, so that the uppermost water layer is removed.
9. Hold the Formvar-coated slide at a 90° angle to the surface of the water in the middle of the glass dish and with the water just touching the bottom of the slide. The Formvar film should start to come away from the glass.
10. Slowly push the slide into the water, watching the film as it lifts off the glass and floats on the water surface.
11. Remove the glass slide from the water and examine the floating film. The incident light should show interference colors in the film. These should be silver or gray; yellow, purple, or green colors indicate that the film is too thick.
12. Place the cleaned grids onto the floating film in groups of 3 grids. Place a small round cover glass (12 mm diameter) over each group of 3 grids.
13. Attach a piece of Parafilm over the film, the grids, and the cover glasses, and remove everything from the water.
14. Leave to dry.

15. Coat the film with a thin carbon layer. Place the grids in the carbon evaporator, and mount the carbon thread between the electrodes. The grids should be at a distance of about 10 cm from the carbon thread. Obtain vacuum and heat the carbon thread by increasing the current according to the manufacturer's instructions.
16. Sterilize the grids by UV radiation for at least 3 h or overnight.

3.3.2. Preparation and Analysis of Cells on a Thin Film

1. Harvest sub-confluent cells with trypsin-EDTA as described above (*see* **Subheading 3.4.1., step 1**).
2. Allow the cells to recover in culture medium in which they have been cultured previously, and seed the cells on the film-covered titanium grids.
3. As described above, 3 grids are placed on a round glass slide, and 3 of these glass slides can be placed in a Petri dish.
4. Place one drop of culture medium with cells on each glass slide, so that the grids are covered.
5. Allow the cells to attach, which takes about 3 h.
6. Add fresh culture medium.
7. Culture the cells for 3–7 d (depending on cell type) at 37°C in a humidified atmosphere of 5% CO_2/95% air in a culture chamber.
8. The following alternative procedure is based on a method published by Warley and coworkers *(25)*.
9. Prepare a film from 0.3% Pioloform and float on double-distilled water.
10. Place grids on the film.
11. Place Thermanox coverslips (circular, 15 mm diameter) over the grids.
12. Lift the preparation from the water surface and dry under a lamp with the Pioloform facing upwards.
13. Then sterilize the coverslip with the grids under UV light.
14. Seed cells at an appropriate density on the coverslips, so that they grow on the grids. The area on the coverslips next to the grids may be used for other types of experiments.
15. Carry out the experiment (e.g., exposure to agonists) and terminate the experiment by washing the cells in one of the solutions described above in **Subheading 3.2., step 7** (*see* **Note 3**).
16. Hold the grids with forceps for 15–20 s in the washing solution, which should be in a beaker placed on a magnetic stirrer.
17. Remove excess washing fluid by blotting with a filter paper.
18. Freeze the grids in liquid propane cooled by liquid nitrogen and freeze-dry them overnight.
19. Coat the grids with carbon to improve conductance in the electron microscope.
20. Analyze the cells on the grid in a STEM (or a transmission microscope with STEM attachment). An accelerating voltage of around 100 kV is appropriate. Acquisition times of around 100 s are required.
21. It is easiest to acquire spectra from the thickest part of the cell, where the nucleus is located, but if of interest, spectra can also be acquired from a peripheral area containing only cytoplasm.

22. Quantitative analysis can be performed by using the ratio (P/B) of the characteristic intensity (peak, P) to the background intensity (B) and comparing this P/B ratio with that obtained by analysis of a standard *(2)*. Alternatively, standardless analysis can be carried out if the microscope is equipped with a thin-window detector that allows the detection of light elements (C, N, and O) (*see* **Note 1**).

3.4. X-Ray Microanalysis of Isolated Human Nasal Epithelial Cells

1. Harvest nasal epithelial cells with cytology brushes from the inferior nasal turbinate of the subject.
2. Ask the subject to blow and thoroughly clean the nose prior to the brushing and visualize the area to be brushed directly through a rhinoscope.
3. The cells can be dislocated from the brush by manually rotating the vertically-held brush along its own axis for 1 min. This procedure should be carried out with the brush in an Eppendorf tube containing 1.5 mL culture medium.
4. Alternatively, the brush can be pulled through the opening of a disposable Eppendorf pipet tip.
5. If needed, the procedure can be repeated, with the other nostril and the cells pooled.
6. Prepare 75 mesh titanium grids with a thin Formvar film and sterilize the grids by UV light, as described in **Subheading 3.3.1.**
7. Treat the grids with Cell-Tak (1–5 µg/cm^2) according to the instructions provided by the manufacturer 30 min prior to seeding, in order to make the cells adhere.
8. Centrifuge the nasal epithelial cells at 800g for 1 min and resuspend in a small volume of culture medium (100 µL) and then seed onto the grids.
9. Incubate the cells for 30 min at 37°C to let them adhere to the grids.
10. Check the viability of the cells prior to the experiment by visualizing cells with beating cilia in a light microscope.
11. Incubate the cells with the experimental solution for the desired time.
12. Terminate the experiment by washing and freezing as in **Subheading 3.3.2., steps 15–17.** The grids are freeze-dried, coated with carbon, and analyzed in the STEM as described in **Subheading 3.3.2., steps 18–21.**

4. Notes

1. Quantitative analysis of thin specimens (thin cryosections of cultured cells, cells cultured on thin films) is generally carried out according to the so-called continuum or Hall method *(31)*. In this method, the ratio of the characteristic counts for a particular element (peak, P) to the background in a peak-free region of the spectrum (white radiation, W) is determined. A correction is made for the contribution of grid (and specimen holder) to the spectrum *(2)*. The P/W ratio for the elements in the specimen is compared to that obtained from a standard, consisting of known concentrations of mineral salts in an organic matrix, frozen, cryosectioned, and freeze-dried in the same way as the specimen. Software for quantitative analysis of thin biological specimens is provided by at least some of

the manufacturers of microanalysis equipment. Pitfalls are discussed in detail in references *(2,32)*. Quantitative analysis of thick biological specimens is generally carried out using a method based on the ratio of the characteristic counts (P) to the background counts in the same energy region as the characteristic counts (the background under the peak, B). Using the background under the peak rather than the background in a peak-free region of the spectrum is done to correct for any absorption of X-rays that may occur in thick specimens. Corrections for the contribution of the specimen holder to the background are not considered to be necessary *(2,32)*. Software for this type of quantitative analysis is supplied with many of the commercially available systems.

2. Different types of solid substrates can be used. For the experimental approach it can be important whether the substrate is permeable or impermeable. With an impermeable substrate, a substance added to the experimental solution can only reach the apical membrane of the cells, whereas if the cells are cultured on a permeable substrate, also the basolateral membrane may be accessed. From a practical point of view, the substrate should be easy to handle, allow the growth of cells, should not show excessive charging in the electron microscope, and should not contain elements that disturb the analysis. Glass is not recommended, since it may contain several elements that could be of interest in the analysis (Na, K). Some plastics used for cell culture show excessive charging in the microscope.

3. The rinsing procedure is possibly the most critical step in the preparation of whole cells for X-ray microanalysis. The procedure should be evaluated for each new cell type investigated. The rinsing procedure is necessary because the salts in the culture medium or the experimental solution, if not completely removed, would, after freeze-drying, cover the surface of the cells and interfere with analysis. Distilled water has the advantage that it does not leave any remnants after freeze-drying. It may, however, cause osmotic shock, and induce efflux of ions either by general damage to the membrane or by specific ion transport mechanisms. Ammonium acetate is volatile, and most or all of this compound will disappear after freeze-drying, leaving little or no remnants. Though a 150 mM ammonium acetate solution is about isoosmotic with the cytoplasm, ammonium acetate may cause pH changes in the cell and thereby induce ion transport. A 300 mM mannitol solution is isoosmotic and is not expected to cause changes in the ionic content of the cells. However, after freeze-drying, the cells are covered with a thin layer of powdery mannitol. Some of this may be removed by careful brushing, but some will remain. This makes visualization of the cells more difficult and also adds a layer of organic substance to the specimen, which "dilutes" the signal from the cell. This can be a problem in quantitative analysis (*see* **Note 5**). In our experience, some cell types withstand washing with ice-cold distilled water or ammonium acetate, and in such a case, these solutions are to be preferred. If the cells obviously lose ions after washing with water or ammonium acetate, then mannitol or a substance with similar properties should be used. (We find sucrose, however, to be even more sticky than mannitol.) The best way to

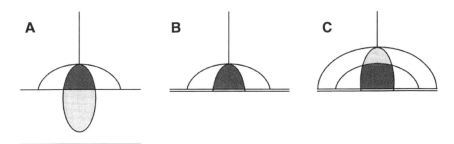

Fig. 5. **(A)** Cells grown on a thick substrate and analyzed in the SEM. The electron beam penetrates the cell completely and excites the substrate. The analyzed volume, which gives rise to the X-ray spectrum, consists of the cell (dark area) and the substrate (light area). **(B)** Cells grown on a thin film, rinsed with water or a volatile buffer, and analyzed in the STEM. The thin substrate (dark) contributes very little to the spectrum, which is mainly due to the cell (light). **(C)** Cells grown on a thin film, rinsed with mannitol, and analyzed in the STEM. The mannitol covering the cell contributes substantially to the spectrum and "dilutes" the signal from the endogenous elements in the cell.

      make sure that the rinsing procedure does not introduce artifacts is to compare whole-mount specimens, rinsed in different washing fluids, with cryosections of the same cells, frozen without rinsing. A good example of such a procedure is given in **ref. 25**.

4. Freezing should be rapid to reduce the damage that ice crystals, which form during the freezing process can do to the cell. Nevertheless, because analysis is carried out at low resolution, there is no reason to assume that the freezing step is very critical. Commercial equipment for freezing can be used as well as simple homemade equipment, and instead of propane, one can use ethane or isopentane.

5. Cells grown on a solid substrate have to be analyzed at low accelerating voltage to avoid overpenetration of the beam, and even then, overpenetration cannot always be avoided. If the cells grow in a single layer, the freeze-dried specimen is, in effect, only about 3 µm thick and is easily penetrated by a 10-kV beam. This means that apart from the cell, the substrate is also excited (**Fig. 5**). The substrate only contains elements with an atomic number <10, which are not seen by a conventional detector, but it "dilutes" the elements present in the specimen. This results in lower peak-to-background ratios. One can analyze the specimen at different values of the accelerating voltage to find an optimum value for the peak-to-background ratio. The lower limit for the accelerating voltage is set by the necessity to have sufficient electron energy to excite the X-rays of the heaviest element of interest in the sample. If overpenetration cannot be avoided, it is possible to carry out semiquantitative analysis by using one element as an "internal standard". In many cases, e.g., where the experiments involve activation of ion fluxes during a few minutes, phosphorus (P) or sulfur (S) are the most suitable

elements for this purpose, because the concentrations of these elements is not likely to change during the experiment. Of these two, phosphorus is usually the most suitable, because it occurs at higher concentrations than sulfur, and thus, the counting statistics are better. If changes in phosphorus and sulfur are suspected to occur during the experiment, e.g., in long-term experiments involving changes in cellular protein and nucleotide content, this procedure should not be used. However, often information on ratios between the concentrations of elements, such as Na/K, Na/Cl, or P/S, provides information that is biologically meaningful and can help to solve the scientific problem posed. The problem, which occurs when mannitol (sucrose, glucose) is present on top of the specimen after freeze-drying and it "dilutes" the concentrations of elements within the cell (**Fig. 5**), is in this respect similar to the problem of overpenetration in which the substrate "dilutes" these concentrations and should be handled in the same manner.

6. Although the electron beam in a SEM or STEM may be very narrow, the incident electrons will spread when they hit the specimen and undergo elastic and inelastic collisions with specimen atoms. The volume within the cell from which X-rays are generated will, therefore, have a much larger diameter than the diameter of the beam. Depending on the thickness of the cell at the site of analysis, the analyzed volume within the cell may actually be a large part of the cell.

7. Some manufacturers of X-ray microanalysis systems have software that allows so-called "standardless" analysis of specimens. Although developed for applications in the materials sciences (analysis of oxides, nitrides, and carbides), this method can be used for biological specimens, provided that the X-ray detector has a thin plastic (rather than a beryllium) window, which allows analysis of light elements, and that the quantitative analysis takes into account the presence of these elements (C, N, and O), which usually make up about 90% of the specimen. A small problem remains in that hydrogen (H) is neglected, because this element is not measured by X-ray microanalysis (it does not produce X-rays). However, the hydrogen concentration in freeze-dried tissue can quite safely be assumed to be in the order of 5%, so a good correction can be made by correcting the concentrations that are obtained by the software for standardless analysis with 5%. The advantage of this procedure is that preparation and analysis of standards *(2,32)* is not necessary. The method has, however, not been tested extensively on biological material.

8. Titanium is used because it is nontoxic, and its X-ray spectrum does not interfere with that of the cells. Gold grids are an alternative from the point of view of toxicity and have been used for this type of study *(25)*. However, the X-rays emitted by gold may partially overlap the peak from phosphorus originating from the cells.

Acknowledgment

The author wishes to acknowledge the contributions of Dr. Romuald Wróblewski, Anca Dragomir, and Marianne Ljungkvist to the techniques described in this paper. The research on which this paper is based was supported by the Swedish Medical Research Council (project no. 07125) and the Swedish Heart Lung Foundation.

References

1. Roomans, G. M. (1988) Introduction to X-ray microanalysis in biology. *J. Electron Microsc. Tech.* **9**, 3–18.
2. Roomans, G. M. (1988) Quantitative X-ray microanalysis of biological specimens. *J. Electron Microsc. Tech.* **9**, 19–44.
3. Zierold, K. and Schäfer, D. (1988) Preparation of cultured and isolated cells for X-ray microanalysis. *Scanning Microsc.* **2**, 1775–1790.
4. von Euler, A., Pålsgård, E., Vult von Steyern, C., and Roomans, G. M. (1993) X-ray microanalysis of epithelial and secretory cells in culture. *Scanning Microsc.* **7**, 191–202.
5. Warley, A. (1994) The preparation of cultured cells for X-ray microanalysis. *Scanning Microsc.* **(Suppl) 8**, 129–138.
6. Wroblewski, R. and Wroblewski, J. (1994) X-ray microanalysis of endocrine, exocrine and intestinal cells and organs in culture: technical and physiological aspects. *Scanning Microsc.* **(Suppl) 8**, 149–162.
7. Roomans, G. M., Hongpaisan, J., Jin, Z., Mörk, A. C., and Zhang, A. (1996) *In vitro* systems and cultured cells as specimens for X-ray microanalysis. *Scanning Microsc.* **(Suppl) 10**, 359–374.
8. Ring, A., Mörk, A.-C., and Roomans, G. M. (1995) Calcium-activated chloride fluxes in cultured NCL-SG3 sweat gland cells. *Cell Biol. Int.* **19**, 265–278.
9. von Euler, A. and Roomans, G. M. (1992) Ion transport in colon cancer cell cultures studied by X-ray microanalysis. *Cell Biol. Int. Rep.* **16**, 293–306.
10. Zhang, W. and Roomans, G. M. (1998) Volume induced chloride transport in HT29 cells studied by X-ray microanalysis. *Microsc. Res. Tech.* **40**, 72–78.
11. Fernández-Segura E., Cañizares, F. J., Cubero, M. A., Warley, A., and Campos, A. (1999) Changes in elemental content during apoptotic cell death studied by electron probe X-ray microanalysis. *Exp. Cell Res.* **253**, 454–462.
12. Salido, M., Vilches, J., Lopez, A., and Roomans, G. M. (2001) X-ray microanalysis of etoposide induced apoptosis in the PC-3 prostatic cancer cell line. *Cell Biol. Int.,* **25**, 499–508.
13. Fernandez-Segura, A., Cañizares, F. J., Cubero, M. A., Revelles, F., and Campos, A. (1997) Electron probe X-ray microanalysis of cultured epithelial tumour cells with scanning electron microscopy. *Cell Biol. Int.* **21**, 665–669.
14. Grängsjö, A., Pihl-Lundin, I., Lindberg, M., and Roomans, G. M. (2000) X-ray microanalysis of cultured keratinocytes: methodological aspects and effects of the irritant sodium lauryl sulfate on elemental composition. *J. Microsc.* **199**, 208–213.
15. Hongpaisan, J. and Roomans, G. M. (1998) Extracellular UTP regulates Na, Cl and K transport in primary cultures from human sweat gland coils. *Cell Struct. Funct.* **23**, 239–245.
16. Sagström, S., Roomans, G. M., Wroblewski, R., Keulemans, J. L. M., Hoogeveen, A. T., and Bijman, J. (1992) X-ray microanalysis of cultured respiratory epithelial cells from patients with cystic fibrosis. *Acta Physiol. Scand.* **146**, 213–220.

17. Zhang, A. L. and Roomans, G. M. (1997) Ion transport in cultured pig tracheal submucosal gland acinar cells studied by X-ray microanalysis. *Eur. Resp. J.* **10,** 2204–2209.

18. Zhang, A. L. and Roomans, G. M. (1999) Multiple intracellular pathways for regulation of chloride secretion in cultured pig trachea submucosal gland cells. *Eur. Respir. J.* **13,** 571–576.

19. Jin, Z. and Roomans, G. M. (1998) X-ray microanalysis of uterine epithelial cells in culture. *Micron* **28,** 453–457.

20. Dragomir, A., Andersson, C., Åslund, M., Hjelte, L., and Roomans G. M. (2001) Assessment of chloride secretion in human nasal epithelial cells by X-ray microanalysis. *J. Microsc.* **203,** 277–284.

21. Abraham, E. H., Breslow, J. L., Epstein, J., Chang-Sing, P., and Lechene, C. (1985) Preparation of individual human diploid fibroblasts and study of ion transport. *Am. J. Physiol.* **248,** C154–C164.

22. von Euler, A. and Roomans, G. M. (1991) X-ray microanalysis of cAMP-induced ion transport in cystic fibrosis fibroblasts. *Cell Biol. Int. Rep.* **10,** 891–898.

23. Hall, S. R., Sigee, D. C., and Beesley, J. E. (1992) Scanning X-ray microanalysis of microcarrier cultured endothelial cells: elemental changes during the transition to confluency and the effect of ionophore A23187. *Scanning Microsc.* **6,** 753–763.

24. James-Kracke, M. R., Sloane, B. F., Shuman, H., Karp, R., and Somlyo, A. P. (1980) Electron probe analysis of cultured vascular smooth muscle. *J. Cell. Physiol.* **103,** 313–322.

25. Warley, A., Cracknell, K. P., Cammish, H. B., Twort, C. H., Ward, J. P., and Hirst, S. J. (1994) Preparation of airway smooth muscle cells for study of element concentrations by X-ray microanalysis. *J. Microsc.* **175,** 143–153.

26. Zierold, K., Hentschel, H., Wehner, F., and Wessing, A. (1994) Electron probe X-ray microanalysis of epithelial cells: aspects of cryofixation. *Scanning Microsc.* **(Suppl) 8,** 117–127

27. Zierold, K. (1997) Effects of cadmium on electrolyte ions in cultured rat hepatocytes studied by X-ray microanalysis of cryosections. *Toxicol. Appl. Pharmacol.* **144,** 70–76.

28. Zierold, K. (2000) Heavy metal cytotoxicity studied by electron probe X-ray microanalysis of cultured rat hepatocytes. *Toxicol. In Vitro* **4,** 557–563.

29. Warley A. (1987) X-ray microanalysis of cells in suspension and the application of this technique to the study of the thymus gland. *Scanning Microsc.* **1,** 1759–1770.

30. Fernandez-Segura, E., Canizares, F. J., Cubero, M. A., Campos, A., and Warley, A. (1999) A procedure to prepare cultured cells in suspension for electron probe X-ray microanalysis: application to scanning and transmission electron microscopy. *J. Microsc.* **196,** 19–25.

31. Hall T. A., Anderson, H. C., and Appleton, T. (1973) The use of thin specimens for X-ray microanalysis in biology. *J. Microsc.* **99,** 177–182.

32. Roomans, G. M. (1990) X-ray microanalysis, p. 347–412. In *Biophysical electron microscopy* (Hawkes, P. W. and Valdrè, U., eds.). Academic Press, London.

23

ENU Mutagenesis of Rat Mammary Epithelial Cells

George Stoica

1. Introduction

Studies of the rat mammary carcinogenesis model have provided useful information on the mechanisms of human breast cancer. The rat model demonstrated that chemical carcinogens are causative agents of mammary cancer and that initiation of cancer requires the interaction of the carcinogen with an undifferentiated and proliferating mammary gland. Comparative studies between humans and rodents have allowed us to determine that mammary cancer originates in undifferentiated terminal structures of the mammary gland. The terminal ducts of the Lob 1 of the human female breast have many points in common with the terminal end buds (TEB) of the rat mammary gland. Both the TEB in the rat and the Lob 1 in women are the site of origin of ductal carcinoma (*1*). Consequently, investigating the mechanisms involved in human breast cancer in an established rat animal model is a necessity. Various in vitro assays have been designed to understand the mechanisms of chemically induced neoplastic transformation of mammary gland epithelial cells.

Successful neoplastic transformation of rat mammary gland epithelial cells in vitro has been reported by only a few laboratories. This was initially described by Brennan et al. (*2*) and Dao and colleagues (*3*) using organ cultures of rat mammae and the carcinogen 7,12-dimethylbenzanthracene (DMBA) and by Richards and Nandi (*4*) and Greiner et al. (*5*) using rat mammary gland cell cultures and the carcinogen DMBA or N-methyl-N-nitrosourea (MNU). It is well known that DMBA and MNU are potent genotoxic rat mammary gland carcinogens in vivo (*6*).

From: *Methods in Molecular Biology, vol. 188: Epithelial Cell Culture Protocols*
Edited by: C. Wise © Humana Press Inc., Totowa, NJ

Previous reports have demonstrated that N-ethyl-N-nitrosourea (ENU) is an active rat mammary gland genotoxic carcinogen in vivo *(7,8)*. ENU, like MNU, is a potent alkylating agent and, in contrast to certain other carcinogens, for example DMBA, it acts directly without the necessity of enzymatic activation. Since the half-life of ENU is very short, it is considered to act relatively rapidly both in vivo and in vitro *(8,9)*. Possible cellular targets for ENU are DNA, various species of RNA and a variety of proteins *(10–13)*.

Because of the well recognized need for the development of an in vitro system of neoplastic transformation of rat mammary epithelium and the acknowledged difficulties encountered to date in the developments of such systems *(14–19)*, we felt it is important to examine whether or not ENU could serve as a model carcinogen in such a system. The impetus for this quest was derived primarily from reports documenting the potency of ENU as a rat mammary gland carcinogen in vivo *(7,8)* and additional reports showing that ENU is an effective in vitro carcinogen when applied to nonepithelial cell types, i.e., rodent fibroblasts and neurogenic cells *(20,21)*.

2. Materials

2.1. Source and Isolation of Cells

1. Female Sprague-Dawley rats, 50 d-old, specific-pathogen-free (Charles River Laboratories, Wilmington, MA).
2. Concave glass plate.
3. Sterile scalpels.
4. 100-mL Erlenmeyer flask.
5. Dissociation media: Dulbecco's modified eagles medium (DMEM) (Life Technologies), supplemented with 0.1% collagenase (Worthington Biochemical Company), 100 I.U. penicillin, 100 µg/mL streptomycin (Life Technologies).
6. Gyratory water bath.
7. Nylon mesh, 74 µm opening (Cistron, Elmsdorf, NY).
8. 60-mm Petri dishes.
9. Growth medium: DMEM supplemented with 25% horse serum, 20 ng/mL hydrocortisone (Sigma), 20 ng/mL ovine prolactin (Sigma), 20 ng/mL insulin (Sigma), 10 ng/mL epidermal growth factor (Collaborative Research), 100 I.U. Pencillin, 100 µg/mL Streptomycin.
10. 0.25% trypsin, 0.02% EDTA (Life Technologies).

2.2. Carcinogen Pulse

1. ENU crystals (Pfaltz and Bauer, Stamford, CT).
2. Phosphate citrate-buffered saline at pH 4.2.
3. Serum-free DMEM.
4. Hank's-buffered saline solution (HBSS) (Life Technologies).
5. Tissue culture flasks (T25 and T75) (Life Technologies).

2.3. Flow Cytometric Determination of Cellular DNA Content

1. 0.05 mg/mL Propidium iodide in 0.1% sodium citrate.
2. Rat peripheral blood leukocytes.
3. Coulter Epics V MDADS system (Hialeah, FL).

2.4. DNA Synthesis

1. (^{3}H)-Thymidine (1 mCi/mL, specific activity 6.7 mCi/mg; New England Nuclear, Boston, MA).
2. 5% Trichloracetic acid (TCA).
3. 0.2 M Sodium hydroxide.
4. Scintillation counter (Beckman).

2.5. Cell Counts

1. Trypan blue.
2. Hemocytometer.

2.6. Chromosome Analysis

1. 0.04 mg/mL Colcemid (Life Technologies).
2. Methyl alcohol, absolute, reagent grade.
3. Glacial acetic acid, reagent grade.
4. Pasteur pipettes with rubber bulbs.
5. Precleaned microslides, 3 × 1 inch thickness 0.96–1.06 mm.
6. Giemsa blood stain.

2.7. Colony Formation

1. Agar solution I: DMEM, 2% sea plaque agarose (FMS, Marine Colloids Division, Rockland, ME), 25% horse serum, 0.2% bicarbonate.
2. Agar solution II: DMEM, 0.33% sea plaque agarose, 25% horse serum, 0.2% bicarbonate.

2.8. Tumorgenicity

1. Female athymic nude mice (Harlan Sprague-Dawley, Madison, WI).

2.9. Histology

1. 10% Buffered formalin.

2.10. Mycoplasma Testing

1. Hoescht Stain 33258 (Calbiochem-Behring).

3. Methods

3.1. Source and Isolation of Cells

1. Obtain epithelial cells from primary normal mammary glands from the whole mammary fat pad (inguinal and axillary) of 50-d-old female rats by previously described techniques (22).

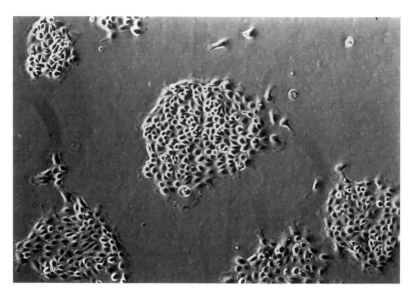

Fig. 1. Inverted microscopic appearance of pure cuboidal epithelial colonies after 2 mo in culture.

2. Transfer the tissue to a concave glass plate and mince with crossed sterile scalpels.
3. Place the finely minced tissue in a 100-mL Erlenmeyer flask containing 50 mL dissociation media and incubate at 37°C in a gyratory water bath for 40 min.
4. Filter the cell suspension through one layer of a 74-μm opening nylon mesh.
5. Plate cells out in a 60-mm Petri dish containing growth medium (*see* **Note 1**).
6. Incubate the cells in a humidified 10% CO_2 atmosphere at 37°C.
7. At 12-h intervals, remove the suspended cells from each dish and place in another dish (*see* **Note 2**).
8. This process should be repeated 5 times (enrichment of epithelial cells).
9. For further separation of epithelial and mesenchymal components, differential trypsinization (gradually increasing trypsin concentrations from 0.01 to 0.20%) can be applied for 2–10 min.
10. A mechanical separation procedure using a rubber policeman should be carried out to remove any mesenchymal components that are unaffected by trypsin.
11. After 2 mo, you should have dishes enriched with pure cuboidal epithelial colonies (*see* **Note 3** and **Figs. 1** and **2**).

3.2. Carcinogen Pulse

1. Dissolve ENU crystals in phosphate citrate-buffered saline. This should be freshly made each time.
2. Add the ENU to passage 3 epithelial cells, in serum-free medium (*see* **Note 4**), at 25, 50, 100, and 500 μg/mL.
3. After 2 h, remove the supernatant and wash the cells twice with HBSS.
4. Plate out in growth medium.

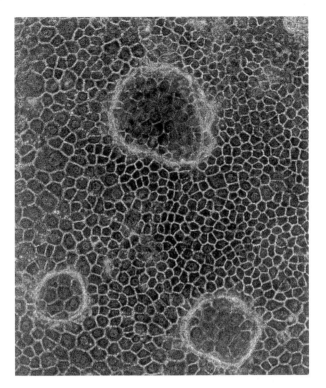

Fig. 2. Inverted microscopic appearance of confluent normal mammary epithelial cell cultures showing a cobble stone-like pattern with dome formation.

5. Monitor the morphologic appearance of the cell cultures by phase contrast micro-scopy and record photographically (*see* **Note 5**). Multiple stage of in vitro neoplastic transformation of rat mammary epithelial cells is schematically represented in **Fig. 3**.

3.3. Flow Cytometric Determination of Cellular DNA Content

1. Dilute primary cultures of passage 3 rat mammary epithelial cells to 1×10^6 in hypotonic propidium iodide solution *(23)*.
2. Treat some peripheral blood leukocytes (PBL) and a suspension of freshly disag-gregated rat mammary tissue cells in an identical manner, to determine where the 2C peak occurs in the DNA histograms.
3. Samples with greater than 1% cell clumps should be discarded.
4. Measure fluorescence using a Coulter Epics V MDADS system.
5. The argon-ion laser should emit light at 488 nm, and the output power should be set so that the 2C peak occurs in channel number 6. The coefficients of variation for the PBL and mammary cells should be 3 and 3.2%, respectively.
6. Collect data for each sample, such that 10,000 cells are counted in the peak expo-sure (1–4 d after ENU treatment), at 0, 50, 100, and 500 µg ENU/mL of culture medium (*see* **Fig. 4**).

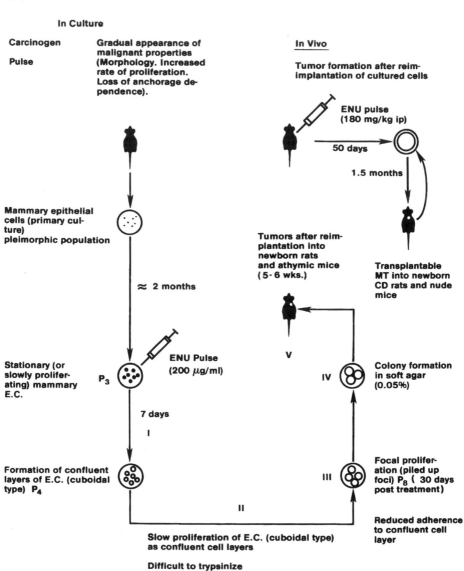

Fig. 3. Diagrammatic representation of the in vitro–in vivo system for ENU-induced mammary epithelial cell neoplastic transformation.

3.4. DNA Synthesis

1. Seed out Primary cultures of rat mammary epithelial cells (passage 3) onto 60 mm Petri dishes at a concentration of 7×10^5/mL.
2. Two days after seeding, when the cells have reached approximately 50–60% confluency, add ENU to the culture media in concentrations of 0, 25, 50, and 100 µg ENU/mL.

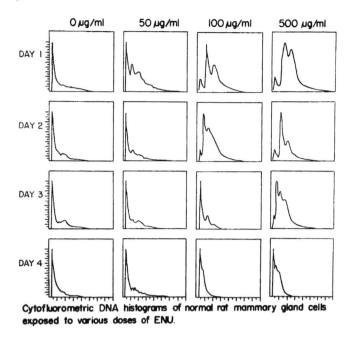

Cytofluorometric DNA histograms of normal rat mammary gland cells exposed to various doses of ENU.

Fig. 4. Temporal cytometric DNA histogram following the addition of ENU to the normal mammary epithelial cultures.

3. Pulse-label 3 dishes from each dose level with (^{3}H) thymidine 1, 2, 3, 4, and 5 d after ENU treatment.
4. One hour after (^{3}H)-thymidine treatment, trypsinize the cells, and process for the (^{3}H)-thymidine analysis.
5. Rinse the cells several times with HBSS.
6. Incubate with 5% TCA at 37°C for 1 h.
7. Centrifuge at 4430g for 15 min at 4°C.
8. Dissolve TCA-insoluble material in 0.2 M NaOH for 15 min at 37°C.
9. Transfer aliquots of the 0.2 M NaOH extract to scintillation vials and count in an aqueous counting scintillation fluid with a scintillation counter.

3.5. Cell Counts

1. Count 3 dishes from each dose level using the Trypan blue exclusion technique and a hemocytometer at 24-h intervals up to 120 h.

3.6. Chromosome Analysis

1. Chromosome analysis should be performed according to established methods *(24–26)* with minor modifications.
2. Briefly, treat cells in a logarithmic phase of growth with colcemid for 1 h.
3. Harvest with trypsin.

4. The cell suspension should then be centrifuged at 114 g for 10 min.
5. Remove the supernatant and, without disturbing the pellet, add distilled water.
6. Resuspend the cell pellet in the water.
7. Incubate at 37°C for 15 min.
8. Fix the cells in methanol:glacial acetic acid (3:1v:v) for 15 min.
9. Prepare slides by dropping the cell suspension from a narrowed Pasteur pipet onto a glass slide.
10. The slide preparation should then be rapidly air-dried.
11. Keep the slides in an oven at 65°C for 2 d.
12. G-banding can be performed by a modification of the method used by Yunis *(26)* with a trypsinization time of approximately 15 s.
13. Chromosomal aberrations should be scored according to World Health Organization standards *(27,28)*.
14. Perform the experiment in duplicate and for each sample of 5×10^6 cells per group, and include controls.
15. For each sample, 100 metaphases should be scored (*see* **Note 6**).

3.7. Colony Formation and Cloning in Semisolid Agar Medium

1. Determine the ability of rat mammary epithelial cells to form colonies in agar by the method described by MacPherson *(29)* with minor modifications.
2. The basal layer should contain 5 mL of agar solution I .
3. A second layer (1.5 mL) agar solution II containing 7.5×10^4 mammary epithelial cells should be added to each dish.
4. Incubate the mammary epithelial cells at 37°C in a 6% CO_2 atmosphere.
5. Five to six weeks after plating, count all colonies greater than 0.1 mm in diameter and greater than 40 cells/colony.
6. Cloned sublines (greater than 1 µm in diameter colonies) can be obtained by aspiration of single colonies from the cloning medium with a Pasteur pipet, followed by tripsinization for 1 to 2 min then transferred to a 60-mm Petri dish for further examination in culture.

3.8. Tumorigenicity

1. Inoculate suspensions of ENU exposed and control cells ($1 \times 10^6/0.05$ mL of culture medium) subcutaneously (s.c.) into the mammary gland fat pad of each of 10 newborn isologous female rats or 2-mo-old female athymic nude mice.
2. All rats and mice must be examined 3× weekly for progressively growing tumors at the site of inoculation.
3. Five to six weeks after cell inoculation, sacrifice the animals, and surgically excise all palpable nodules and tumors.
4. Prepare these for cell culture, electron microscopy, and/or histological analysis .

3.9. Histology

1. Fix tissues in 10% buffered formalin.
2. Embed in paraffin and section at 5 µm.
3. Stain with hematoxylin and eosin (H & E).

3.10. Mycoplasma Testing

1. All cell cultures must be screened with the use of Hoechst 33258 stain for the presence of mycoplasma contamination by the procedures used by Chen *(29)*.

3.11. Statistics

1. Quantitative changes must be assessed for significance by the 2-way analysis of variance followed by Duncan's multiple range post-test. Changes are considered significant at $p<0.05$.

4. Notes

1. Hormonal and epithelial growth factor supplementation of primary mammary tissue cultures is necessary to maintain and stimulate cell replication in vitro. The DMEM media contains 25% horse serum for the first 5 cell passages. This horse serum concentration greatly increases the epithelial cell replication when compared with the fetal bovine serum supplementation.
2. Initially, the cells and cell aggregates should be plated at high density into 60-mm Petri dishes. After 10 h, the dishes should be examined under an inverted microscope. There will be cells in suspension, aggregates, and ductular structures, some of them resembling closely rat mammary TEB. From these structures, the mammary epithelial cell colonies will later develop.
3. At 12-h intervals, the suspended cells, aggregates, and TEB should be removed by decanting to another dish. This process can be repeated several times. The initial dishes usually contain (attached) mesenchymal cells, but in the subsequent dishes, epithelial colonies start growing. Most of the epithelial colonies develop from cell aggregates and TEB, which attach to the bottom of the dishes between 24–72 h post-seeding. Ten days later, multiple epithelial colonies of various sizes surrounded by mesenchymal cells can be recognized in several dishes, mostly in dishes that have been seeded at later time periods. Using a marker objective mounted on the inverted Nikon microscope, the epithelial colonies can be identified, and then mesenchymal cells can be removed using a rubber policemen and differential trypsinization. These procedures should be repeated several times until only epithelial colonies remain. Confluency in culture dishes will be reached in 2 mo. Once growth is established, the cells are transferred to T_{75} flasks and maintained as previously described. Epithelial cells strongly attach to the dishes for the first passages and, therefore, are difficult to remove by trypsinization entirely. The mammary epithelial cells are not totally removed from the parental flasks initially, remaining colonies are maintained as an original source for future subcultures in case of cell loss. The medium should be changed every other day. The epithelial cells are characterized by a cuboidal shape forming a typical "cobblestone" appearance with dome formation (*see* **Figs. 1** and **2**).
4. ENU is a genotoxic chemical carcinogen, and safety procedures should be considered for human protection and proper neutralization and disposal of chemical and objects used during this procedure. A container with 2% sodium hydroxide

solution for neutralization of carcinogen and contaminated instruments should be at hand. Individuals handling this carcinogen should use plastic gloves, mask, goggles and protective gown.

5. Morphological changes characteristic of rat epithelial cell transformation are related to increased rates of proliferation, temporal increases in multinucleated cells, and loss of anchorage dependence and dome formation.

6. Exposure of mammary epithelial cells to ENU results in many cytogentic changes, most abundant are chromatid and isochromatid exchanges, trisomy of chromosome 10, double minutes, and loss of sex chromosomes (*see* **Table 1**). These changes are carcinogen dose-dependent, and the higher the concentration, the more abundant the chromosomal changes. However, after recovery from the carcinogen treatment, the neoplastic transformed mammary epithelial cells maintain a near diploid chromosomal pattern.

References

1. Russo, J. and Russo, I. H. (1993) Developmental pattern of the human breast and susceptibility to carcinogenesis. *Eur. J. Cancer Prev.* **3,** 85–100.
2. Brennan, M. J. (1976) Murine and rat mammary tumors as models for the immunological study of human breast cancer. *Cancer Res.* **36,** 728–733.
3. Dao, T. L. and Sinha, D. (1972) Mammary adenocarcinoma induced in organ culture by 7,12dimethybenzanthracene. *J. Natl. Cancer Inst.* **49,** 591–593.
4. Richards, J. and Nandi, S. (1978) Neoplastic transformation of rat mammary cells exposed to 7,12-dimethylbenzanthracene or N-nitrosomethylurea in cell culture. *Proc. Natl. Acad. Sci. USA* **75,** 38–68.
5. Greiner, J. W., Dipaolo, J. A., and Evans, C. H. (1983) Carcinogen-induced phenotypic alterations in mammary epithelial cells accompanying the development of neoplastic transformation. *Cancer Res.* **43,** 273–278.
6. Welsch, C. W. (1985) Host factors affecting the growth of carcinogen induced rat mammary carcinomas: a review and tribute to Charles Brenton Huggins. *Cancer Res.* **45,** 3415–3443.
7. Stoica, G., Koestner, A., and Capen, C. (1983) Characteristics of N-ethyl-N-nitrosourea induced mammary tumors in the rat. *Am. J. Pathol.* **110,** 161–169.
8. Stoica, G., Koestner, A., and Capen, C. (1984) Neoplasms induced with high single doses of N-ethyi-N-nitrosourea in 30–day-old Sprague-Dawley rats with special emphasis on mammary neoplasia. *Anticancer Res.* **4,** 5–12.
9. Gichner, T. and Veleminsky, J. (1982) Genetic effects of N-methyl-N'-nitro-N-nitrosoquanidine and its homologs. *Mutation Res.* **99,** 129–242.
10. Singer, B. (1979) N-nitroso alkylating agents: formation and persistence of alkyl derivatives in mammalian nucleic acids as contributing factors in carcinogenesis. *J. Natl. Cancer Inst.* **6,** 1329–1339.
11. Druckrey, H. (1973) Chemical structure and action in transplacental carcinogenesis and teratogenesis, p. 45. In *Transplacental carcinogenesis, publication no. 4.* International Agency for Cancer Research, Lyon.
12. Magee, P. N., Barnes, J. M. (1969) Carcinogenic nitroso compounds. *Adv. Cancer Res.* **10,** 163–246.

Table 1
Effect of ENU Treatment In Vitro on Chromosomes of Rat Mammary Epithelial Cells (P$_4$ and P$_5$)

Dose ENU (μm/mL)	Modal Number or Chromosomes (range)	Percent of Cells with Chromosome Aberrations (range)	Types of Chromosome Abberations/100 cells				
			Single Chromatid Breaks	Isochromatid Breaks	Chromosomal Exchanges	Multiple Cromosomal Breaks	Double Minutes
Control	38(36–60)	9(8–10)	4	5	0	0	0
ENU added 6 h before harvest							
25	38(28–60)	15(14–16)	6	9	0	0	0
50	38(26–80)	25(20–30)	5	10	5	3	2
100	48(28–90)	45(40–50)	20	10	5	5	5
200	40(26–90)	50(48–52)	30	15	0	5	5
ENU added 24 h before harvest							
25	38(28–60)	10(9–11)	10	0	0	0	0
50	44(24–60)	12(10–14)	5	3	2	0	2
100	50(28–90)	25(24–26)	10	2	10	0	3
200	52(26–96)	27(17–29)	12	4	10	0	1
500	MI	0	0	0	0	0	0

MI = Mitotic inhibition.

13. Rice, J. M. (1973) An overview of transplacental chemical carcinogenesis. *Teratology* **8,** 113–135.

14. Franks, L. M. and Wigley, C,B. (1979) *In vitro* transformation in the respiratory tract, p. 137–162. In *Neoplastic transformation in differentiated epithelial cell systems in vitro* (Franks and Wigley, eds.). Academic Press, New York.

15. Fusenig, N., Breitkreutz, D., Boukamp, P., Lueder, M., Irmscher, G., and Worst, P. K. M. (1979) Chemical carcinogenesis in mouse epidermal cultures: altered expression of tissue specific functions accompanying cell transformation, p. 37–98. In *Neoplastic transformation in differentiated epithelial cell systems in vitro* (Franks and Wigley, eds.). Academic Press, New York.

16. Indo, K. and Maivaji, H. (1979) Neoplastic transformation and abnormal differentiation in foetal rat keratinizing epidermal cells in culture, p. 99–112. In *Neoplastic transformation in differentiated epithelial cell systems in vitro* (Franks and Wigley, eds.). Academic Press, New York.

17. Kuroki, T., Drevon, C., Saint Vincent, L., and Montesano, R. (1979) Properties of the IAR-series of liver epithelial cells transformed by chemical carcinogens, p. 173–188. In *Neoplastic transformation in differentiated epithelial cell systems in vitro* (Franks and Wigley, eds.). Academic Press, New York.

18. Stimmerhaves, I. C. (1979) Influence of donor a-c on *in vitro* transformation of bladder epithelium, p. 137–162. In *Neoplastic transformation in differentiated epithelial cell systems in vitro* (Franks and Wigley, eds.). Academic Press, New York.

19. Wigley, C. B. (1979) Transformation *in vitro* of adult mouse salivary gland epithelium; a system for studies on mechanisms of initiation and promotion, p. 3–6. In *Neoplastic transformation in differentiated epithelial cell systems in vitro* (Franks and Wigley, eds.). Academic Press, New York.

20. Au, W., Soukup, S. W., and Mandybur, T. I. (1977) Excess chromosome #4 in ethylnitrosourea-induced neurogenic tumor lines of the rat. *J. Natl. Cancer Inst.* **59,** 1709–1716.

21. Laerum, O. and Rajaewsky, M. E. (1975) Neoplastic transformation of fetal rat brain cells in culture after exposure to ethylnitrosourea *in vivo*. *J. Natl. Cancer Inst.* **5–5,** 1177–1187.

22. Stoica, G., Koestner, A., and O'Leary, M. (1985) Characteristics of normal rat mammary epithelial cells and N-ethyl-N-nitrosourea-induced adenocarcinoma cells grown in culture. *Anticancer Res.* **5,** 499–510.

23. Krishan, A. (1975) Rapid flow cytofluorometric analysis of mammalian cell cycle by propidium iodide staining. *J. Cell Biol.* **66,** 188–193.

24. Levan, G. and Mitleman, F. (1976) G-banding analysis in a serially transplanted Rous rat sarcoma. *Hereditas* **80,** 140–145.

25. Wooranooj, U. and Hsu, T. C. (1972) The C- and G-banding patterns of *Rattus norvegicus*. *J. Natl. Cancer Inst.* **49,** 1425–1431.

26. Yunis, J. J. (1981) New chromosome techniques in the study of human neoplasia. *Hum. Pathol.* **12,** 450–549.

27. Buckton, K. E. and Evans, H. J. (1973) Methods for the analysis of human chromosome aberrations. *World Health Organization,* 18–22.
28. Commitee for a Standard Karyotype of *Rattus norvegicus.* (1973) Standard karyotype of the Norway rat *Rattus norvegicus. Cytogenet. Cell Genet.* **12,** 199–205.
29. Chen, T. R. (1977) In situ detection of mycoplasma contamination in cell cultures by Hoechst 33258 stain, *Cell Res.* **104,** 255–262.

24

ENU-Induced Ovarian Cancer

George Stoica

1. Introduction

Carcinogenesis, in both humans and experimental animals, is recognized to represent a multistep process involving a sequence of morphophenotypical changes, which may lead to malignant transformation. Various in vivo and in vitro models were developed to better mechanistically understand specific aspects of carcinogenic process. N-Ethyl-N-nitrosourea (ENU) is recognized as a potent direct-acting neurocarcinogen in a variety of rat strains *(1)*. One rat strain, Berlin Druckrey (BD-IV), has been observed to be relatively resistant to the development of neural tumors following transplacental administration of ENU *(2,3)*. Few data have been reported on the effect of ENU in young BD-IV rats. It was reported that ENU administered intraperitoneally (i.p.) (90 mg/kg) to BD-IV 30-d-old female rats increased the incidence to up to 50% of an uncommon ovarian tumor with testicular characteristics (Sertoli cell tumor of the ovary) compared to controls (3%) *(4)*. The ovarian tumors in BD-IV rats exceeded in incidence all other tumors encountered in this strain.

Similar tumors have been described in the ovary of humans *(5)* and animals *(6)*, including mice, rats, agoutis, shrews, mares, Indian Deshi hens, and cats. In mice, mares, and Indian Deshi hens, these ovarian tumors have been associated with virilizing changes. In rats, these tumors were reported to be associated with an excess of sex steroid hormone secretion *(4)*.

Sertoli cell tumors are classified as sex cord stromal tumor with uncertain histogenesis. In general, it is believed that this type of tumor developed from pluripotential stem cells located in the hilus region of the ovary. In tissue culture, these tumor cells show an epithelial phenotype that resembles that of granulosa cells of the ovary. Although granulosa cells are considered epitheliod rather than epithelial cells (because they do not line a body surface or lumen

From: *Methods in Molecular Biology, vol. 188: Epithelial Cell Culture Protocols*
Edited by: C. Wise © Humana Press Inc., Totowa, NJ

that is continuous with the external surface), the facts that they are avascular, are formed by layers of cells that rest on a basal lumina, and function as epithelial cells make them a valid model for carcinogenesis studies.

In vitro characterization of rat Sertoli cell tumors of the ovary has not been reported. One of the ENU-induced Sertoli cell tumors of the ovary in BD-IV rats (adenoma), derived from a nonsteroid hormone-producing tumor was cultured and maintained as a continuous cell line.

This chapter describes the procedures used to monitor in vitro malignant transformation of these cells (derived from an ENU-induced adenoma of the ovary) with regard to their growth requirements, morphological characteristics, DNA content, karyotype, and transplantation potential.

2. Materials

2.1. Animals and Treatments

1. Female BD-IV rats, 30 d old (Harlan Industries) (*see* **Note 1**).
2. ENU crystals (Fluka).
3. Phosphate/citrate-buffered saline, pH 4.2.

2.2. Isolation of Cell Cultures

1. Sterile scalpel blades.
2. Scissors .
3. Concave glass.
4. Hank's-buffered saline solution (HBSS), pH 7.0–7.2.
5. Erlenmayer flask (50 mL).
6. Enzyme solution: Dulbecco's modified Eagle's medium (DMEM) (Life Technologies), 0.1% collagenase (Sigma), 1% penicillin–streptomycin.
7. 37°C Gyratory water bath.
8. Nylon mesh (74 µm).
9. Centrifuge tubes (15 mL).
10. Growth medium for primary cultures: DMEM, 25% horse serum (Life Technologies), 20 ng/mL hydrocortisone (Sigma), 20 ng/mL insulin, 20 ng/mL prolactin, penicillin–streptomycin.
11. Growth medium for established cell lines: DMEM, 10% horse serum, glutamine, 1% penicillin–streptomycin.
12. 0.25% Trypsin, 0.02% EDTA.
13. 60-mm Plastic Petri dishes.
14. T_{75} Tissue culture flasks.
15. Needles (18 G).

2.3. Flow Cytometric DNA Distribution Analysis

1. Coulter Epics V MDADS system (Hialeah, FL).
2. 0.05 mg/mL Propidium iodide in 0.1% sodium citrate.

2.4. Chromosome Analysis

1. 12.5 µg/mL Colcemid stock (Life Technologies).
2. Methanol, alcohol, absolute, reagent grade.
3. Glacial acetic acid, reagent grade.
4. Pasteur pipets with rubber bulbs (*see* **Note 3**).

2.5. Anchorage-Dependant Growth

1. Agar solution I: DMEM, 2% sea plaque agarose (FMS Corporation, Marine Colloids Division, Rockland, ME), 25% horse serum, 0.2% bicarbonate.
2. Agar solution II: DMEM, 0.33% sea plaque agarose, 25% horse serum, 0.2% bicarbonate.

2.6. Oncogenicity

1. Pentobarbital.
2. Ketamine hydrochloride.

3. Methods
3.1. Animals and Treatments

1. Innoculate a group of 30 female, 30-d-old, specific-pathogen-free BD-IV rats, i.p. with 90 mg/kg of ENU crystals freshly prepared before administration in phosphate/citrate-buffered saline at pH 4.2 *(4)* (*see* **Notes 1** and **2**).

3.2. Isolation of Cell Cultures

1. After a latency period of 320 d post ENU inoculation, isolate the Sertoli cell tumor (adenoma) from the rat. The histology of this tumor is illustrated in **Fig. 1**.
2. Tissue (about 50 mg) from the core of this nonsteroid hormone-producing Sertoli cell tumor should be removed and transferred to a concave glass.
3. Mince the tissue in 0.5 mL of HBSS with crossed scalpels.
4. The finely minced tissue should then be placed in a 50-mL Erlenmayer flask containing 25 mL enzyme solution.
5. Place the flask in a 37°C gyratory water bath for 40 min.
6. Filter the cell suspension through one layer of 74–µm nylon mesh.
7. Centrifuge the filtrate at 100g twice to remove cell debris.
8. Resuspend the resulting pellet in 4 mL of growth medium for primary cultures.
9. Plate the cells at 5×10^5 into 60-mm dishes and incubate in a humidified 6% CO_2 incubator at 37°C.
10. Once growth is established, the cells need to be transferred to T_{75} flasks.
11. At later passages (after P_{10}), the established Sertoli cell tumor line (SCTL-1) should be maintained in growth medium for established cell lines.
12. To subculture, dissociate the cells with 0.25% trypsin containing 0.02% EDTA.
13. Incubate with trypsin for 3 to 5 min at 37°C.
14. Study the morphology of the cultured cells (*see* **Fig. 2**) using an inverted microscope.

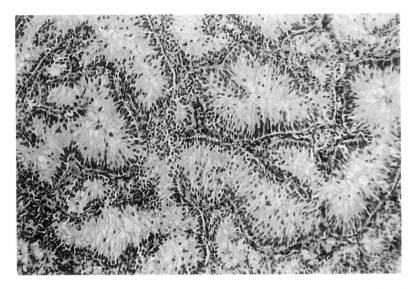

Fig. 1. Characteristic histologic tubular pattern of ENU-induced Sertoli cell tumor of the ovary in BD-IV rats. (H&E, ×40).

15. Calculate the population doubling time by expressing the cell number as a function of $\log_2$ by the multiplication of the common logarithm of the cell count by the factor 3.33. The formula used for the calculation of population doubling time is:

$$\text{Number of population doublings} = \log_{10}(N/N_0) \times 3.3$$

where N is the number of cells in the growth plate at the end of a period of growth, and N_0 is the number of cells planted in the growth plate *(7)(see* **Note 4**).

3.3. Flow Cytometric DNA Distribution Analyses

1. This can be carried out on the nonsteroid cell line (SCTL-1) at various passages from 1 to 20.
2. Obtain monocellular suspensions by syringing.
3. Propidium iodide at a working concentration of 0.05 mg/mL in 0.1% sodium citrate is used as the DNA intercalating fluorochrome *(8)*.
4. Measure fluorescence using a Coulter Epics V MDADS system.
5. Use normal nonstimulated rat lymphocytes from peripheral blood as standards.
6. The frequency distribution histograms of cellular DNA content obtained from cultured SCTL-1 cell line is illustrated in **Fig. 3**.

3.4. Chromosome Analysis

1. Chromosome analysis can be performed on cell line SCTL-1 at various passage numbers (for example passages 2, 10, and 20).
2. Add colcemid (0.4 mg/mL) to cells grown in T_{75} flasks in a logarithmic phase of growth for 1 h.

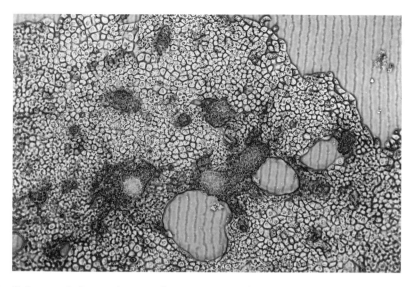

Fig. 2. Inverted phase microscopic appearance of cultured SCTL-1 at passage 20. The cells form a monolayer with densely packed cells in a cobblestone-like appearance.

3. Harvest with trypsin solution.
4. Centrifuge the cell suspension at 600*g* for 10 min.
5. Remove the supernatant and add a hypotonic solution (distilled water) without disturbing the cell pellet (*see* **Note 5**).
6. After adding the hypotonic solution, resuspend the pellet and incubate at 37°C for 15 min.
7. Fix the cells in methanol:glacial acetic acid (3:1, v/v) for 15 min.
8. To make the slides, drop the cell suspension onto the slides with a narrowed Pasteur pipet.
9. Air-dry the preparation (*see* **Note 6**).
10. G-banding was should be carried out by modifying the method used by Yunis *(9)* and using a trypsinization time of 15 s.
11. The chromosomes which are identified, should conform to the classification of normal rat chromosomes *(10)*.
12. Select a total of 50 metaphases from the SCTL-1 at random from various passage numbers and photograph (*see* **Note 7** and **Fig. 4**).

3.5. Anchorage-Independent Growth

1. The ability of the cultured Sertoli cell tumor of the ovary to form colonies in agar can be assessed by using the techniques described by MacPherson *(11)* with minor modifications.
2. Form the basal layer by placing of 5 mL agar solution I in 60-mm plastic dishes.
3. Add 1.5 mL of agar solution II, containing 7.5×10^4 cells/plate, to form the second layer.

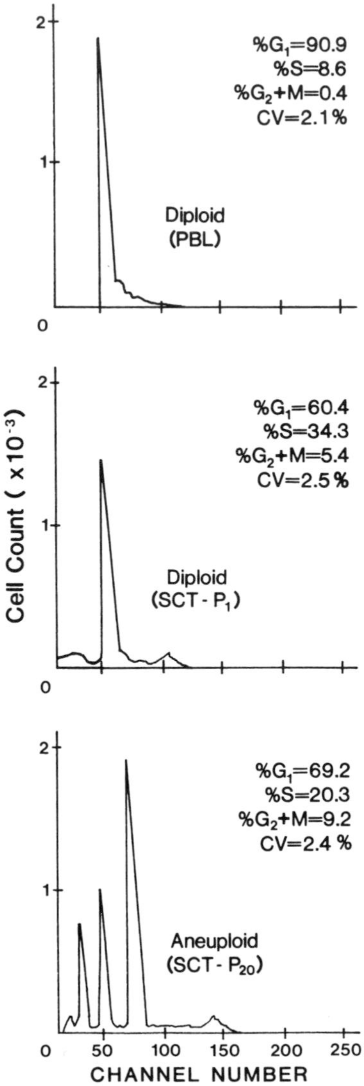

Fig. 3. Frequency distribution histograms of cellular DNA content obtained from cultured SCTL-1 at two passages; P_1, near diploid and aneuploid P_{20}. PBL = peripheral blood lymphocytes as a standard. Cellular DNA content is directly proportional to channel number.

4. Incubate plates at 37°C in an atmosphere of 10% CO_2.
5. After 5 to 6 wk, colonies greater then 40 cells can be counted using an inverted phase microscope.

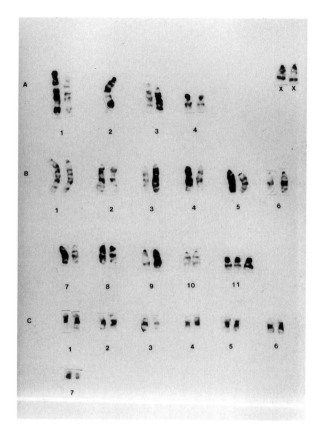

Fig. 4. Karyotyping of SCTL-1, P_{20}, G-banding. Nonrandom changes in 30% of the metaphases revealed the absence of one chromosome at the subtelocentric pair, two additional pairs of chromosomes, and a trisomy of 11 in the acrocentric group.

3.6. Oncogenicity

1. Innoculate newborn rats i.p. and nude mice with a subcutaneous (s.c.) injection of $1 \times 10^6/0.2$ mL cells at various passage numbers.
2. The animals inoculated with early passage cells should be observed for a period of 4 mo.
3. The animals inoculated with SCTL-1 after P_{10} will start to develop tumors after 2 to 4 wk (*see* **Fig. 5**).
4. Sacrifice the animal after a period of 4 wk, under anesthesia (80 mg/kg pentobarbital).
5. Record the intra-abdominal and subcutaneous tumors.
6. Save tissues for routine histology and culture (*see* **Notes 7–9**).

3.7. Morphological Studies

1. Sacrifice the experimental rats using pentobarbital overdose (180 mg/kg).
2. Perform a complete necropsy on each animal.

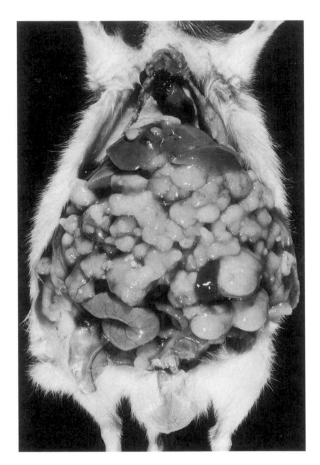

Fig. 5. Intra-abdominal disseminated nodular appearance 4 wk post-inoculation (ip) of transplanted SCTL-1, P_{20} into BD-IV rats.

3. Tissues for examination under light microscopy should be fixed in 10% buffered formalin or Bouin's solution.
4. Section at 4 to 6 μm, and stain with hematoxylin and eosin (H&E).
5. The morphohistologic characterization of Sertoli cell tumor has been previously reported *(13)*.
6. Tissue cultures should be examined and photographed under an inverted microscope.

4. Notes

1. The BD-IV breeding colony of rats is available in the laboratory of Dr. G. Stoica and is maintained at Texas A&M University, Lab Animal Facility.
2. ENU is a chemical carcinogen used in experimental animal carcinogenesis studies. These procedures are hazardous and should not be undertaken without the proper safeguards. Preparation of ENU solution should take place in a chemical hood. The investigators should wear gloves, a mask, and have a solution of

sodium hydroxide (2%) to neutralize the ENU, instruments, and other materials used in preparing the carcinogenic solution.

3. To obtain a better chromosomal spread, it is important to narrow the Pasteur pipets lumen at a flame of a Bunsen burner.

4. Spontaneous immortalized nontumorigenic rat (BD-IV) granulosa cells lines were also obtained and characterized and are available for future studies *(12)*. One cell line (SIGC) was transfected with early region genes of simian virus 40 (SV40) to generate fully transformed cell lines to study in vitro neoplastic transformation of granulosa cells.

5. Swelling of the cells is a critical step and is essential to achieve well-spread chromosomes. A variety of hypotonic solutions can be used. One of the most commonly used hypotonic solutions is 0.075 M potassium chloride, but in our hands, distilled water worked just fine. Treatment time can varies from one cell line to another, but 15–20 min was enough to obtain a good chromosomal spread.

6. Fixation is another critical step, and it always follows the hypotonic treatment. The fixative is usually made fresh and kept cold until use. It is recommended that half of the hypotonic solution should be removed, and then slowly add the fixative solution to prevent the cells from clumping. To insure complete fixation, the fixative is changed 3 to 4 times before drying the cells onto a slide. Cells are dropped onto slide with a Pasteur pipet, and the optimal height can be adjusted after several trials. Cells are spread by drying them onto a slide. Drying time can be manipulated by blowing on the slide or fanning the slide in the air.

7. Karyotyping of SCTL-1, P_{20}, G-banding revealed nonrandom changes in 30% of the metaphases. These changes consisted of the absence of one chromosome at the second subtelocentric pair, two additional pairs of chromosomes, and a trisomy of 11 in the acrocentric group.

8. The rat's earliest clinical sign post SCTL-1 cell inoculation is enlargement of the abdomen and ascites. Inoculated nude mice showed a nodular subcutaneous growth at the site of inoculation (back).

9. The inoculated rats or nude mice with cells under P_{10} did not develop any tumors after a 4-mo period of observation. Animals inoculated with cells after P_{10} developed tumors 2–4 wk post-inoculation. The rats developed multiple intra-abdominal tumors disseminated throughout the serosal surfaces of the peritoneum, diaphragm, and parenchymal organs (*see* **Fig. 4**). Usually, these fast growing tumors killed the hosts in 4 wk post-inoculation. Histologies of transplanted tumors were that of undifferentiated anaplastic carcinomas (*see* **Fig. 5**).

References

1. Rajewsky, M. F., Augenlicht, L. H., Biessmann, H., Goth, R., Husler, D. E., Lacrum, O. D., and Lomakina, L. Y. (1977) *Nervous-systemic-specific carcinogenesis by ethylnitrosourea in the rat: molecular and cellular aspects*, p. 709–726. (Hiatt, H. H., Watson, J. D., Winsten, J. A., eds.). CSH Laboratory Press, Cold Spring Harbor, NY.

2. Druckrey, H., Landschultz, C. H., and Ivankovic, S. (1970) Transplacentare erzeugung maligner tumoren des nervensystems. II. Ethyl-nitrosoharnstoff ein 10 genetisch definierten rattenstammen. *Z. Krebsforsch.* **73,** 371–386.

3. D'Ambrosio, S. M., Su, C., Channg, M. J. W., Oravec, C., Stoica, G., and Koestner, A. (1986) DNA damage, repair, replication, and tumor incidence in the BD-IV rat following administration of N-Ethyl-N-Nitrosourea. *Anticancer Res.* **6,** 49–54.

4. Stoica, G., Koestner, A., and Capen, C. C. (1985) Testicular (Sertoli's cell) like tumors of the ovary induced by N-ethyl-N-nitrosourea (ENU) in rats. *Vet. Pathol.* **22,** 483–491.

5. Ashley, D. J. B. (1978) *Evan's histological appearances of tumors, 3rd ed.,* p 663–672. Churchill, Livingston.

6. Cotchin, E. (1977) *Pathology of the female genital tract,* p. 836–838. (Blaustein, ed.). Springer, Berlin.

7. Pastan, T. H. (1973) Cell culture. Methods in enzymology, vol LVIII, p. 150. (Jakoby, ed.). Academic Press, New York.

8. Krishan, A. (1975) Rapid flow cytofluorometric analysis of mammalian cell cycle by propidium iodine staining. *J. Cell. Biol.* **66,** 188–193.

9. Yunis, J. J. (1981) New chromosome techniques in the studies of human neoplasia. *Hum. Pathol.* **12,** 540–549.

10. Unakul, W. and Hsu, T. C. (1972) The C- and G-banding patterns of *rattus norvegicus* chromosomes. *J. Natl. Cancer Inst.* **49,** 1425–1431.

11. MacPherson, I. (1972) Soft agar techniques, p. 276–280. *Tissue culture methods and applications.* (Kruse and Patterson, eds.). Academic press, New York.

12. Stein, L. S., Stoica, G., Tilley, R., and Burghardt, R. C. (1991) Rat ovarian granulosa cell culture: a model system for the study of cell-cell comunication during multistep transformation. *Cancer Res.* **51,** 696–706.

13. Stoica, G. and O'Leary, M. (1988) In vitro malignant transformation of in vivo ENU-induced rat ovarian Sertoli cell tumor (adenoma). *J. Cancer Res. Clin. Oncol.* **114,** 142–148.

25

Measurement of Membrane Capacitance in Epithelial Monolayers

Carol A. Bertrand and Ulrich Hopfer

1. Introduction

Biological membranes serve as physical barriers and electrical insulators to separate different aqueous compartments, such as the intracellular and extracellular environments. In electrical terms, membranes that separate highly conductive aqueous media represent capacitors. What makes this definition particularly useful to biologists is that the capacitance of a capacitor is proportional to its area. By measuring membrane capacitance, one can get an estimate of the actual area of a cell membrane. The proportionality constant sufficient for most biological membranes is 1 $\mu F/cm^2$ *(1)*.

Monolayers of epithelial cells, following the formation of tight junctions between adjacent cells, serve as macroscopic physical barriers and electrical insulators between different extracellular compartments in higher animals. The epithelial monolayer is a compound barrier because it consists of individual cells with their surrounding plasma membrane and specialized intercellular junctions (**Fig. 1A**). In culture, epithelial cells usually grow in a polarized fashion on a basement lamina of collagen or other matrix material. The tight junction between adjacent cells divides the plasma membrane of each polarized epithelial cell into an apical (or luminal) portion on the free surface and a basolateral one corresponding to the nutrient (or blood or serosal) side in vivo. The basolateral plasma membrane includes the surface in contact with the basement lamina and the lateral surface between cells. The space between cells is part of the paracellular route for transport and is termed the lateral intercellular space (LIS) (**Fig. 1A**). Macroscopic monolayers of epithelial cells forming barriers between aqueous compartments can be readily grown in cell culture

From: *Methods in Molecular Biology, vol. 188: Epithelial Cell Culture Protocols*
Edited by: C. Wise © Humana Press Inc., Totowa, NJ

A

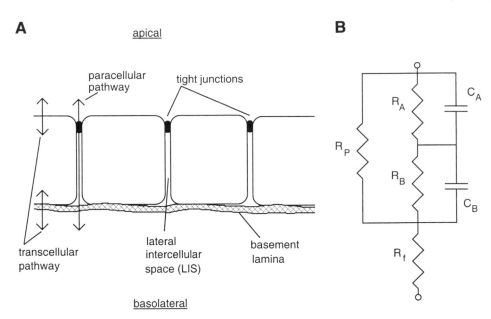

Fig. 1. Simplified model of an epithelial monolayer. (**A**) The apical membrane is shown at top, basolateral at bottom. Tight junctions connect the apical membranes of the individual cells, forming a barrier between the apical and basolateral environments. Movement of solutes and water may occur through a transcellular or a paracellular pathway. The basement lamina is a layer of connective tissue to which the cells attach; in cell cultured monolayers, this is typically a porous filter that has been coated with collagen. (**B**) Lumped-model of the intact epithelial monolayer. A refers to apical, B to basolateral, and P to paracellular pathways; R_f is the extracellular fluid resistance.

using inserts with porous filters. As the permeability or electrical conductivity of the monolayer (flow perpendicular to the plane of the monolayer) is proportional to monolayer area, it is common to normalize appropriate monolayer properties in terms of macroscopic filter area. The macroscopic area needs to be distinguished from the true microscopic area of apical or basolateral plasma membranes.

The technique for determining membrane or monolayer capacitance utilizes basic electrophysiology equipment and involves measuring voltage and current signals in response to an appropriate electrical stimulus. An understanding of basic transepithelial electrophysiology (*2*) is required during experimental setup. The equipment and protocol defined here are specific for confluent epithelial monolayers using external nonimpaling electrodes. The measurements allow the study of the dynamics of electrical properties of monolayers, including the short-circuit current (Isc), the DC resistance (R_{DC}), and monolayer capacitance. The methodology is applicable to monolayers that exhibit an R_{DC} of ≥200 Ωcm^2 (macroscopic area).

Measurement of monolayer membrane area can be performed under static or dynamic conditions. Static measurements are used to determine the actual microscopic areas of the basolateral and apical membranes. Dynamic measurements are used to track changes in membrane area, such as occur during exocytosis and endocytosis. The primary difference between the two is how quickly a measurement needs to be performed, or how constant the monolayer must remain during the course of the measurement. This is crucial: all current methods of measuring membrane capacitance assume the value remains constant during the measurement cycle. When this assumption fails, erroneous data can be produced even though the system may appear to be functioning correctly. A review of different methods for measuring capacitance *(3–8)* reveals a wide range of complexity in describing the monolayer and generating an appropriate measurement scheme, some suitable for static measurements and others suitable for dynamic tests. The technique described below has been designed specifically to measure dynamic changes in membrane capacitance and utilizes a fast measurement cycle.

1.1. Impedance Analysis Theory

The technique of measuring membrane capacitance is more commonly referred to as impedance analysis because the monolayer contains ion channels and other alternate pathways for ionic flux in addition to capacitance. These components act together as an impedance that shapes the time-dependence (or in its equivalent expression the frequency-dependence) of the current-voltage relationship of the monolayer. As an epithelial monolayer is a compound barrier, the first step in impedance analysis is the definition of a suitable model that accounts for the components. These models use resistors to define conductive pathways through the monolayer and capacitors to define the membranes of the monolayer. The model used by our system is shown in **Fig. 1B**. It consists of 3 resistors to describe pathways of ionic flux through the monolayer (apical, basolateral, and paracellular) and 2 capacitors to describe the membranes across which a potential exists (apical and basolateral). The paracellular resistance (R_p) is the sum of the tight junction and LIS resistances, which can change independently. The component R_f is also included in our model to account for the resistance of the fluid between the electrodes and monolayer. The value of R_f can be measured; the other 5 components are parameters to be calculated from the impedance measurements.

The impedance of the model (Z_T) can be mathematically calculated without ambiguity from its 5 known components and R_f (*see* **Note 1**). It can be described in two equivalent ways, either as a function of time or complex frequency. Complex frequency expressions transform time domain derivatives to simple multiplications and are used in this technique. We can calculate the impedance of the monolayer by measuring simultaneously and over time the current I(t) through and voltage V(t) across it in response to a suitable electrical pulse:

$$Z_x(s) = FFT\ [V(t)]/FFT\ [I(t)]$$

where FFT = fast Fourier transform. Having defined Z_T and measured V and I, the parameters of Z_T can be determined using a nonlinear least squares parameter estimation routine. The routine compares the error between the model-derived $Z_T(s)$ and the experimental $Z_x(s)$ and then determines the magnitude and direction to adjust each parameter of $Z_T(s)$ to reduce the error, proceeding iteratively to the best-fit parameters.

The stimulus signal needs to provide frequency information in the range of maximum component sensitivity, and be of short duration to meet the demands of a dynamic measurement. Component sensitivity can be determined by plotting the partial derivatives of $Z_T(s)$, or Jacobians, with respect to each parameter using approximate component values of real monolayers (3); typically epithelial monolayers fall within the range of 10 Hz – 10 kHz. To achieve this frequency range in a short measurement cycle, the stimulus signal should be a composite of different frequencies generated simultaneously (5). A simple way to generate a wide band of frequencies in a short time interval is to use a square pulse as a stimulus signal.

1.2. Practical Impedance Analysis

The application of impedance analysis to capacitance measurement involves several practical considerations. The most serious of these involves the number of parameters that can be uniquely estimated. The model described by **Fig. 1B** is perhaps the simplest model for an intact epithelial monolayer, yet all 5 of its parameters cannot be estimated from transcellular measurements alone. We are missing information about the intracellular potential, the critical node that involves 4 of our 5 parameters. This limitation can be demonstrated mathematically by examining the impedance equation Z_T. Z_T depends on 3 polynomial coefficients (N1, N0, and D1; *see* **Note 1**) that, in turn, involve sums and products of parameters. We can estimate the polynomial coefficients, but additional information would be required to uniquely identify all of the parameters (*see* **Note 2**). It is not necessary to identify the parameters in many circumstances, however, as the coefficient N1 is directly related to total monolayer capacitance.

When the 5 parameter model of **Fig. 1B** adequately describes the epithelial monolayer, $N1^{-1}$ gives the serial combination of apical and basolateral capacitance (C_T). Because of this serial arrangement, C_T will be dominated by the smaller of the 2 capacitances, typically the apical membrane (C_A). In cases where the basolateral capacitance (C_B) $\geq 5 \times C_A$, C_T provides a good measure of the changes in apical membrane area. The 5 parameter model is adequate for epithelial monolayers that meet the following criteria (3): (i) the parameters do not vary as a function of the voltage, frequencies, or duration of the stimulus signal; (ii) the cell monolayer is a homogeneous population of cells; (iii) the LIS do not contribute significantly (< 10%) to the paracellular resistance.

Electrical noise is always present during transepithelial measurements, causing deviations in voltage and current readings that result in noisy experimental data. While the calculation of impedance from component or polynomial values is straightforward and unambiguous, the inverse process of estimating polynomials from noisy experimental data is difficult and can give erroneous results. Noise will cause a finite difference to exist between $Z_T(s)$ and $Z_x(s)$ even when the estimated parameters are exact. Noise is dealt with by first minimizing external and equipment sources. Next, multiple measurements are taken, and these results are averaged to improve signal to noise ratio. Finally, the remaining noise is measured as a standard deviation at each of the measurement frequencies ($\sigma[s]$), and these values are used as weights in parameter estimation. Weights are used to normalize the errors between $Z_T(s)$ and $Z_x(s)$, which are due to noise (9):

$$\text{normalized error} = [Z_T(s) - Z_x(s)]/\sigma(s)$$

The number of measurements to average in a dynamic system is a trade-off between improving signal to noise and maintaining a short measurement interval.

Data collected on voltage clamped monolayers will exhibit an offset or bias value whenever Isc $\neq 0$, which is typically the case for dynamic measurements. Isc is effectively a constant during the measurement interval, and its value will cause an error in the DC component of $Z_x(s)$. To correct for this error, R_{DC} is measured with a simple pulse and its value is substituted for the DC component of $Z_x(s)$. This has the additional benefit of simplifying the model equations (see **Note 1**).

2. Materials

2.1. Basic Electrophysiology Equipment

1. Capacitance measurement is performed using a transepithelial electrophysiology rig controlled with a data acquisition card (see **Subheading 2.2.**). The standard rig consists of a University of Iowa Bioengineering Model 558-C-5 epithelial voltage clamp and pulse generator modules with separate preamplifier (Department of Biomedical Engineering, University of Iowa, Iowa City, IA; http://www.engineering.uiowa.edu/~bme/contact.html).

2. Ussing-type chamber for horizontally mounted filter inserts (Analytical Bioin-strumentation, c/o Department of Physiology and Biophysics, Case Western Reserve University, Cleveland, OH, 44106–4970) with a conventional 4-electrode system.

3. Shielded cables for all signal connections especially between the Ussing chamber, preamplifier, and voltage clamp. Maintaining a low-noise environment is important for accurate membrane capacitance measurements, and a grounded work area or Faraday cage is highly recommended. Auxiliary equipment (i.e., perfusion pump) may also contribute noise and should be isolated if possible; the easiest solution if auxiliary equipment noise is a problem is to shut it down during the measurement cycle (approximately 5 s). Monolayers of cultured cells are routinely tested for adequate R_{DC} and potential before experiments under sterile conditions using a Millicell ERS Voltohmmeter (Millipore, Bedford, MA).

2.2. Impedance Data Acquisition

1. Measuring capacitance requires a stimulus pulse and acquisition pattern not typically provided with standard electrophysiology. The 558-C-5 permits external control, and this feature is exploited to use the voltage clamp and its interface to the monolayer with minimal additional hardware (see **Note 3**). The basic components needed are a multifunction data acquisition (A/D) card, an interface between the A/D card and the 558-C-5, a computer, and software to control the card. A suitable A/D card is the National Instruments PCI-6024E (Austin, TX); a terminal box that allows easy connection to the A/D card can also be purchased. Four connections are made between the 558-C-5 and the A/D card, three directly and the fourth through a filter and attenuator (see **Note 4**). The voltage clamp's measured voltage and current are connected to analog input channels, and the pulse generator external trigger is connected to a counter. The stimulus pulse, also generated by a counter on the A/D card, is low-pass filtered (4-pole Butterworth filter with $f_c = 11$ kHz) and attenuated (-36 dB, from 5 V to 80 mV) before connection to the voltage clamp external command input. It is possible to assemble a filter and attenuator from standard components, however a commercial filter–attenuator could be used (i.e., Frequency Devices Model ASC-50, Haverhill, MA). The personal computer requires a PCI slot to accept the A/D card, but other requirements are minimal. Processor speed and storage requirements will depend on the software design and whether analysis is to be performed on the same computer.

2. There is no commercial source of software for performing data acquisition for monolayer impedance analysis at this time, and most users generate their own custom program (see **Note 5**). The specific program requirements are as follows. The overall sample rate for analog acquisition is 49,152 samples/s (see **Note 6**); with 2 channels sampled, the individual channel rate is half the overall rate. The total number of points collected is 4500, or 2250/channel; 2^N points will be used in the FFT. The stimulus pulse is started after a delay of 400 samples and lasts 2 samples, for an effective pulse width of 40.69 μs. After the 4500 points are collected, the data is converted to voltages and stored in temporary arrays. This

sequence is repeated 8 times, with each additional data sweep summed with the previous data. Once completed, the values in the temporary arrays are divided by 8 to compute the average of the sweeps. During each sweep, the order of channel acquisition is reversed to average out the phase error caused by the finite sampling interval. Once the impedance measurement is completed, measurement of R_{DC} is performed. First a pulse is generated to trigger the 558-C-5 pulse generator. A 500 μs pulse is sufficient. Following a trigger, the 558-C-5 delays pulse generation for a time interval equal to the set pulse duration; 1 s is required for the acquisition settings below (a bipolar pulse is used, for a total pulse time of 2 s). After an 800-ms wait, analog acquisition is started with an overall sample rate of 80 samples/s. Total samples (200) are collected or 100/channel. After data collection, the values are converted to voltages and concatenated with the impedance data, then stored to disk. The process is repeated at a user-adjustable interval, with a minimum interval of 5 s. The data is saved in raw form and processed off-line.

2.3. Impedance Data Analysis

Data analysis is performed using commercial math-processing software such as MathCAD (Mathsoft, Cambridge, MA) or Matlab (Mathworks, Natick, MA). The program used must be able to read the raw data files, perform FFT, and perform weighted nonlinear least squares parameter estimation. Complex numbers are used in the estimation routine. It is highly desirable for the program to have graphing capabilities and macro or programming options for simplifying repeated tasks. Note that spreadsheet programs are not usually sophisticated enough to handle the required mathematics without extensive user-written programs.

3. Methods

The performance of a new capacitance measurement system must be validated. This involves ensuring that the epithelia to be studied comply with model limits, tests to assess and minimize noise, and optimization of the parameter estimation routine. These preliminary tests are only required following major changes to equipment, type of epithelium or cell line, or environment. Once the system is validated, a typical experiment involves 2 stages: (*i*) collecting data during the desired experiment with an epithelial monolayer; and (*ii*) performing the parameter estimation to extract monolayer and possibly membrane capacitance values. With a fast computer and some programming skill, these 2 stages can also be interleaved to provide membrane capacitance values in real time.

3.1. Preliminary Tests

1. The epithelia to be tested should be well characterized by conventional means prior to capacitance measurements *(3)*.

2. Electron micrographs of sectioned monolayers provide information on the appearance of the LIS and relative membrane areas, and how these may be affected during a specific protocol.
3. Transepithelial electrophysiology will determine the variation of R_{DC} and Isc during a specific protocol; when combined with membrane permeabilization, the relative contributions of R_A or R_B to R_{DC} can be assessed. These data can be used to determine an expected range of component values that will assist in optimizing the parameter estimation.
4. A dummy load should be constructed using resistors and capacitors in the expected ranges to further validate the system.
5. Using the dummy load in place of the monolayer, collect data as described in **Subheading 3.2.** for noise assessment. Be sure all equipment that would normally be used (heater, perfusion pump) is operating.
6. Process the data through **Subheading 3.3., step 2**. A plot of the standard deviations (σ) vs frequency will indicate any noise problems that exist. By repeating the test with or without specific equipment, noise sources can be identified. For optimum performance, (σs) should be <5% of $Z_x(s)$, although greater σ at 2 or 3 frequencies (i.e., power line) will be accounted for by weighting.
7. The parameter estimation routine can be tested and optimized at 2 levels with known data: using equation-generated data and dummy load data. Because equation-generated data is inherently noisefree, it is primarily used to test that the algorithm is correctly implemented. Dummy load data should be used to assess the impact of noise and starting guesses on algorithm performance *(3)*. With noisy data, it is usually necessary to incorporate limits on the range of solutions the parameter estimation routine may try. Limits are assigned based on physical laws and preliminary tests of the epithelia: (*i*) parameters must be positive; (*ii*) R_P and the sum of $R_A + R_B$ must each be >R_{DC}; (*iii*) C_A and C_B must be > macroscopic monolayer area; and (*iv*) $C_A < C_B$. Starting guesses will also impact the estimation success, and viable ranges can be determined with dummy load data. During a typical experiment, only the first data set needs a starting guess; succeeding data sets should use the last set's results as a starting point.
8. The parameter estimation routine will require tolerance criteria to determine when it has successfully determined the parameters. Noisy data should use both a relative and function tolerance. Relative tolerance specifies the allowable difference between $Z_T(s)$ and $Z_x(s)$, while function tolerance specifies the difference between successive parameter guesses. Both should be minimal, 10^{-5}, or better. Once a set of parameters is estimated, the overall fit of the data must be assessed *(9)*. This involves examining the residuals or error terms between $Z_x(s)$ and $Z_T(s)$ with the given parameter set. The sum of the weighted residuals squared should be approximately the number of residuals minus the number of parameters for a good fit *(9)*. The weighted residuals should have a normal distribution, and a runs test should indicate no patterns in the distribution of residuals versus frequency *(10)*. If the runs test or distribution consistently deviates for dummy load data, a voltage clamp or processing bias error should be suspected and corrected for. If this occurs

with monolayer data, it usually signifies that the model is inadequate to describe the epithelia. This may occur at specific points in a given protocol, for example, when monolayer parameters are changing too rapidly for the measurement interval. Estimated results that fail any of these tests lack statistical significance.

3.2. Data Collection

1. Verify that the monolayer to be tested has sufficient R_{DC} (≥ 200 Ωcm^2, macroscopic area).
2. Before inserting the monolayer in the Ussing chamber, measure fluid resistance (R_f) of the solutions to be used and compensate for electrode offsets. R_f can be recorded from the 558-C-5, but *Fluid Res Comp* must be set to zero during the experiment.
3. Set the 558-C-5 voltage clamp time constant to 0.5 ms, the pulse generator period to 50 s, the duration to 1 s, the amplitude to 2.0 mV, and mode to bipolar.
4. Mount the monolayer in the Ussing chamber.
5. Apply short-circuit voltage clamp, and allow Isc and R_{DC} to stabilize. It is convenient to use a strip chart recorder to monitor Isc during the course of the experiment; this avoids hardware and software conflicts with the capacitance measurement system.
6. Set the 558-C-5 pulse generator period to manual, and start the capacitance measurement software.
7. Collect at least 10 measurements under baseline conditions over the course of several min to use in calculating noise weights (e.g., use a measurement interval of 30 s).
8. Proceed with the desired experimental protocol, e.g., stimulation of exocytosis. At this stage, the capacitance measurement software controls the voltage clamp and is continuously sampling and saving data at the desired intervals and requires no user intervention.

3.3. Parameter Estimation

1. Calculate $Z_x(s)$ and R_{DC} for each data set (the 2 separate measurements are concatenated into one data set during acquisition and should be separated first).
2. To calculate $Z_x(s)$, take the FFT of $V(t)$ and $I(t)$ and divide the array $V(s)$ by $I(s)$. Optimally, the FFT should be performed on arrays of size 2^N *(9)*; $V(t)$ and $I(t)$ should be truncated from their original length of 2250 points to 2048 points by discarding the first 196 and last 6 points. Note that the first 196 points occur before the stimulus pulse is applied. $Z_x(s)$ will be a complex array of 1025 points, including a zero (DC) element and 1024 frequency elements ranging from 12 Hz to 12 kHz in 12 Hz increments (*see* **Note 6**). R_{DC} is calculated from the averaged voltage and current levels occurring during the steady-state portions of the bipolar pulse; in performing the averaging, use both the positive and negative excursions to eliminate bias errors:

$$R_{DC} = |(\Sigma V^+ - \Sigma V^-)/(\Sigma I^+ - \Sigma I^-)|$$

Substitute the value of R_{DC} for the zero element of $Z_x(s)$ to eliminate its bias error.

3. Calculate the standard deviations of the 10 baseline measurements using the corresponding arrays of $Z_x(s)$, and assign as weights.

4. Determine a suitable starting guess for the first data set. The estimation routine will require guesses for N1, N0, and D1. Since preliminary information is usually in the form of component values, the corresponding coefficients should be calculated from the equations in **Note 1**. Viable starting guesses depend on the type of tissue being studied. A manual fit of the data can be helpful in determining a starting guess: compare curves of $Z_x(s)$ and $Z_T(s)$ while adjusting the parameter values. An initial guess could be $C_A = 1.5 \times$ macroscopic area; $C_B = 10 \times C_A$; $R_P = 2 \times R_{DC}$, $R_A = R_B = R_{DC}$. Approximate relative ratios between components should be known from preliminary tests and substituted accordingly.

5. Estimate the parameters N1, N0, and D1 for all the data sets. The Levenberg-Marquardt nonlinear weighted least squares algorithm *(9)* is well suited for this purpose. Both the real and imaginary components of the complex impedance must be used; the components can be concatenated. Include the weights calculated in step 2, and the limits determined from preliminary tests. Some packaged algorithms may give the option of estimating the Jacobians (partial derivatives) of the model equation rather than having the user derive and supply them. The algorithm will run quicker and potentially with fewer errors if given the actual Jacobians; use a symbolic processor to calculate them from the equation for $Z_T(s)$ in **Note 1**. The Jacobians will also indicate the range of frequencies over which the polynomial coefficients are most sensitive, given a set of parameter values. If the parameters exhibit no sensitivity past a certain frequency, including higher frequency data will not improve the quality of the data fit. Optimally, the algorithm should be run in a loop for all data sets, with each set's results passed on as a starting guess for the next data set.

6. Verify the fits as described in **Subheading 3.1. step 8.** Plots of C_T and R_{DC} versus time can be generated.

7. Nyquist or Bode plots of the impedance of any particular data set can be plotted using the $Z_x(s)$ data array; these types of plots do not require parameter estimation results. These plots can also be used to determine the accuracy with which additional processing, such as range analysis or parameter calculations may be performed.

8. If additional information has been gathered about one component (*see* **Note 2**), the others can be solved from the polynomial coefficient equations (*see* **Note 1**) using a nonlinear equation solver. This is especially true when Nyquist plots indicate that 2 distinct semicircles or poles are evident. In these cases, the apical parameters are distinct from the basolateral parameters.

9. Note that the appearance of more than 2 distinct semicircles in a Nyquist plot indicates that the model (**Fig. 1B**) is insufficient.

10. Be aware that whatever tolerances apply to the "known" component must be applied to all components solved using its value. Caution should be exercised in assuming that any component remains constant throughout the course of a dynamic measurement protocol.

4. Notes

1. The model equations used by this method are listed below *(3)*. Note that no capacitance is assigned to the tight junction membrane area, as its contribution is typically negligible compared to the apical membrane area. Measurement of R_{DC} reduces the unknown parameters to 4, but also reduces the number of unique polynomial coefficients to 3.

$$Z_T(s) = (N1 \times s + N0)/(s^2 + D1 \times s + [N0/R_m]) + R_f$$

where

$$N1 = (1/C_A) + (1/C_B)$$

$$N0 = ([1/R_A] + [1/R_B])(1/C_A C_B)$$

$$D1 = N1 \times ([1/R_m] - [1/\{R_A + R_B\}]) + (1/R_A C_A) + (1/R_B C_B)$$

$$R_m = ([1/R_P] + [1/\{R_A + R_B\}])^{-1} = R_{DC} - R_f$$

2. In order to estimate the individual components, the value of at least one must be known. This is typically accomplished through an auxiliary measurement involving permeabilization of one membrane *(11)* or a microelectrode measurement of intracellular potential *(6,7)*, or even an educated guess. These techniques are problematic when applied to a dynamic protocol, where parameters are expected to change during the course of the experiment. If the auxiliary measurement is performed at the end of an experiment, the user must verify that the result is applicable during dynamic behavior. Applying an auxiliary measurement throughout the course of an experiment may perturb the normal response of the monolayer. Useful information about individual parameters is often available by using range analysis *(3)*, which can be performed without additional measurements.

3. A substitute for the 558-C-5 can be used if it meets the following. As a minimum, the voltage clamp must have an external command input and measured voltage and current outputs. It must have a reasonably constant frequency response from DC to 10 kHz, i.e., the measured voltage signal divided by the measured current signal must equal a constant resistance over this frequency range. The voltage clamp should have a pulse generator that can be externally triggered for performing DC measurements. The pulse generator function can be implemented in the software, which controls the A/D card, and applied to the external command signal in lieu of triggering an external device. If performed in software, additional interface hardware may be required to change the R_{DC} pulse amplitude independent of the stimulus pulse amplitude. Differences to be aware of when substituting voltage clamps include scaling factors of the input and output signals and delays in the response to external triggers. All signals on the 558-C-5 are scaled 10×.

4. The physical connections between the 558-C-5 front panel BNC connectors and the PCI-6024E connector are as follows. E OUT connects to analog input channel 0 (ACH < 0,8> for differential input), connector pin 68 (+) and 34 (–). I OUT

connects to analog input channel 1 (ACH <1,9>), connector pin 33 (+) and 66 (–). Unused analog input channels should be grounded to avoid spurious noise transmissions, connect pins 23–32, 57–61, and 63–65 together. TRIG IN connects to the output of counter 1 (GPCTR1_OUT), pin 40 (+) and 39 (ground). The stimulus signal is output from counter 0 (GPCTR0_OUT), pin 2 (+), and 36 (ground). The above signal names and pin numbers are derived from the connector schematic in the documentation accompanying the PCI-6024E A/D card.

5. The authors have posted their program code (in Microsoft Visual C++) for performing the basic measurement procedure on the Internet site: (http://physiology. cwru.edu/~hopfer/model.htm.) This code uses the National Instruments program NIDAQ, a library of functions for programming National Instruments A/D cards. The program uses NIDAQ functions to generate a delayed counter pulse and perform a scanned analog acquisition. It achieves synchronization by assigning SCANCLK, a signal generated during each analog acquisition, to the stimulus pulse counter's clock. The counter will wait until the analog acquisition starts, then generate a pulse at precisely the same moment during analog acquisition each time it is called. This synchronization allows averaging the measurements of consecutive scans to decrease noise. Because of this dependency, the width of the stimulus pulse is set by the scan rate used for analog acquisition. This value is critical, as it determines the frequency content applied to the monolayer. After impedance data acquisition, a trigger pulse and acquisition cycle for R_{DC} data are performed.

6. The sample rate of 49,152 samples/se is used to achieve a frequency interval of 12 Hz, which results in frequency samples at the fundamental and harmonic components of a 60 Hz power system. Sampling at the power system frequencies combined with weighted estimation allows us to minimize power line noise. The sampling rate should be adjusted for different power line systems, i.e., 40,960 samples/s for a 50 Hz power line. The stimulus pulse width should be changed accordingly (a stimulus pulse of 2 samples at 40,960 samples/s = 48.8 μs).

Acknowledgments

We thank Dr. Mike Butterworth and Chris Sciortino for helpful discussions during the preparation of this manuscript. The research was supported by a grant from the Cystic Fibrosis Foundation to U.H. and the National Instutes of Health training grant no. T32 DK07678.

References

1. Cole, K. S. (1968) *Membranes, ions, and impulses*. University of California Press, Berkeley.
2. Lewis, S. A. (1996) Epithelial electrophysiology, p. 93–117. In *Epithelial transport: a guide to methods and experimental analysis* (Wills, N., Reuss, L., and Lewis, S. A., eds.), Chapman & Hall, London.

3. Bertrand, C. A., Durand, D. M., Saidel, G. M., Laboisse, C., and Hopfer, U. (1998) System for dynamic measurements of membrane capacitance in intact epithelial monolayers. *Biophys. J.* **75,** 2743–2756.
4. Clausen, C. and Fernandez, J. M. (1981) A low-cost method for rapid transfer function measurements with direct application to biological impedance analysis. *Pflügers Arch.* **390,** 290–295.
5. Clausen, C. and Wills, N. K. (1981) Impedance analysis in epithelia, p. 79–92. In *Ion transport* (Schultz, S. G., ed.), Raven Press, New York.
6. Kottra, G. and Frömter, E. (1984) Rapid determination of intraepithelial resistance barriers by alternating current spectroscopy II: test of model circuits and quantification of results. *Pflügers Arch.* **402,** 421–432.
7. Kottra, G. and Frömter, E. (1984) Rapid determination of intraepithelial resistance barriers by alternating current spectroscopy I: experimental procedures. *Pflügers Arch.* **402,** 409–420.
8. Lewis, S. A. and Alles, W. P. (1984) Analysis of ion transport using frequency domain measurements. *Curr. Top. Membr. Transport* **20,** 87–103.
9. Press, W. H., Flannery, B. P., Teukolsky, S. A., and Vetterling, W. T. (1986) *Numerical recipes: the art of scientific computing,* first ed. Cambridge University Press, Cambridge.
10. Straume, M. and Johnson, M. L. (1992) *Analysis of residuals: criteria for determining goodness-of-fit.* Methods in enzymology, vol. 210. Academic Press, New York.
11. Wills, N. K., Lewis, S. A., and Eaton, D. C. (1979) Active and passive properties of rabbit descending colon: a microelectrode and nystatin study. *J. Membr. Biol.* **45,** 81–108.

26

Assessing Epithelial Cell Confluence by Spectroscopy

Simon A. Lewis

1. Introduction

There is an increasing use of epithelial cells grown on tissue culture supports. Such tissue culture systems are used to study the cellular mechanisms involved in protein and lipid sorting between the two series membranes, which comprise the polarized epithelia cell, the molecular biology of transporter assembly, and the study of transporter associated proteins. By necessity, these studies start after the tissue culture cells reach confluence and form tight junctions.

Tight junction formation, as a function of time post-seeding, can be assessed using a number of techniques. All techniques rely on the measurement of the movement of selected substances from one tissue culture compartment (e.g., the lumen) to the opposing compartment (the plasma). The method used should be noninvasive, simple to implement and measure, accurate, low cost, and with minimal risk of contaminating the tissue culture cells. Thus, the use of radioisotopes is precluded due to cost of the isotopes and risk of contamination (multiple sampling and multiple washes to remove isotopes from both sides). In addition, long-term ionizing radiation might alter gene expression in these cells. The most frequently used method is electrical in nature. In brief, one passes a square current pulse (ΔI) across the epithelium and measures the resulting voltage response (ΔV). Using Ohm's law, one then calculates the conductance ($\Delta I/\Delta V$). This method is rapid and simple to implement. However, it can be inaccurate and can increase the chance of infection of the culture system. The increased probability of contamination is introduced by placing voltage measuring and current passing electrodes into both the lumen and plasma compartments. The inaccuracy of the measurement is due to nonuniform current fields caused by the point source nature of the current passing electrodes (for a

From: *Methods in Molecular Biology, vol. 188: Epithelial Cell Culture Protocols*
Edited by: C. Wise © Humana Press Inc., Totowa, NJ

more complete description, see Fig. 7 of **ref. *1***). The extent of the inaccuracy is a function of the positioning of the voltage measuring electrodes around the circumference of the tissue culture insert, as well as the positioning of the current passing electrodes. It is important to stress that the transepithelial conductance represents the tight junction conductance in parallel with the transcellular conductance. Thus, the transepithelial conductance is an overestimate of the tight junction conductance. In addition, the transepithelial conductance gives an estimate of the ability of small ions to move across the epithelium, but does not permit the measurement of low concentrations of large molecules.

The purpose of this chapter is to describe in detail a simple and inexpensive method for determining the formation of tight junctions in tissue culture epithelial monolayers. In addition, the data collected from the described method will allow for the calculation of fluid flow across the epithelium.

This paper will attempt to describe not only the method of using phenol red as an indicator of epithelial confluence, but also the assumptions that are inherent in the method. The advantages of the method are speed, expense, and low probability of contamination. The disadvantage is poor time resolution (particularly for low conductance epithelia).

2. Materials

The underlying principle of the method is the measurement of the movement of a substance between the two compartments formed by the epithelium. The substance to be used to measure tight junction formation should meet the following criteria: (*i*) the substance must be non-toxic to the epithelial cells; (*ii*) the tissue culture cells should not metabolize or synthesize the substance; (*iii*) the presence or absence of the substance in the tissue culture medium should not alter cell growth or viability; and (*iv*) the measuring system for the substance must be simple, possess a high signal-to-noise ratio, and be highly selective for the substance. Most (if not all) of the above criteria can be met by phenol red. Phenol red, a pH indicator, is used in almost all commercially available tissue culture medium. There are no reports that it is toxic to epithelial cells. Phenol red-free tissue culture medium does not alter tight junction formation or growth of A6 epithelial cells (*S. A. Lewis, personal communication*). Phenol red is not metabolized or synthesized by epithelial cells (no reports), nor does it alter cell growth or viability (*see* above). The concentration of phenol red in solution can be determined by measuring solution absorbance using a spectrophotometer, and then dividing the measured absorbance by the extinction coefficient for phenol red (*see* below). Alternately, one can generate a standard curve of phenol red absorbance vs concentration (by measuring the absorbance of known concentrations of phenol red), and then use this curve and measured absorbance of the sample to determine the phenol red concentration.

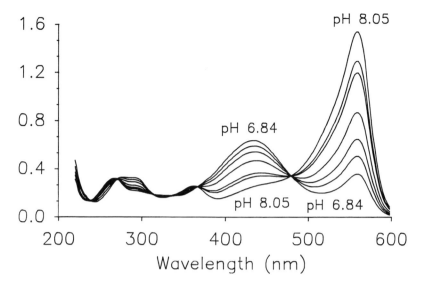

Fig. 1. This figure shows the effect of pH on the absorbance properties of phenol red. Note that pH alters the absorbance magnitudes at all visible wavelengths (wavelength greater than 390 nm) except for 479 nm. It is this wavelength at which one measures the absorbance of the luminal solution. The absorbance was measured on a LKB Ultraspec II using the LKB scan program (reproduced from Jovov et al., 1991, *[1]* with permission from *Am. J. Physiol.*).

Because phenol red is a pH indicator, its absorbance properties will be a function of the pH of the solution. This is shown in **Fig. 1**, where the absorbance spectrum for phenol red was measured at a number of solution pH values. Of interest, there is one wavelength (479 nm) in the visible spectrum at which the absorbance of phenol red is not pH sensitive, this is the isosbestic point. To avoid the problem of pH-dependent absorbance, one should make all absorbance measurements at 479 nm. The extinction coefficient (a constant that relates absorbance to concentration) for phenol red is 8450 L/mol/cm. The extinction coefficient allows one to calculate the concentration of phenol red in a solution from the absorbance measured in a spectrophotometer using a cuvet with a known path length. Cuvettes typically have path lengths of 1 or 0.5 cm, thus the longer the path length the larger the measured absorbance.

The question of signal-to-noise ratio is readily addressed. The absorbance spectrum of tissue culture medium (containing phenol red) at wavelengths greater than 450 nm is not different than a saline solution containing the same concentration of phenol red. In addition, epithelia cells do not seem to produce any substance with a significant absorbance at 479 nm. Thus, the signal-to-noise ratio is very favorable for phenol red measurements at 479 nm.

2.1. Cell Culture

1. Amphibian DMEM: Dulbecco's modified Eagle's medium (DMEM) containing 8 mM NaHCO$_3$ (Life Technologies) supplemented with 40 mU/mL penicillin, 40 µg/L streptomycin, and 10% fetal bovine serum (FBS) (Hyclone Laboratories). This medium contains phenol red.
2. Phenol red-free solution: either of the following can be used:
    a. NaCl bathing solution: 74.4 mM NaCl, 5.36 mM KCl, 1.36 mM CaCl$_2$, 1.66 mM MgSO$_4$, 8 mM NaHCO$_3$, 0.91 mM NaH$_2$PO$_4$, 5.55 mM glucose, 1 mM sodium pyruvate, 1 mM HEPES, pH 7.4.
    b. DMEM without phenol red (Life Technologies, special order), supplemented as amphibian DMEM.
3. A6 Cells: renal epithelial cells from *Xenopus Laevis*.
4. Plastic disposable cuvets (quartz cuvets can also be used).
5. Permeable supports: Millicell-HA, Millicell-CM (Millipore) and Anocell (Anotek Separations, Banbury, UK).

3. Method

3.1. Cell Culture

This section will describe the method in a stepwise manner and will assume that you have the appropriate expertise in tissue culture methods.

1. Seed A6 epithelial cells onto a permeable support *(2)*, bathed in amphibian DMEM.
2. Place in the tissue culture incubator and allow to attach and start growing.
3. The medium contains phenol red. The absorbance of this tissue culture medium should be measured.
4. Twenty four hours post-seeding, remove the luminal medium.
5. Wash the luminal compartment 4 to 5 times with phenol red-free solution.
6. Incubate for 10 min in phenol red-free solution.
7. Over the 10-min period, phenol red will diffuse from the plasma compartment into the luminal compartment.
8. After 10 min, remove both the luminal solution and plasma solution.
9. Place in separate cuvets and measure the absorbance of the luminal solution and plasma solution at 479 nm in a spectrophotometer.
10. Record the individual values.
11. Wash both lumen and plasma compartments fresh amphibian DMEM (which contains phenol red) and place the cells back into the incubator.
12. Follow the above protocol for the next few days.
13. As an example, in A6 cells **steps 4–11** can be performed every day for the first 4 d.
14. For d 5 and 6, the incubation time in luminal phenol red-free solution should be increased to 1 h.
15. On d 6, replace the lumen solution with phenol red-free tissue culture medium, while the plasma compartment should remain in the amphibian DMEM with phenol red (*see* **Note 1**).

16. After 6 d, remove the lumen solution and plasma solution for absorbance measurements during the normal feeding schedule of the cultured cells.
17. Thus, after d 6, the luminal medium used to feed the cells does not contain phenol red.
18. In experiments on A6 cells, this feeding schedule is typically every 2 or 3 d (*see* **Note 2**).
19. For a quantitative estimate of the phenol red flux and phenol red permeability, the absorbance of the luminal compartment should not exceed 3–10% of the plasma compartment.

3.1. Phenol Red Flux and Permeability

Using the above procedure, the flux of phenol red can be calculated from the absorbance measured in the spectrophotometer, using the equation that relates absorbance to flux:

$$J_{pr} = (A_{479}{}^l \times Vol_l)/(t \times A \times EC \times Pl) \qquad [Eq. 1]$$

where J_{pr} is the phenol red flux (units: mol/cm^2/h), $A_{479}{}^l$ is the absorbance of the luminal solution at 479 nm, Vol_l is the volume of the luminal solution (the volume of solution in the luminal compartment at the time of the measurement; liters), t is time in h, A is the surface area of the epithelium (area of the tissue culture insert: cm^2), EC is the extinction coefficient (8450 L/mol/cm), and Pl is the path length (cm) of the measuring cuvet.

The permeability of the epithelial monolayer to phenol red can be calculated using the flux equation:

$$P_{pr} = J_{pr}/[PR] \qquad [Eq. 2]$$

Where P_{pr} is the permeability to phenol red (units: cm/s), J_{pr} is the calculated phenol red flux (*see* above), and [PR] is the phenol red concentration in the plasma compartment (for the tissue culture medium for A6 cells this was approximately 40 µ*M*/L). The concentration of phenol red in tissue culture media is dependent on the type of tissue culture medium used.

3.1.1. The Units

In calculating permeability one must take care that all units are correct.

1. Units for permeability: cm/s.
2. Units for concentration of phenol red: mol/cm^3 (mol/mL).
3. Units for phenol red flux: mol/cm^2/s.

3.2.2. An Example

An example calculation is as follows. Epithelial cells are seeded onto a filter with an area of 4.2 cm^2. On d 6, the luminal solution is replaced with a phenol

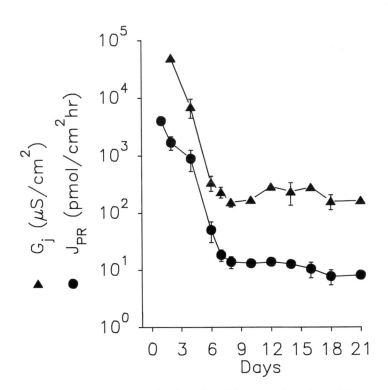

Fig. 2. Example of the decrease in phenol red flux as a function of time post-seeding. In this example, the transepithlial conductance (the inverse of the resistance) was also measured. The vertical bars are the standard error. Each point is the mean of 4 (d 1–7), 3 (d 8), and 2 (d 10–21), (reproduced from Jovov et al., 1991, [1] with permission from *Am. J. Physiol.*).

red-free solution and after a 24-h incubation (d 7 post-seeding), the absorbance of the luminal solution is 0.004 U and the volume is 0.0015 L. The permeability is calculated in the following steps:

From **Eq. 1**:

$$J_{pr} = (0.004 \times 0.0015 \text{ L})/(24 \text{ h} \times 4.2 \text{ cm}^2 \times 8450 \text{ L/mol/cm} \times 1 \text{ cm})$$

The calculated $J_{pr} = 7.04 \times 10^{-12}$ mol/cm^2/h.

From **Eq. 2**:

$$P_{pr} = 1.96 \times 10^{-15} \text{ mol/cm}^2\text{/s} / 40 \times 10^{-9} \text{ mol/cm}^3$$

The calculated $P_{pr} = 49 \times 10^{-9}$ cm/s. An example of the decrease in phenol red permeability as a function of time post-seeding is shown in **Fig. 2**. This example is from the renal epithelial cell line A6. In this particular example, the junctional conductance was measured at the same time as the phenol red flux. **Fig. 2** shows that both conductance and phenol red flux decreases over time and reach a steady state some 8 d post-seeding. It also demonstrates that phenol red flux is a good marker for epithelial confluence and a good estimate of the junctional conductance.

3.2.3. Estimating Transepithelial Conductance from P_{PR}

To many, the value for the permeability is a small and perhaps meaningless number. To put this value into perhaps more meaningful terms, we can estimate the transepithelial conductance from the P_{pr} value. This calculation assumes that the ratio of the diffusion coefficient of phenol red to sodium or chloride through the paracellular pathway is the same as the ratio of the free solution diffusion coefficients of these substances. Using the equation of Delamere and Duncan (3):

$$G_t = (F^2/RT) \times P_{pr} \times \sqrt{w} . y$$

$$w = ([Cl]_l \, P_{Cl}/P_{pr} + [Na]_l \, P_{Na}/P_{pr}) \text{ and } y = ([Cl]_p \, P_{Cl}/P_{pr} + [Na]_p \, P_{Na}/P_{pr})$$

where F is faradays constant (96500 coulombs/mol), R is the gas constant (8.314 J/°C/mol) and T is temperature in degree Kelvin (310°K), P_{pr} is as defined above, $[X]_i$ is the concentration of chloride or sodium in the luminal (l) or plasma (p) compartment (140×10^{-6} mol/cm^3), and P_X/P_{pr} is the ratio of free solution diffusion coefficient of chloride or sodium to phenol red. This ratio is calculated as the square root of the ratio of molecular mass of phenol red (354.4) to cither chloride (35.5) or sodium (22.9). The calculated conductance is 176×10^{-6} S/cm^2, which is a resistance of about 5680 $\Omega.$cm^2.

3.2.4. Net Solution Movement

To accurately determine the flux or permeability of the epithelium to phenol red we must know the volume of the luminal compartment at the time of the measurement. If we use the volume added during cell feeding, we assume that there is no net solution transport across the epithelium. By measuring phenol red absorbance in the tissue culture media, the luminal, and the plasma compartment, and knowing the initial volume of each compartment, one can calculate the volume of each compartment at the time of the measurement of phenol red flux. This method is based on two conditions. First, the sum of the luminal and plasma compartment volume is constant over time (loss of volume from one compartment is equal to the gain in volume in the other compartment). Second, the cells do not metabolize or synthesize phenol red (the quantity of phenol red is constant over time). These conditions lead to the following equation:

$$A_{479}{}^{tcm} \times iVol_p = A_{479}{}^{l} \times (iVol_l - x) + A_{479}{}^{p} \times (iVol_p + x)$$

where the superscripts tcm, l, and p refer to the tissue culture medium, luminal, and plasma solutions, respectively; $A_{479}{}^{tcm}$ is the absorbance of the phenol red in the respective solutions; iVol is the initial volume (in mL or L) in the indicated compartment; x is the volume of solution lost or gained from either compartment. The units for x is then the same as iVol. Net solution movement is then determined by solving the above equation for x. A positive value for x indicates that solution has moved from the luminal compartment to the plasma compartment. It is important to note that this method is not dependent on the mechanism of movement of phenol red between the two compartments, and the method is not valid when phenol red is in equilibrium across the epithelium. The validity of this method has been tested on the A6 tissue culture system *(1)*.

4. Notes

1. To optimize the measurement, the compartment to which phenol red is moving should have as small a volume as is feasible for the tissue area.
2. The time-line was found to be optimal for A6 cells. The investigator will have to empirically determine the optimal time for **Subheading 3.1., steps 3** and **4**. The time will dependent on the cell type, seeding density, growth conditions etc.

References

1. Jovov, B., Wills, N. K., and Lewis, S. A. (1991) A spectroscopic method for assessing confluence of epithelial cell culture. *Am. J. Physiol.* **261,** C1196–C1203.
2. Wills, N. K. (1996) Epithelial cell culture, p. 236–255. In *Epithelial transport: a guide to methods and experimental analysis.* (Wills, N. K., Reuss, L., and Lewis, S. A., eds.). Chapman and Hall, London.
3. Delamere, N. A. and Duncan, G. (1977) A comparison of ion concentrations, potentials and conductances of amphibian, bovine and cephalod lenses. *J. Physiol.* **271,** 167–186.

27

Co-Cultivation of Liver Epithelial Cells with Hepatocytes

Rolf Gebhardt

1. Introduction

Primary hepatocytes from rat and other species maintained in pure monolayer culture undergo phenotypic changes within a few days (1–3). This is particularly pronounced with respect to the cytochrome P450-dependent biotransformation capacity, but may also involve other metabolic pathways and, eventually, the switch from adult to fetal isozymes and proteins (4–6). Many such changes are due to nutritional and/or hormonal deficiencies of the culture media and to inadequate extracellular matrix conditions (7,8). In 1983, Guguen-Guillouzo and coworkers, in an attempt to create a more liver-like environment, observed that co-cultivation of rat hepatocytes with rat liver epithelial cells stimulated maintenance and reversibility of hepatocellular albumin secretion (9). Subsequently, it became well documented through many studies that co-cultivation provides a promising culture approach for extending the life span and for maintaining the differentiated phenotype of liver parenchymal cells (10,11). This not only concerns the capacity of hepatocytes for carrying out complex biotransformation reactions of xenobiotics (12–15), but also many other features, such as production of acute phase proteins, transport phenomena, and proliferation (16–18). Thus, co-cultured hepatocytes can be considered as a valuable equivalent to hepatocytes in situ with respect to many metabolic and regulatory aspects and can be used in various biological and toxicological fields (19). However, it should be noted that certain functions or enzymes may still deviate from normal. For instance, epoxide hydratase activity remains diminished (12). On the other hand, the spontaneous induction of glutamine synthetase has been noted in hepatocytes co-cultured with some, but not all, epithelial cell lines (20,21), reflecting that there is a specific exchange of signals between hepatocytes and epithelial cells

From: *Methods in Molecular Biology, vol. 188: Epithelial Cell Culture Protocols*
Edited by: C. Wise © Humana Press Inc., I otowa, NJ

(22). Such signals and cell interactions may provide a clue to the heterogeneity of hepatocytes in liver parenchyma *(23)*.

   This leads directly to the important question of what might be the cause of the spectacular phenotypic stabilization of the primary hepatocytes. Firstly, it has been noted that in co-cultures, a special extracellular matrix is produced *(22)*, the composition of which is not yet completely known. Secondly, there is evidence against a direct coupling of the co-cultured cells via gap junctions *(24)* and in favor of membrane-bound and membrane-soluble signals and factors, which may be exchanged between these cell types *(25–27)*. Since these factors are still unknown, co-cultures between these liver cell populations may provide an important system to identify and characterize signals involved in cell–cell communication within organs such as the liver *(22)*.

2. Materials

2.1. Isolation of Rat Hepatocytes

1. Pentobarbital sodium (75 mg in 2.5 mL saline), prepare fresh.
2. Perfusion media (*see* **Note 1**).
    a. Medium A: 145 mM sodium chloride, 5.4 mM potassium chloride, 0.77 mM magnesium sulfate, 0.93 mM magnesium chloride, 0.44 mM potassium dihydrogenphosphate, 0.34 mM disodium hydrogenphosphate, 10 mM HEPES, adjusted to pH 7.4.
    b. Medium B: 145 mM sodium chloride, 5.4 mM potassium chloride, 0.77 mM magnesium sulfate, 0.93 mM magnesium chloride, 0.44 mM potassium dihydrogenphosphate, 0.34 mM disodium hydrogenphosphate, 10 mM HEPES, 0.2% glucose, and 0.2% bovine serum albumin (BSA) (defatted), adjusted to pH 7.4.
    c. Medium C: 137 mM sodium chloride, 5.4 mM potassium chloride, 1.2 mM magnesium sulfate, 0.15 mM potassium dihydrogenphosphate, 0.79 mM disodium hydrogenphosphate, 1 mM calcium chloride, 10 mM HEPES, and 0.1% glucose, adjusted to pH 7.4.
3. Collagenase (units determined with z-glycyl-L-propyl-glycyl-glycyl-L-propyl-L-alanine). Can be stored at –20°C for up to 1 yr, if kept dry (*see* **Note 2**).
4. 500 M Calcium chloride in distilled water, sterilize by passing through a 0.22-µm filter, dilute 1:100.
4. 0.5% Trypan blue (in saline). Stable for 3 wk when refrigerated. If solution is clumpy, clear by filtration.

2.2. Preparation of Co-Cultures

1. Williams' medium E: the formulation without glutamine can be stored at 4°C for several months.
2. Culture medium: Williams' medium E supplemented with 10% newborn calf serum, 2 mM L-glutamine, 50 U/mL penicillin, 50 µg/mL streptomycin.

3. Hank's buffer A (with HEPES): 8 g/L sodium chloride, 0.4 g/L potassium chloride, 0.1 g/L magnesium sulfate (7 H_2O), 0.1 g/L magnesium chloride (6 H_2O), 0.06 g/L disodium hydrogen phosphate (2 H_2O), 0.06 g/L potassium dihydrogenphosphate, 0.01 g/L calcium chloride, 0.48 g/L HEPES in double-distilled water, adjusted to pH 7.4. The buffer is sterilized by passing through a 0.22-μm filter and can be stored at 4°C for 6 mon.
4. Hank's buffer B (without calcium, magnesium, and HEPES): omit calcium chloride, magnesium sulfate, magnesium chloride, and HEPES from the formulation given above.
5. Accutase: 3 mL/75-cm^2 flask (PAA Laboratories).

2.3. Staining of Co-Cultures for Glycogen (see Note 3)

1. Methanol.
2. % Periodic acid.
3. Schiff's reagent (for detection of aldehydes) (Fluka).
4. Sodium azide.
5. Nylon mesh: 250 and 100 μm pore size.
6. Equipment: basic cell culture laboratory specially equipped for the isolation of hepatocytes with CO_2 incubator, centrifuge, shaking water bath, inverse light microscope, sterile scalpels, hemocytometer, sterile pipets, disposable plastic culture flasks, and Petri dishes.

3. Methods
3.1. Isolation of Rat Hepatocytes
3.1.1. Surgery and Preperfusion of the Liver

1. Anesthesize rat by intraperitoneal injection of sodium pentobarbital (60 mg/kg body weight) (*see* **Note 4**).
2. Shave the abdomen of the rat, disinfect the animal, and immobilize it on the surgery table.
3. Open the peritoneal cavity, ligate the vena cava inferior and the portal vein, and insert a cannula into the portal vein using the standard technique.
4. Cut the vena cava below the ligation and flush the liver free of blood with calcium-free medium A at a rate of 35 mL/min (*see* **Note 5**).
5. Continue liver perfusion until about 900 mL of medium A are flushed through.
6. While perfusion is in progress, open the thorax, and place a second cannula in the vena cava superior.
7. Close the ligation at the vena cava inferior, such that the perfusate drains from the cannula at the vena cava superior.
8. Shortly before medium A is used up, remove the liver from the rat carefully, while it is still connected to the perfusion tubing.
9. Place liver into an insulated chamber allowing recirculated perfusion at constant temperature (37°C) and hydrostatic pressure (30 cm water column) (*see* **Note 6**).

3.1.2. Recirculating Perfusion of the Liver with Collagenase

1. Switch from perfusion with medium A to medium B containing collagenase (70 U in 80 mL) for recirculating perfusion. Perfusion is continued at a flow rate of 35 mL/min.
2. After 2 min, add calcium chloride to medium B to reach a final concentration of 5 mM.
3. Continue perfusion with collagenase for 15–20 min until liver tissue is softened (*see* **Note 7**).
4. Stop the perfusion and transfer the liver to a beaker containing 50 mL of medium C.
5. Perforate the liver capsule with a pair of scissors several times without cutting off the different lobes.
6. Hold the liver with forceps at the remainder of the hepatic vein and gently shake the tissue in medium C to liberate the hepatocytes (*see* **Note 8**).

3.1.3. Purification of the Hepatocytes

1. Filter the resulting cell suspension through double layers of gauze to remove undissociated tissue and large aggregates of cells.
2. Repeat filtration first through nylon mesh of 250 µm pore size and then through nylon mesh of 100 µm pore size.
3. After filtration, centrifuge the cell suspension at 50g for 5 min. Discard the supernatant containing primarily cell debris and nonparenchymal cells (*see* **Note 9**).
4. Resuspend the pellet gently and recentrifuge at 50g for 3 min and then discard the supernatant.
5. Repeat step for 3 times.
6. Finally resuspend the cells in the pellet in medium C.

3.1.4. Determination of Cell Viability and Number

1. Mix 100 µL of Trypan blue solution with 250 µL of cell suspension (*see* **Note 10**).
2. Count the viable (uncolored) and dead (blue) cells using a hemocytometer under a light microscope (*see* **Note 11**).
3. Calculate the mean number of viable and dead cells as well as the viability index (*see* **Note 12**).
4. Use only cell suspensions with a viability of more than 85%.

3.2. Preparation of Co-Cultures (see Note 13)

3.2.1. Seeding of Hepatocytes

1. Dilute the hepatocyte suspension with culture medium to a concentration of 6.25×10^6 cells/mL (*see* **Note 14**).
2. Seed out cells at a density of 62.5×1000 cells/cm^2 onto tissue culture grade plastic (*see* **Notes 15** and **16**).
3. Incubate plates in a CO_2 incubator at 37°C for 2 h to allow viable hepatocytes to attach to the substratum.

4. Remove culture medium together with nonattached cells and discard.
5. Add new culture medium, or immediately proceed with the addition of the epithelial cells (*see* **Subheading 3.2.2.**).

3.2.2. Seeding of Liver Epithelial Cells (see **Note 17**)

1. Take a culture of pure epithelial cells in the log growth phase and remove the culture medium (*see* **Note 18**).
2. Add 1 mL of Hank's buffer B and incubate cultures for 10 min in an incubator.
3. Aspirate Hank's buffer B.
4. Add accutase (1 mL/25 cm^2 of culture area) (*see* **Note 19**).
5. Maintain at room temperature for 2–5 min until cells lift off (control under microscope).
6. Flush all cells from the bottom of the Petri dish by means of a pipet.
7. Transfer cell suspension to a centrifuge tube and centifuge at 150g for 3 min.
8. Discard supernatant and add fresh culture medium.
9. Add suspension of liver epithelial cells prepared with fresh culture medium to the previously prepared hepatocyte cultures. Gently shake the flasks to ensure equal distribution of the epithelial cells (*see* **Note 20**).
10. Incubate the cells in a humidified CO_2-incubator at 37°C. Change culture medium each day (*see* **Note 21**).

3.3. Staining of Co-Cultures for Glycogen (see **Note 22**)

1. Aspirate the medium from the co-cultures and wash the monolayer twice with Hank's buffer A.
2. Fix the cells by adding ice-cold methanol. Leave for 5 min, then discard.
3. Add 0.5% periodic acid for 10 min.
4. Wash with distilled water.
5. Add Schiff's reagent and keep for 30 min at room temperature.
6. Wash for 30 min under running tap water. Glycogen containing hepatocytes should be colored red-violet (*see* **Note 23**).
7. Add 0.05% sodium azide for conservation.

4. Notes

1. In this protocol, the 2-step isolation procedure described by Seglen (*28*) is used with slight modifications. Although successful isolation achieved by perfusion with bicarbonate-buffered media has been described, in our hands, HEPES-buffered media and 100% oxygen as used by Seglen were superior.
2. Because pure collagenase is insufficient, the choice of collagenase is of utmost importance for successful isolation of the hepatocytes. The collagenase must be contaminated with other (unknown) proteolytic activities. It is recommended that different batches from various suppliers be tested and compared. A large quantity of an optimal batch can then be ordered and stored in appropriate aliquots at –20°C.
3. Glycogen staining is performed with the so-called PAS method, which is a widely used in pathology. Since glycogen is found in hepatocytes only, these cells can

be easily distinguished in the co-cultures with this staining. Furthermore, the staining intensity will tell about the performance of the hepatocytes after prolonged cultivation.

4. Rats (adults or pups) should be maintained and treated according to ethical standards and the specific national regulations for animal care. Rats should be anesthesized with pentobarbital sodium according to international ethical rules. It is of utmost importance that the animals are cleaned with a disinfectant after anesthesia and that sterile equipment is used for removal of the liver.

5. A flow rate of at least 35 mL/min is required to ensure minimal oxygenation. The perfusate is discarded.

6. A common device for recirculating liver perfusion suitable also for the isolation of hepatocytes is described by Mehendale *(29)*. The liver should be protected from drying at its surface and from being perfused at temperatures below or above 37°C.

7. The correct time for stopping perfusion with collagenase may be determined by touching the liver capsule with a spatula. If the digestion is complete, small fissures will form at the site of touching. Avoid perfusing the liver longer than necessary.

8. Alternatively, cells can be liberated by gentle combing.

9. The supernatant can be used for the isolation of nonparenchmal cells according to techniques described in the literature. Such cells, e.g., endothelial cells, are also suitable for co-cultivation with hepatocytes.

10. Staining of the cells with Trypan blue is a simple viability test. It should be noted that good viabilities indicated with this method do not always result in appropriate cell cultures.

11. It is advised that the mixture of Trypan blue and the cell suspension should stand for 3 min to complete staining of the nuclei of nonviable hepatocytes.

12. Viability index (in%) = (no. viable cells × 100)/[(no. viable cells) + (no. dead cells)].

13. In principle, co-cultures can be established simultaneously with or at any time after plating of the hepatocytes. The earlier the co-culture is prepared, the stronger is the effect on longevity and performance of the hepatocytes. However, sometimes mixing suspensions of hepatocytes and liver epithelial cells and simultaneous plating may result in bad attachment of hepatocytes. Thus, seeding of the epithelial cells 2 h after plating of the hepatocytes was found a good compromise to obtain optimal and reproducible results.

14. The cell density of hepatocytes for co-cultures may vary considerably and should be chosen as required for each experiment. For best results, the cell density should range within half (62.5 × 1000 cells/cm^2) and one-fifth (12.5 × 1000 cells/cm^2) of that required for monolayer formation.

15. Precoating of Petri dishes or culture flasks with collagen (type I, or better, type 4) is recommended *(9,15)*.

16. Equal distribution of the hepatocytes should be ensured by gently shaking the plates.

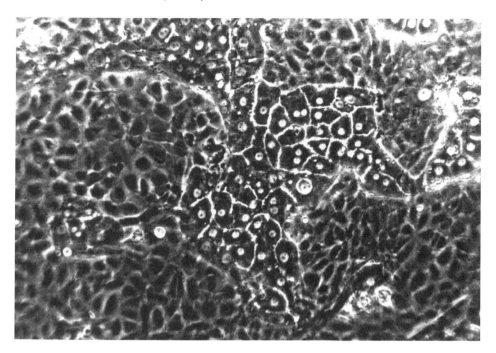

Fig. 1. Appearance of a co-culture between primary rat hepatocytes and rat liver epithelial cells (line RL-ET-14, *[6]*) after 1 wk of cultivation. Note the polygonal shape of the hepatocytes (lucid round nuclei) and the formation of an anastomosing network of slender lucid channel at their periphery which correspond to newly formed bile canaliculi. Phase contrast micrograph; magnification, 40×.

17. Rat liver epithelial cells can be obtained by following the protocol described in **Chapter 6** of this text. If cells have to be thawed from frozen stocks, they should be maintained for one passage before using them for co-cultivation.

18. Note that the culture medium for propagating the epithelial cells is different from that described here for hepatocyte cultures and co-cultures (*see* **Chapter 6**).

19. Accutase was found to give optimal results by less harming the epithelial cells during detachment. Alternatively, 0.1% trypsin can be used.

20. The concentration of the epithelial cell suspension for preparing the co-cultures must be high enough for filling the free spaces between the hepatocytes, i.e., a slight excess of epithelial cells has to be used. Thus, when hepatocytes are cultured at half confluency (62.5×1000 cells/cm^2), the concentration of the epithelial cells should be 10^6 cells/mL, i.e., a final cell density of 10^5 cells/cm^2.

21. In co-culture, rat hepatocytes may survive for several weeks. They should maintain their polygonal morphology and should reform an anastomosing network of slender bile canaliculi (*see* **Fig. 1**). It should be taken into account that even though the phenotype of the hepatocytes is quite stable during co-cultivation, there are nonetheless changes in many functions that need to be monitored carefully.

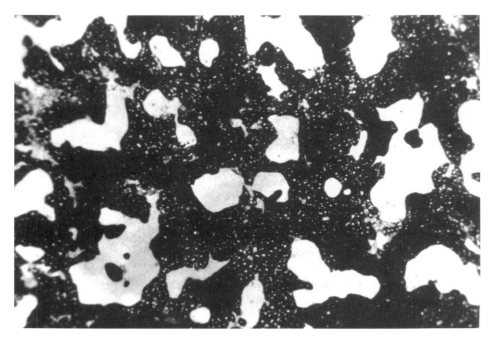

Fig. 2. Photomicrograph of a co-culture between primary rat hepatocytes and rat liver epithelial cells maintained for 1 wk stained with PAS for cellular glycogen. The culture was kept under 20 m*M* glucose and 0.1 μ*M* insulin 24 h prior to fixation. Note the presence of high amounts of glycogen in the cytoplasm (not nuclei) of hepatocytes, but not in epithelial cells. Magnification, 25×.

22. Staining of hepatocytes for glycogen usually leads to a randomized pattern of strongly and weakly stained cells in pure hepatocyte cultures, while in co-cultured hepatocytes, a more homogeneous staining is obtained. If higher levels of glycogen and, thus, stronger staining is wanted, 20 m*M* glucose and 0.1 μ*M* insulin should be added to the culture medium 24 h prior to staining. This will result in a homogeneous strong staining for glycogen only in the co-cultured hepatocytes (*see* **Fig. 2**). The staining can be used for determining the amount of hepatocytes by using computerized image analysis.
23. Avoid direct contact of the plates with the stream of tap water. This may wash away parts of the cell layer. Use a container filled with water where the stream is entering at one corner, while the plates are placed in the diagonal corner.

References

1. Gebhardt, R., Bellemann, P., and Mecke, D. (1978) Metabolic and enzymatic characteristics of adult rat liver parenchymal cells in non-proliferating primary monolayer cultures. *Exp. Cell Res.* **112,** 431–441.
2. Guguen-Guillouzo, C. and Guillouzo, A. (1983) Modulation of functional activities in cultured rat hepatocytes. *Mol. Cell. Biochem.* 53/54, 35–36.

3. Guillouzo, A. and Guguen-Guillouzo, C. (eds.) (1986) *Isolated and cultured hepatocytes*. John Libbey Eurotext Ltd/INSERM, London.
4. Paine, A. J. (1990) The maintenance of cytochrome P450 in rat hepatocyte culture: some applications of liver cell cultures to the study of drug metabolism, toxicity and the induction of the P-450 system. *Chem. Biol. Interact.* **74**, 1–31.
5. Isom, H. C., Secott, T., Georgoff, I., Woodworth, C., and Mummaw, J. (1985) Maintenance of differentiated rat hepatocytes inprimary culture. *Proc. Natl. Acad. Sci. U.S.A.* **82**, 3252–3256.
6. Gebhardt, R. (guest ed.) (1997) International Congress on Hepatocytes. *Cell Biol. Toxicol.* **13**, 215–386.
7. Gebhardt, R. and Mecke, D. (1979) The role of growth hormone, dexamethasone and trijodothyronine in the regulation of glutamine synthetase in primary cultures of rat hepatocytes. *Eur. J. Biochem.* **100**, 519–525.
8. Schuetz, E. G., Li, D., Omieciniski, C. J., Muller-Eberhard, U., Kleinman, H. K., Elswick, B., and Guzelian, P. S. (1988) Regulation of gene expression in adult rat hepatocytes cultured on a basement membrane matrix. *J. Cell. Physiol.* **134**, 309–323.
9. Guguen-Guillouzo, C., Clement, B., Baffet, G., Beaumont, C., Morel-Chany, E., Glaise, D., and Guillouzo, A. (1983) Maintenance and reversibility of active albumin secretion by adult rat hepatocytes co-cultured with another liver epithelial cell type. *Exp. Cell Res.* **143**, 47–54.
10. Begué, J.-M., Guguen-Guillouzo, C., Pasdeloup, N., and Guillouzo, A. (1984) Prolonged maintenance of active cytochrome P-450 in adult rat hepatocytes co-cultured with another liver cell type. *Hepatology* **4**, 839–842.
11. Lescoat, G., Pasdeloup, N., Kneip, B., and Guguen-Guillouzo, C. (1987) Modulation of alpha-fetoprotein, albumin and transferrin gene expression by cellular interactions and dexamethasone in co-cultures of fetal rat hepatocytes. *Eur. J. Cell Biol.* **44**, 128–134.
12. Ratanasavanh, D., Beaune, P., Baffet, G., Rissel, M., Kremers, P., Guengerich, F. P., and Guillouzo, A. (1986) Immunocytochemical evidence for the maintenance of cytochrome P450 isoenzymes, NADPH cytochrome C reductase and epoxide hydratase in pure nad mixed primary cultures of adult human hepatocytes. *Food Chem. Toxicol.* **24**, 577–578.
13. Rogiers, V. and Vercruysse, A. (1993) Rat hepatocyte cultures and co-cultures in biotransformation studies of xenobiotics. *Toxicology* **82**, 193–208.
14. Akrawi, M., Rogiers, V., Vandenberghe, Y., Palmer, C. N. A., Vercruysse, A., Shephard, E. A. and Phillips, I. R. (1993) Maintenance and induction in co-cultured rat hepatocytes of components of the cytochrome P-450 mediated monooxygenase. *Biochem. Pharamacol.* **45**, 1583–1591.
15. Gebhardt, R., Wegner, H. and Alber, J. (1996) Perifusion of co-cultured hepatocytes: optimization of studies on drug metabolism and cytotoxicity *in vitro*. *Cell Biol. Toxicol.* **12**, 57–68.
16. Lebreton, J.-P., Daveau, M., Hiron, M., Fontaine, M., Biou, D., Gilbert, D. and Guguen-Guillouzo, C. (1986) Long-term biosynthesis of complement component

C3 and alpha-1 acid glycoprotein by adult rat hepatocytes in a co-culture system with an epithelial liver cell-types. *Biochem. J.* **235**, 421–428.

17. Foliot, A., Glaise, D., Erlinger, S. and Guguen-Guillouzo, C. (1985) Long-term maintenance of taurocholate uptake by adult rat hepatocytes co-cultured with a liver pithelial cell line. *Hepatology* 5, 215–219.

18. Karam, W. G. and Ghanayem, B. I. (1997) Induction of replicative DNA synthesis and PPAR alpha-dependent gene transcription by Wy-14 643 in primary hepatocytes and non-parenchymal cell co-cultures. *Carcinogenesis* 18, 2077–2083.

19. Gebhardt, R.. and Hartung, T. (1996) Cokulturen in der *in vitro*-toxikologie. *Biospektrum* **2**, 36–39.

20. Schrode, W., Mecke, D. and Gebhardt, R. (1990) Induction of glutamine synthetase in periportal hepatocytes by cocultivation with a liver epithelial cell line. *Eur. J. Cell. Biol.* **53**, 35–41.

21. Gebhardt, R., Schrode, W., and Eisenmann-Tappe, I. (1998) Cellular characteristics of epithelial cell lines from juvenile rat liver: selective induction of glutamine synthetase by dexamethasone. *Cell Biol. Toxicol.* **14**, 55–67.

22. Gebhardt, R. and Gaunitz, F. (1997) Cell-cell interactions in the regulation of the expression of hepatic enzymes. *Cell Biol. Toxicol,* **13**, 263–273.

23. Gebhardt, R. (1992) Cell-cell-interactions: clues to hepatocyte heterogeneity and beyond? *Hepatology* **16**, 843–845.

24. Mesnil, M., Fraslin, J. M., Piccoli, C., Yamasaki, H., and Guguen-Guillouzo, C. (1987) Cell contact but not junctional communication (dye coupling) with biliary epithelial cells is required for hepatocytes to maintain differentiated functions. *Exp. Cell Res.* **173**, 524–533.

25. Corlu, A., Kneip, B., Lhadi, C., et al. (1991) A plasma membrane protein is involved in cell contact-mediated regulation of tissue-specific genes in adult hepatocytes. *J. Cell Biol.* **115**, 505–515.

26. Haupt, W., Schrode, W., and Gebhardt, R. (1998) Conditioned medium from cultured rat hepatocytes completely blocks induction of GS by dexamethasone in several liver epithelial cell lines. *Cell Biol. Toxicol.* **14**, 69–80.

27. Gebhardt, R., Schuler, M., and Schörner, D. (1998) The spontaneous induction of glutamine synthetase in pig hepatocytes co-cultured with RL-ET-14 cells is completely inhibited by trijodothyronine and okadaic acid. *Biochem. Biophys. Res. Commun.* **246**, 895–898.

28. Seglen, P. O. (1976) Preparation of isolated rat liver cells. *Methods Cell Biol.* **13**, 29–83.

29. Mehendale, H. M. (1982) Application of isolated organ techniques in toxicology, p. 509–559. In *Principles and methods of toxicology* (Hayes, A. W., ed.). Raven Press, New York.

28

Co-Culture and Crosstalk between Endothelial Cells and Vascular Smooth Muscle Cells Mediated by Intracellular Calcium

Wee Soo Shin, Chieko Hemmi, and Teruhiko Toyo-oka

1. Introduction

This chapter aims to describe the basic procedure needed to establish primary cultures of vascular smooth muscle cells (VSMCs) (*1*), and vascular endothelial cells (ECs) (*2*). Direct visualization of crosstalk between two types of cell was first accomplished by means of 2-dimensional Ca^{2+} image analysis of co-cultured smooth muscle cells and ECs (*3*). In order to carry out image analysis of intracellular calcium ions, these two cell types need to be grown in co-culture, and the methods for that are also described. Since Tsien's group developed calcium-sensitive fluorescent dyes, outstanding progress has been made in the field of intracellular calcium dynamics and cellular functions. These dyes are suitable for longer and repetitive experiments and much improve signal-to-noise ratios without foregoing calcium-sensitive photoprotein (aequorin) or metallochromic dyes for measurement of intracellulcar calcium concentration (*4*). Progress made includes excitation-contraction coupling of several muscle cells, excitation–secretion coupling in endocrine cells, and intra- and intercellular signaling mechanisms (*5*). More recently, progress has been made in elucidating the behavior of nitric oxide, a multifunctional effector molecule, which not only conveys signals for vasorelaxation, neurotransmission, and cytotoxicity, but plays a critical role in atherosclerosis, apoptosis, and cellular redox states (*6,7,8*). All of this progress has been greatly aided by the image analysis system first described by Fay and coworkers (*9*). Therefore, this chapter also describes the basic principle of intracellular calcium image analysis. We have used the term isoculture to refer to one type of cells that were grown in isolation

From: *Methods in Molecular Biology, vol. 188: Epithelial Cell Culture Protocols*
Edited by: C. Wise © Humana Press Inc., Totowa, NJ

and the term co-culture to designate that two types of cells coexisted in the same dish.

2. Materials

2.1. Isolation of VSMCs

1. Wistar-rats, 5 to 6 wk old (*see* **Note 1**).
2. Glass culture chambers for Ca^{2+} measurement (*see* **Note 2**).
3. Dental wax plates (GC Corporation).
4. 21-Gauge needles.
5. Disposable 10-mL syringes.
6. Disposable scalpel.
7. Plastic dishes for tissue culture.
8. Autoclaved disposable Pasteur pipets.
9. 10-mL Sterile plastic pipets.
10. 50-mL Sterile conical tubes.
11. Paper filters (100 µm pore size) and a filter holder.
12. Dissection kit (scissors and forceps in two sizes).
13. Alcohol swabs (70% ethanol).
14. Medium A: Dulbecco's modified Eagle's medium (DMEM) (Life Technologies).
15. Medium B: DMEM supplemented with 10% heat-inactivated fetal bovine serum (FBS) (Cell Culture Technologies), 1% antibiotic–antimycotic cocktail (Life Technologies). Store at 4°C and prewarm to 37°C before use.
16. Enzyme solution 1: to make 20 mL, dissolve 30 mg collagenase type 1 (Worthington) (final concentration: 1.5 mg/mL) and 7.5 mg soybean trypsin inhibitor type 1-S (Sigma) (final 0.375 mg/mL) in 20 mL of medium A, mix well, and sterilize through 0.22-µm bacteriofilter (Millipore). Aliquot it into 2 sterile conical tubes (10 mL each). Keep at 4°C until use.
17. Lens cleaning tissue.

2.2. Primary culture of Bovine Descending Aorta ECs

1. A ring of bovine descending aorta (10 cm in length) (*see* **Note 3**).
2. 23-Gauge needles.
3. Disposable 20-mL syringes.
4. Medium C: DMEM supplemented with 1% antibiotic–antimycotic cocktail.
5. Enzyme solution 2: to make 20 mL, dissolve 2000 U dispase powder (Godo Shusei, Japan) in 20 mL of medium A (final concentration 1000 U/mL), and sterilize the enzyme mixture through a 0.22-µm bacteriofilter. Dispase (1000 U/mL) is optimal to strip off ECs without injuring underlining VSMCs.
6. Phosphate-buffered saline (PBS), Ca^{2+}- Mg^{2+}-free (–) (Life Technologies).

2.3. Co-Culture of ECs and VSMCs

1. Trypsin-EDTA (0.05% trypsin, 0.53 *M* EDTA), liquid (Life Technologies).

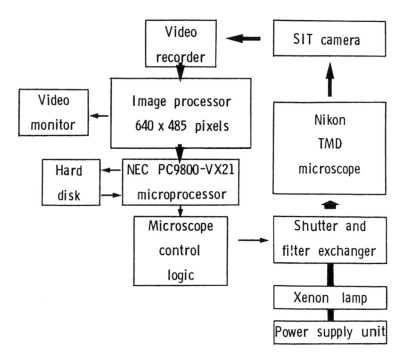

Fig 1. Two-dimensional calcium image analysis system. Cells on the fluorescence-free glass chamber are excited with UV light (340 or 380 nm), and the Ca^{2+}_i image expressed as fura-2 fluorescence is detected through a SIT camera and stored on a video-tape. Reproduced Ca^{2+}_i image is digitized by an image processor for 2-dimensional image analysis (*see* **Notes 4** and **11–13**).

2.4. Ca²⁺ Measurement with 2-Dimensional Image Analysis System (see Fig. 1)

1. 1 mM Fura-2 acetoxymethyl form (fura-2 AM) (Dojin Chemical, Japan) dissolved in dimethyl sulfoxide (DMSO) (Wako Pure Chemical, Japan). This is the stock solution.
2. PBS(–) containing 1 mM CaCl$_2$
3. Computer hardware for the 2-dimensional Ca²⁺ measurement and image analysis (**Fig. 1**) (*see* **Note 4**).
   a. An inverted fluorescence microscope (Diaphot, Nikon) with UV-fluor objective lens (×20, ×40, or ×100 by fluorescence-free glycerin immersion).
   b. A xenon lamp (75-W, Nikon).
   c. An interference filter (340 or 380 nm, 10 nm bandwidth) automatically switched by a computer-assisted controller (Sankei, Japan).
   d. An attenuation filter and a heat-cut filter (Nikon).
   e. A silicon target (SIT) camera (C2400; Hamamatsu Photonics, Japan).
   f. An on-line image processor (DVS-3000; Hamamatsu Photonics, Japan).

2.5. Protocol Example for Reagent Applications

1. Adenosine triphosphate (ATP) (Sigma).
2. High potassium solution: to make 100 mL of 80 mM potassium solution, add 884 mg KCl (118.53 mM), 20 mg KH$_2$PO$_4$ (1.47 mM), 124 mg NaCl (21.15 mM), 100 mg Na$_2$PO$_4$ (8.37 mM), 10 mg MgCl$_2$ (0.49 mM), 10 mg CaCl$_2$ (0.9 mM) to 100 mL of distilled water. Mix and autoclave. The final concentration used in the assay is 40 mM after half volume replacement.
3. Angiotensin II (Ang II) (Sigma).
4. PBS with Ca^{2+} and Mg^{2+}(+): to make 40 mL PBS(+) solution, gradually add 400 μL of 100 mM CaCl$_2$ stock solution (1 mM CaCl$_2$), 20 μL of 1 M MgCl$_2$ stock solution (0.5 mM MgCl$_2$) into 40 mL of PBS(−) (Life Technologies). Mix well.

3. Methods

3.1. Isolation of VSMCs

1. Dissect rat thoracic aortas and place in a culture dish containing 10 mL medium C.
2. Gently remove the blood from the aortic tubes using small forceps. Avoid excess tension on the aortas.
3. Place the aortas into a tube containing enzyme mixture 1 and incubate it for 10 min at 37°C with vigorous shaking.
4. Transfer the aortas to a second culture dish containing medium C.
5. Remove the adventitia from the aorta with forceps. They can be easily stripped off.
6. Cut the aortic tube longitudinally with small scissors to make an aortic strip.
7. Rub the inner surface of the aorta (the endothelial side) with an autoclaved cotton ball to remove the ECs.
8. Mince the aortic strip with a disposable scalpel blade (*see* **Note 5**).
9. Place the minced aortic pieces into a tube containing enzyme solution 1 and incubate for 90 min at 37°C with continuous gentle shaking at 100 rpm.
10. Detach cells from the aortic pieces by passing through a 21-gauge needle several times.
11. Filter the enzyme-dissolved aortic pieces through lens cleaning tissue, folded double in a plastic funnel.
12. Place the filtered solution into a fresh 50-mL conical tube and add approx 2 to 3 volumes of medium B to the tube.
13. Centrifuge at 300g for 10 min at room temperature.
14. Aspirate supernatant with vacuum (*see* **Note 6**).
15. Resuspend in 4 mL of medium B.
16. Place a 1-mL aliquot of the suspended cells into a pre-autoclaved glass chamber.
17. Examine cells under an inverted microscope to confirm that all dispersed cells keep long spindle shapes and that no distince cellular debris is seen.
18. Incubate them at 37°C in 95% air plus 5% CO$_2$.
19. Change the culture medium every 2 d (*see* **Note 7**).
20. Confluent primary cultures of VSMCs are shown in **Fig. 1A**.

3.2. Primary Culture of Bovine Descending Aorta ECs

1. Obtain a fresh bovine aortic ring from a slaughter house and place in a 50 mL tube containing medium A.
2. When back in the laboratory, remove the medium using a Pasteur pipet connected to vacuum suction.
3. Wash the aorta with PBS twice and then aspirate off the PBS.
4. Add 20 mL enzyme solution 2.
5. Incubate at 37°C for 60 min with shaking at medium speed (100 rpm).
6. Place the enzyme solution (containing the dispersed cells) into a 20-mL syringe and force through a 23-gauge needle (*see* **Note 8**).
7. Rinse the inner surface (the endothelial side) of the aortic ring with the aspirated enzyme solution several times (*see* **Note 9**).
8. Remove the aortic ring with sterile forceps.
9. Add approx 1 to 2 volumes of medium B to the 50-mL tube of enzyme solution.
10. Centrifuge the cells at room temperature for 10 min at 300g.
11. Aspirate supernatant with vacuum (*see* **Note 6**).
12. Add 10 mL of medium B to the tube and resuspend the pellet well.
13. Transfer the medium containing cells to a new culture dish.
14. Examine cells under an inverted microscope to confirm that enzyme-dispersed cells look lemon- or rugby ball-shaped and not round.
15. Incubate them at 37°C in 95% air plus 5% CO_2.
16. Change the culture medium every 2 d (*see* **Note 10**).
17. Confluent primary cultures of ECs are shown in **Fig. 2A**.

3.3. Co-Culture of ECs and VSMCs

1. Seed VSMCs (**Subheading 3.1.**) onto a culture dish at a density of $1.5\text{Å} \times 10^3/cm^2$. The cell number is counted by hemocytometer. Maintain the cell culture for 4 d.
2. Grow the ECs (**Subheading 3.2.**) until confluent.
3. Rinse ECs with PBS twice and aspirate the PBS.
4. Add 2 mL of trypsin-EDTA solution to EC culture. Incubate at 37°C for 5 min in 95% air plus 5% CO2 (*see* **Note 11**).
5. Add 5 mL of medium B to the dish to inactivate the trypsin.
6. Pipet several times to detach the cells.
7. Transfer to a 50-mL centrifuge tube.
8. Add another 20 mL of medium B.
9. Centrifuge cells at room temperature for 5 min at 300g.
10. Aspirate supernatant with vacuum (*see* **Note 6**).
11. Add 10 mL of medium B to the tube and resuspend the pellet well.
12. Seed ECs at a density of $1.5\text{Å} \times 10^3/cm^2$ on culture dishes containing semiconfluent cultures of primary VSMCs (*see* **Note 12**).
13. Both VSMCs and ECs are cultured together in the same dish.
10. Change the culture medium (medium B) every 2 d.
11. Co-cultures of VSMCs and ECs can be used for the following experiments on the 7th day after seeding the VSMC (*see* **Fig. 4A**).

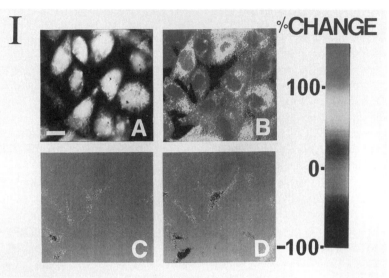

Fig 2. Two-dimensional images of the Ca^{2+}_i response in isocultured bovine aortic endothelial cells (×1000) *(3)*. Fura-2 loaded cells in the resting state illuminated at an excitation wavelength (340 nm) **(A)**, peak F_{340}/F_{380} divided by resting F_{340}/F_{380} ratio image after stimulation by 1 μ*M* ATP **(B)**, after stimulation by 40 m*M* KCl **(C)**, or after stimulation by 30 n*M* Ang II **(D)**. Scale bar length indicates 20 μm.

3.4. Ca²⁺ Measurement with 2-Dimensional Image Analysis System (see Fig. 1)

1. Add fura-2 AM dissolved in DMSO to the culture medium of cells at a final concentration of 4 μ*M*
2. Incubate ECs and/or VSMCs in fura-2 AM for 40 min at 37°C in 95% air plus 5% CO_2.
3. Rinse the cells twice with PBS plus 1 m*M* $CaCl_2$ to remove residual fura-2 AM.
4. Allow to stabilize for 20 min at room temperature before taking fluorescence measurements.
5. Place the glass culture chamber with fura-2-AM treated cells on a prewarmed stage (37°C) of an inverted fluorescence microscope.
6. Excitation wavelengths at 340 or 380 nm can be obtained using interference filters switched automatically by a controller at 2-s intervals. A shutter between the filters and lamp condenser lens controls the exposure time.
7. An emission spectrum of fura-2 AM should be filtered through a dichroic mirror above 500 nm and focused on a SIT camera.
8. Store the fura-2 AM images of VSMCs on a video recorder throughout the experiments.
9. Digitize the recorded fluorescence images of these cells at 640 × 485 pixels and 8 bits using an on-line image processor *(see* **Note 13**).

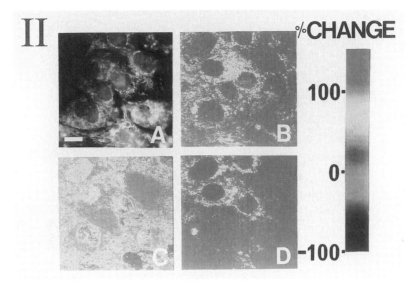

Fig 3. Two-dimensional images of the Ca^{2+}_i response in isocultured rat aortic vascular smooth muscle cells ($\times 1000$) *(3)*. Fura-2-loaded cells in the resting state illuminated at an excitation wavelength (340 nm) (**A**), peak F_{340}/F_{380} divided by resting F_{340}/F_{380} ratio image after stimulation by 1 µ*M* ATP (**B**), after stimulation by 40 m*M* KCl (**C**), or after stimulation by 30 n*M* Ang II (**D**). Scale bar represents 20 µm.

10. After subtracting background at 340 or 380 nm, reconstruct the 2-dimensional ratio (340/380 nm) image by dividing on pixel by pixel basis and convert to Ca^{2+} concentration (*see* **Notes 14** and **15**).

3.5. Protocol Example for Reagent Applications (see Figs. 2–5)

1. After equilibrating cells at 37°C for 10 min, stimulate ECs and/or VSMCs with 1 µ*M* adenosine triphosphate (ATP) and perform Ca^{2+} image measurement for 3 min (*see* **Note 16**).
2. Remove the ATP by washing with PBS(+) and leave the cells for 10 min at room temperature.
3. Add a high potassium solution to permit both the identification of VSMCs with voltage-dependent Ca^{2+} channels and the loading of sarcoplasmic reticulum Ca^{2+} in VSMCs.
4. Rinse the cells with PBS(+) and add Ang II (30 n*M*) to the medium to detect VSMCs with a receptor-operated Ca^{2+} channel.

4. Notes

1. One aorta from a Wistar rat is suitable for one fluorescence-free glass chamber slide for Ca^{2+} measurement.
2. Seed cells at a density of $1.5 \text{Å} \times 10^3/cm^2$ on the fluorescence-free glass chamber slide.

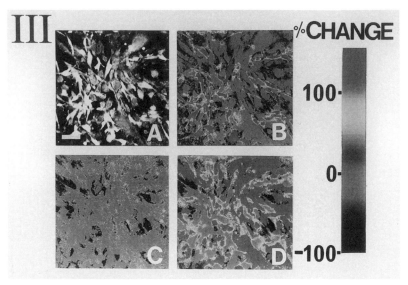

Fig 4. Two-dimensional images of the Ca^{2+}_i response in co-cultured bovine ECs and rat VSMCs (×200) *(3)*. Each experiment shows fura-2-loaded cultured cells in the resting state at an excitation wavelength (340 nm) **(A)**, peak F_{340}/F_{380} divided by resting F_{340}/F_{380} ratio image after stimulation by 1 μ*M* ATP **(B)**, 40 m*M* KCl **(C)**, or 30 n*M* Ang II **(D)**. Scale bar represents 100 μm.

3. Rinse to shear off the inside of the descending aorta in the same centrifuge tube. Cell clumps consisting of 10 to 100 ECs may be obtained.
4. To increase S/N ratio and to avoid image persistence, 32 successive videoframes at 1 s within 2-s recording time were accumulated, and its average was calculated at each excitation wavelength.
5. Cut the aortic tube (2 to 3 cm length, intrathoracic descending aorta) open to make a sheet using scissors and mince it into pieces (20 pieces or more) with a sterile scalpel.
6. Carefully remove supernatant from a 50-mL conical tube. Leave 0.5 mL of supernatant to prevent detachment of the fragile small cell pellet from the bottom of the tube.
7. VSMCs are recognized by the following three criteria: (*i*) a "hill and valley" pattern in confluent culture; (*ii*) immunological staining of myosin filaments after disrupting the sarcolemma by fluoresein isothiocyanate (FITC)-conjugated polyclonal antibody against smooth muscle myosin heavy chain; and (*iii*) the documentation of Ca^{2+}_i elevation to high K^+ (40 m*M*) depolarization or Ang. (30 n*M*) application.
8. Rinse the bovine aortic tube in the same tube. Using a smaller size than 23-G results in excess injury to the cells, and larger than a size 23-G lowers the yield of cells.

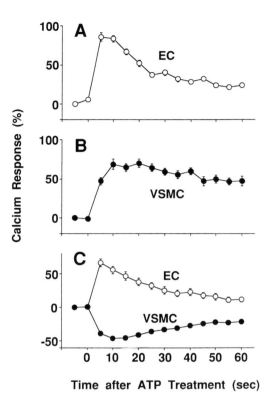

Fig 5. Time course of the F_{340}/F_{380} response to ATP (1 μM) in isocultured ECs (EC, n = 30) (**A**), in isocultured VSMCs (VSMC, n = 21) (**B**), in co-cultured ECs (open circles, n = 27) (**C**) and in co-cultured VSMCs (closed circles, n = 26) (**C**) (*3*). Each point denotes mean ± SE.

9. Rinse to shear off the inside of the descending aorta in the same centrifuge tube. Cell clumps consisting of 10 to 100 ECs may be obtained.
10. ECs are identified as follows: (*i*) "cobblestone" appearance in confluency; and (*ii*) immunological detection of von Willebrand factor, by FITC-labeled polyclonal antibody against human factor-related antigen. Monolayers of ECs ($6 \times 10^5/cm^2$) were used for the experiments. Prepare primary ECs culture after passage 20 or whenever cell shape becomes flat or the cellular response to an agonist is not prompt.
11. Monitor the status of cell dispersion under a microscope. Cells may look as if they are floating or flowing freely. Minimize the time the cells spend in the trypsin solution.
12. Cell clusters consisting of 5–10 cells are desirable for optimal co-culture. Seeding of ECs with VSMCs on the same day of primary VSMC culture results in an incorrect ratio of ECs to VSMCs. Seeding of ECs with VSMCs on the next day of

primary culture of VSMCs or later is recommended. The ratio of ECs to VSMCs varies depending the proliferation of VSMCs. This is quite an important point in co-culture of ECs/VSMCs for the Ca^{2+}_i image analysis. The inadequate ECs/VSMCs ratio does not exhibit clear Ca^{2+}_i reduction in VSMCs (*see* **Fig. 4B**) to agonists, which release nitric oxide from ECs. Modify the ratio to find out the most suitable condition (*see* **Fig. 4A** for the optimal ratio of ECs to VSMCs).

13. To increase S/N ratio and to avoid image persistence, 32 successive videoframes at 1 s within 2-s recording time were accumulated, and its average was calculated at each excitation wavelength.

14. Since the fura-2 method contains several intrinsic problems in estimating the absolute Ca^{2+}_i concentrations, the amplitude of Ca^{2+}_i elevation in response to each stimulant was evaluated by a percentage of increase in F_{340}/F_{380} with reference to F_{340}/F_{380} at the resting state (the percent increase of F_{340}/F_{380}) in the present study.

15. The relative increase of F_{340}/F_{380} at the peak after stimulation was displayed as a percent increase image in pseudo-color from blue to green, yellow, and brown corresponding to the increment of F_{340}/F_{380}. The mean percent increase of F_{340}/F_{380} at all pixels within each cell was defined as the percent increase of F_{340}/F_{380} of the cell.

16. **Figs. 2–4** for isoculture of VSMCs, of ECs, and co-culture of ECs and VSMCs, respectively. Time courses of Ca^{2+} response in each type of cells are shown in **Fig. 5**.

References

1. Gunther, S., Alexander, R. W., Atkinson, W. J., and Gimbrone, M. A., Jr. (1982) Functional angiotensin II receptors in cultured vascular smooth muscle cells. *J. Cell Biol.* **92,** 289–298.

2. Tokunaga, O., Fan, J., and Watanabe, T. (1989) Atherosclerosis- and age-related multinucleated variant endothelial cells in primary culture from human aorta. *Am. J. Pathol.* **135,** 967–976.

3. Shin, W. S., Sasaki, T., Kato, M., et al. (1992) Autocrine and paracrine effects of endothelium-derived relaxing factor on intracellular Ca^{2+} of endothelial cells and vascular smooth muscle cells: identification by two-dimensional image analysis in coculture. *J. Biol. Chem.* **267,** 20377–20382.

4. Grynkiewicz, G., Poenie, M., and Tsien, R. Y. (1985) A new generation of Ca^{2+} indicators with greatly improved fluorescence properties. *J. Biol. Chem.* **260,** 3440–3450.

5. Berridge, M. J. (1993) Inositol trisphosphate and calcium signaling. *Nature* **361,** 315–325.

6. Moncada, S, Palmer, R. M. J., and Higgs, E. A. (1991) Nitric oxide: physiology, pathophysiology, and pharmacology. *Pharmacol. Rev.* **43,** 109–142.

7. Nathan, C. Nitric oxide as a secretory product of mammalian cells. *FASEB J.* **6,** 3051–3064.

8. Michel, T. and Feron, O. (1997) Nitric oxide synthases: which, where, how, and why? *J. Clin. Invest.* **100,** 2146–2152.

9. Williams, D. A., Fogarty, K. E., Tsien, R. Y., and Fay, F. S. (1985) Calcium gradients in single smooth muscle cells revealed by the digital imaging microscope using Fura-2. *Nature* **318,** 558–561.

29

Establishing Epithelial–Immune Cell Co-Cultures

Effects on Epithelial Ion Transport and Permeability

Derek M. McKay and Mary H. Perdue

1. Introduction

The epithelial lining of the gastrointestinal tract is constantly exposed to a vast array of antigenic and potentially disease-evoking material derived from the diet and gut microflora. Thus, this single cell thick layer of cells (mainly transporting enterocytes, but also mucin-secreting goblet cells, enteroendocrine cells, and defensin-producing Paneth cells) stands as sentinel at the boundary between the external world and the body proper, where it must restrict the entry of potentially noxious substances while simultaneously absorbing nutrients. While regulation of the homeostatic role of the enteric epithelium has been traditionally considered the remit of the neuroendocrine system, it has become increasingly apparent that immune cells can directly, and indirectly, affect many aspects of epithelial function, including electrolyte transport, nutrient absorption, permeability, and the synthesis and release of messenger molecules *(1)*. Much of our current knowledge of immunomodulation of epithelial function has been obtained from in vitro co-culture studies, where model epithelia are juxtaposed to different immune cell types or immune mediators *(2–5)*.

The direct effects of immune mediators or the influence of activated immune cells on epithelia are difficult to examine in vivo or in isolated tissue segments ex vivo because of the inherent complexity of gut tissue. This issue has been addressed by the introduction of rodent and human-derived enteric epithelial cell lines, which has facilitated a reductionistic research approach. Thus, the potential of a given immune cell type to directly affect the epithelium can be examined under controlled culture (i.e., environmental) conditions *(6–11)*.

From: *Methods in Molecular Biology, vol. 188: Epithelial Cell Culture Protocols*
Edited by: C. Wise © Humana Press Inc., Totowa, NJ

Here, we outline a methodological approach that we have used extensively to assess the impact of T cells and/or monocytes on epithelial function, most notably ion transport (which creates the driving force for directed water movement) and permeability.

The advent of immortalized epithelial cell lines and improvements in maintaining primary isolates of epithelia in culture has impacted significantly on awareness of immune regulation of epithelial physiology. It is now clear that all the major classes of immune cells can directly affect one, or more, aspects of epithelial function, either via direct cell–cell contact of the release of a variety of messenger molecules *(19)*. Thus, using a reductionist in vitro co-culture approach the direct potential of T cells and monocytes to increase epithelial permeability, and at the same time perturb active ion transport events, has been established *(7,14)*. These model systems allow for the precise dissection of intercellular signaling pathways and also present themselves as a convenient means to screen new putative therapeutics (e.g., improved corticosteroids *[20]*). The transfer of information gleaned from an analysis of epithelial-immune cell interaction in vitro to the in vivo and clinical setting has the potential to considerably enhance awareness of physiological signaling pathways and pathophysiological mechanisms.

2. Materials

2.1. Epithelial Cells

A variety of enteric epithelial cell lines are commercially available—human (T84, Caco-2, HT-29) and rodent (MODE-K, KATO3, IEC-4.1, IEC-6, IEC-18). These cell types display different phenotypes that reflect the nature of gastric, small intestinal (villus or crypt), or colonic transporting epithelium. The choice of cell type will be determined by the nature of the research investigation (*see* **Note 1**). Another consideration may be the use of primary isolates of gut epithelium, which are suitable for short-term (i.e., hours) culture studies, but generally display low viability rates in extended culture periods. For isolation procedures for intestinal epithelial cells *see* Pang et al. *(12)*.

2.2. Cell Culture

1. Epithelial growth medium: 1:1 mixture of Dulbecco's modified Eagle's medium (DMEM) : Hams F12, substituted with 2% $NaHCO_3$, 200 mM L-glutamine, 2% penicillin–streptomycin, 1.5% HEPES, 10% newborn calf serum.
2. Sterile Phosphate-buffered saline (PBS).
3. Trypsin-EDTA.
4. Additional growth factors may be required on a cell-specific basis.
5. Assorted plasticware (culture flasks, 12-well plates, pipet tips, 15- and 50-mL tubes).
6. Pasteur pipets.

7. Transwell plates with microporous filters (e.g., 1 cm² diameter, 0.4 µm (Costar)) size of filter, pore size, and filter composition will be determined by the nature of the investigation.

2.3. Blood Immune Cell Isolation and Activation

1. Hepranized blood collection tubes.
2. Sterile PBS.
3. Ficoll-Paque® (Pharmacia Biotech).
4. 50-mL Sterile plastic tubes.
5. Pasteur pipets.
6. Oxygenated Kreb's buffer: 115 mM NaCl, 8.0 mM KCl, 1.25 mM CaCl$_2$, 1.2 mM MgCl$_2$, 2.0 mM KH$_2$PO$_4$, 25.0 mM NaHCO$_3$, pH 7.35 ± 0.02, to which 10 mM glucose is added as an energy source.
7. 10-mL Syringes and needles.
8. Magnetic beads: magnetic cell sorting (MACS) (Miltenyl Biotec, Auburn, CA, USA).
9. Hemocytometer.
10. Bacterial products: lipopolysaccharide, *Staphylococcus aureus* enterotoxin B (SEB).
11. 1 µg/mL Anti-CD3 antibodies, made up in PBS.
12. Saturated KCl.
13. Mitogens.
14. Petri dishes.
15. Sterile 12- or 6-well plates.

2.4. Major Pieces of Apparatus

1. Centrifuge.
2. Ussing chambers (World Precision Instruments [WPI]) plus assorted tubing and agar bridges.
3. Voltage clamp (model DVC-100; WPI) and matched pre-amplifiers and calomel electrodes.
4. Heating pump.
5. Aeration regulator.
6. Chart recorder or computerized data acquisition system.
7. Voltmeter and associated chopstick electrodes (Millicel-ERS; Millipore).
8. Sterile laminar flow hood.
9. Sterile incubator.
10. Microscope.
11. Inverted microscope.
12. Heated water bath.

3. Methods
3.1 Epithelial Cell Culture

1. For the analysis of immune regulation of epithelial cell ion transport and barrier functions, we have used the human colonic crypt-line T84 epithelial cell line.

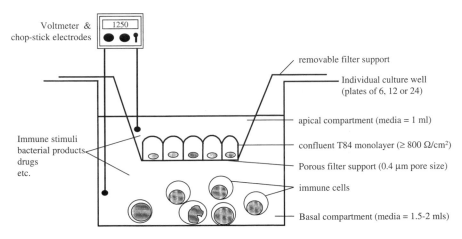

Fig 1. Standard setup for co-culture experiment, in which the epithelial monolayer has grown for 5–7 d and will be used when transepithelial resistance is ≥800 Ω/cm^2 as determined by the voltmeter. Monolayers can be grown on the underside of the filter, to give inverted cultures (*see* **Note 3**).

2. Grow T84 cells under standard culture conditions in epithelial growth medium, at 37°C, 5% CO_2 in 75-mL sterile flasks.
3. To subculture, remove culture medium and rinse the attached cells twice with warm (37°C) sterile PBS.
4. Add 5–10 mL of trypsin-EDTA to the flask.
5. After a 10–30 min incubation at 37°C, pipet the detached cells into a 50-mL tube.
6. Add 20 mL of fresh culture medium and centrifuge at 100g (500 rpm) for 5 min.
7. Aspirate the culture media and resuspend the cells by gentle pipetting in a known volume of fresh culture medium.
8. Count the cells using a hemocytometer and adjust the volume of the culture media to give 10^6 T84 cells/mL.
9. Place 1 mL of the cell suspension (i.e., 10^6 T84 cells) (*see* **Note 2**) onto the filter support.
10. Add 1.5–2.0 mL of fresh culture media to the basal compartment of the co-culture plate.
11. Return plates to the incubator.
12. Change media, both basal and apical, 24 h later and every 1 to 2 d thereafter until the epithelial monolayer is to be used (**Fig. 1**) (*see* **Notes 3** and **4**).

As with all cell culture experiments, preventing contamination is of the utmost importance, and all investigators should be trained in the proper use of the laminar flow hood and sterile technique (*see* **Note 5**).

3.2. Isolation of Blood Immune Cells

The following technique is for the retrieval of peripheral blood mononuclear cells (PBMC). For isolation of gut-derived lymphocytes *see* **ref. 13**.

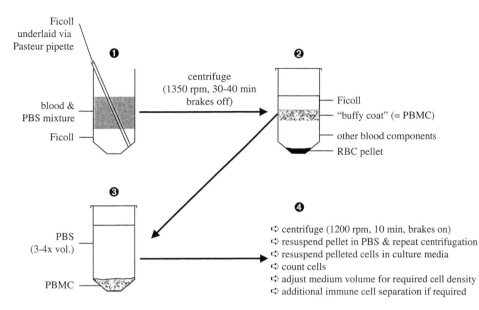

Fig 2. Diagramatic representation (not to scale) of the 4 basic procedural steps to isolate PBMCs from blood (RBC, red blood cells; PBS, sterile phosphate-buffered saline).

1. Collect approximately 10 mL of blood by venipuncture into hepranized tubes (*see* **Note 6**).
2. In a sterile hood, transfer the blood to a 50-mL tube and mix with 10 mL of warm (37°C) PBS.
3. Underlay with 10 mL of warm Ficoll via a syringe, delivered down a Pasteur pipet (**Fig. 2**) (*see* **Note 7**).
4. Taking care not to disturb the layering, cap the tube(s) and centrifuge for 30–40 min at 400 g (1350 rpm) with the <u>brakes off</u> (*see* **Note 8**).
5. Pipet off the "buffy coat" at the interface (this contains predominantly the PBMC) into a new tube.
6. Add approx 3–4 times the volume of warm PBS
7. Cap and centrifuge at 200–900*g* (1000–1200 rpm) for 10 min with the brakes on.
8. Discard the PBS and resuspend the pellet in fresh PBS.
9. Centrifuge again—this is a second washing, and a third may be conducted if judged necessary.
10. Resuspend the immune cells in fresh culture medium, count, and readjust cell number to the desired density. We have typically used 10^6 cells/mL. This whole PBMC population (approx 70% T cells, 15–25% B cells, 5–15% monocytes) can be used as a mixed immune cell population or fractionated into: (*i*) T and B cells, (*ii*) T cells only, and (*iii*) monocytes.
1. For the removal of monocytes, plate PBMC onto sterile Petri dishes and incubate at 37°C for at least 4 h. The nonadherent cells can be collected as the source of T and B cells.

2. Further isolation of a pure T cell fraction, or subpopulations of T cells, can most easily be obtained by using surface antigen-specific antibodies conjugated to magnetic beads following the manufacture's instructions.
3. For co-cultures examining monocyte–epithelial interactions, PBMC, at the desired density (based on analysis of the number of monocytes in the population), should be plated onto 12-well plates and incubated at 37°C for at least 4 h, at which time the nonadherent cells can be removed leaving the adherent monocytes only (*see* **Note 9**).

3.3. Epithelial–Immune Cell Co-Cultures and Immune Activation

1. Aspirate apical and basal culture medium from co-culture plates containing confluent T84 cell monolayers.
2. Replace with desired concentration of immune cells in the basal (immune cell–epithelial cell contact does not occur) or apical (allowing immune cell contact with the epithelial apical cell membrane) compartment.
3. Alternatively, the confluent epithelial monolayers can be transferred to a new sterile 12-well plate. Immune cells can then be activated by addition of the stimulus of interest, for example, bacterial products, mitogens, or activating antibodies.
4. If T cells are to be activated via the T cell receptor-CD3 complex, then the basal compartment of the co-culture well must first be coated with the anti-CD3 antibodies to allow immobilization of the antibody.
5. Add antibodies to the plate for 4 h, then remove PBS and unattached antibody.
6. T cells and filter-grown epithelial monolayers can subsequently be added to the antibody-coated wells (*see* **Note 10**).
7. Following co-culture, remove the epithelium and assess for changes in ion transport and barrier functions and compare with time-matched naive epithelial preparations (**Fig. 3**) (*see* **Note 11**).
8. Other additional aspects of epithelial form and function can also be assessed by applying standard methodologies, such as biochemical analyses for enzyme activities, electron microscopical assessment of ultrastructure, immunohistochemical detection of surface molecules, etc.
9. In addition, the immune cells can be retrieved and compared to nonactivated cells or those activated in the absence of an overlying epithelial monolayer.

3.3.1. Conditioned Medium

1. As a modification of the model, the immune cells can be activated in the absence of the epithelium and the conditioned medium collected.
2. Centrifuge the conditioned media at 200*g* (1000 rpm) for 5 min to pellet out immune cells.
3. Apply this to the basal or apical compartment of culture wells containing filter-grown epithelium (*11,14*).
4. This approach offers 3 advantages that complement the co-culture approach. First, the exact amount of soluble mediators (e.g., cytokines) can be measured in the medium, and dose-response experiments done with 0–50% conditioned medium

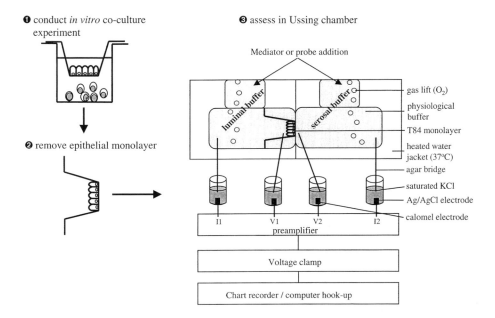

❶ conduct *in vitro* co-culture experiment

❷ remove epithelial monolayer

❸ assess in Ussing chamber

Mediator or probe addition

gas lift (O₂)

physiological buffer

T84 monolayer

heated water jacket (37°C)

agar bridge

saturated KCl

Ag/AgCl electrode

calomel electrode

luminal buffer

serosal buffer

I1 V1 V2 I2

preamplifier

Voltage clamp

Chart recorder / computer hook-up

Fig 3. Diagramatic representation of co-culture experiment and setup of epithelial monolayer in the Ussing chamber–voltage clamp apparatus to allow assessment of epithelial active ion transport and permeability (I, current; V, voltage).

can reveal the threshold level required to elicit a response. The effects of graded doses of conditioned medium can be compared with a dose response of a target cytokine, which may highlight additive or synergistic effects of mediators in the mixed milieu of the conditioned medium.

5. Second, specific inhibitors of mediators, such as neutralizing antibodies, can be applied to the conditioned medium to identify the active components in the medium.
6. Third, the immune cells can be treated with immunosuppressive agents (e.g., steroids, cyclosporine, inhibitors of arachidonic acid metabolism) prior to stimulation, and the ability of the conditioned medium from these cells to alter epithelial function can be assessed.

3.3.2. Pretreatment of Cells

1. The active involvement of the epithelium in the regulation of its' own barrier and transport function can be assessed.
2. First, the epithelium should be pretreated with an appropriate dose of an inhibitory agent (e.g., steroids *[15]*, protein synthesis inhibitors, inhibitors of phosphorylation, etc.) and then either co-cultured with the activated immune cells, or exposed to conditioned medium retrieved from the activated immune cells.
3. Thus, by the application of the approaches in **Subheadings 3.3.–3.3.2.**, the immune cells that regulate epithelial ion transport and permeability can be identified, the

mediators the respective immune cells produce, and any active participation of the enterocyte itself following immune activation elicited by a defined agent, can be precisely defined.

3.4. Ussing Chamber Analysis of Epithelial Ion Transport and Permeability

1. Vectorial electrolyte transport and maintenance of a regulated barrier are two of the primary functions of the enteric epithelium: both of these epithelial properties can be conveniently assessed by mounting the preparation (tissue segments, or in this instance, a filter-grown epithelial monolayer) in an Ussing chamber (*16*).
2. Mount the epithelium between the two leucite halves of the Ussing chamber.
3. Add an equal volume of Krebs Buffer (or other physiological buffers) to both sides of the preparation, so that any hydrostatic, chemical, and osmotic gradients across the epithelium are negated (*see* **Note 12**).
4. Each half of the chamber is equipped with two ports for agar bridges, which should be connected via a reservoir of saturated KCl to either calomel reference electrodes or silver–silver chloride electrodes for measuring potential difference and injecting current, respectively.
5. The pair of bridges placed closest to the apical and basal membranes of the epithelium monitor the spontaneous potential difference across the epithelium, while the bridges that are more distant from the epithelium are used for the injection of current (**Fig. 3**).
6. When the voltage clamp is set to automatically clamp the spontaneous potential difference across the epithelium to zero volts (i.e., elimination of any electrical driving forces), the injected current required to maintain this zero potential difference is the short-circuit current (Isc; expressed in $\mu A/cm^2$) and is indicative of net active ion transport across the preparation. Thus, the Isc value indicates basal active transport, and evoked changes in Isc are used to assess the impact of putative pro-secretory or pro-absorptive agents, which can be added to the appropriate epithelial surface to mimic physiological exposure.
7. Bacterial products such as cholera toxin should be added to the apical aspect of the monolayer, whereas immune mediators such as histamine should be added to the buffer bathing the serosal side of the epithelium.
8. It should be remembered that electrolyte transport creates the driving force for directed water movement, which can result in a diarrheal response or constipation.
9. It should also be noted that the Isc indicates net charge movement, but does not reveal the identity of the charge carrying ion (*see* **Note 13**).
10. In addition, since the voltage clamp apparatus provides potential difference and current values, the application of the Ohmic relationship allows for the calculation of epithelial (or tissue) electrical resistance (expressed in Ω/cm^2), or its converse, conductance (expressed in mS/cm^2) (*see* **Note 14**).
11. The transepithelial resistance is an indication of the passive ion flux across the preparation and is generally accepted as a reflection of the paracellular shunt pathway that is gated by the tight junctions.

12. Also, because mounting of the preparation in the Ussing chamber effectively separates the luminal (or mucosal) side of the epithelium from the basolateral (or serosal) side of the epithelium, it is ideal for assessing the unidirectional, or bidirectional, transepithelial flux of marker molecules.

13. Thus, probes of a specified size (e.g., ^{3}H-mannitol, ^{51}Cr-EDTA, fluorescent markers, proteins) can be added to one side of the Ussing chamber, designated the "hot" side, and after a suitable equilibrium period (i.e., 20–40 min), samples are taken from the opposing side of the chamber ("cold" side) at, for example, 30-min intervals over a 90-min period, and are replaced with an equal volume of the appropriate physiological buffer (*see* **Note 15**). Samples taken from the hot side at the beginning and end of the experiment are used to calculate the specific activity of the probe, and standard flux formulas are applied to the counts and/or amounts measured in the samples from the cold buffer. The transepithelial flux of the probe is expressed as amount per unit area per time or, in the case of ion fluxes, converted to electrical microequivalents and expressed as μE.h.cm^2 (*16*).

4. Notes

1. The nature of the investigation determines the choice of cell line to be employed. The human gut epithelial cell lines (Caco-2, HT-29, T84) establish monolayers with high electrical resistance (i.e., >200 Ω/cm^2, and in the case of T84 cell, up to 3000–4000 Ω/cm^2) and display ion transport responses to secretagogues similar to isolated tissue segments, and hence, are well suited for analysis of immune-mediated changes in epithelial ion transport and permeability. Also, varying the culture conditions for Caco-2 cells facilitates their differentiation into a villus-like cell expressing the brush border enzyme sucrose (*17*). This allows the comparison of Caco-2 crypt-like cells with villus-like cells. In addition, subclones of the HT-29 cell line have proven useful as a model of a mucus-producing cell. Also, if ion transport and/or permeability are not the focus of interest, then other epithelia may be a better choice. For example, in an examination of epithelial cytokine production, the rodent intestine-derived epithelial cells can be used, with the additional advantage that gut-derived immune cells (lamina propria lymphocytes [LPL] or intraepithelial lymphocytes [IEL]) can be obtained from normal mice or animals with a variety of secretory and/or inflammatory enteropathies for use in co-culture studies.

2. Other investigators have seeded T84 cells at lower densities (2.5–5 $\times$ 10^5 cells) onto filter support for use in Ussing chamber studies. Thus, should the yield of cells from the culture flasks be low, or a large number of monolayers required, the investigator may opt to start with a lower cell seeding density.

3. When using T84 cells, the investigator must define what a control monolayer is. This may be determined by the number of days in culture (i.e., ≥7 d) or a minimum baseline transepithelial electrical resistance (i.e., ≥800 Ω/cm^2, in the case of T84 cell monolayers). The latter is the preferred approach, with daily monolayer resistance values being conveniently recorded by use of a voltmeter and

asymmetrical chopstick electrodes (**Fig. 1**). Care must be exercised not to disturb or puncture the monolayer with the electrodes.

4. A modification of this procedure has been used by Madara et al. *(8)* and other investigators, where the T84 cells are seeded onto the under side of the filter support (**Fig. 1**). For this procedure, the sterile filter baskets are inverted in small beakers, an aliquot of cell suspension (e.g., 10^5 cells/100 µL) is added onto the filter, and the beaker is then sealed with parafilm and placed in the incubator. Following an attachment period (e.g., 4 h) additional culture medium is added to the inside well of the beaker and onto the filter. The filter, with attendant T84 monolayer, can subsequently be placed in a 12-well plate. Thus, the epithelium is now on the underside of the filter, with its apical surface facing the bottom of the culture. Immune cells can be added into the apical compartment of the Transwell (i.e., exposed to basal membrane of the epithelial), and the model can be used to assess transepithelial immune cell migration; immune cells being collected from the basal compartment of the Transwell plate.

5. Bacterial and/or fungal contamination is the bane of cell culture, and the investigator should be familiar with the tell-tale signs. Characteristically, the culture media becomes opaque and cloudy and will have a pungent aroma. All infected cultures should be destroyed, and the incubator decontaminated with bleach. Cultures can be tested for bacterial LPS using the *Limulus* amebocyte assay, and mycoplasma infections can be detected using commercially available kits. As a cautionary measure, we will routinely incubate samples of new culture medium and calf serum for 24 h to check for contamination.

6. When using normal volunteer blood, there will be variability in the exact composition of the PBMC retrieved. To minimize this, volunteers should be rejected if they have recently, or are currently, taking medication, and if they are suffering from any common ailments (e.g., colds, allergies).

7. Prior to use, the Ficoll should be shaken well.

8. Care should be taken that the Ficoll/blood/PBS mixture is centrifuged with the centrifuge brakes in the off position. If the centrifuge is used with the brakes on at this stage, the sample has been lost, as a subsequent spin with the brakes off will not fractionate the blood sample to allow PBMC collection.

9. When isolating monocytes, we have found that the initial adherence to plastic activates the monocytes, presumably as they become more macrophage-like. Thus, we would recommend that after the 4-h adhesion period, the cells are given fresh media and incubated overnight at 37°C ("rested"). The following day, after a change of culture medium, the cells can be used in co-culture studies *(7)*.

10. Immobilization of anti-CD3 antibodies is important as it enhances CD3 cross-linkage and capping on the T cell surface, which will activate the cells. Use of the anti-CD3 antibodies as a soluble product results in little, if any, T cell activation.

11. We and others have noted variability in T84 monolayer transepithelial resistance and secretory responses to Ca^{2+}- and cAMP-mediated Cl^- secretagogues between different batches of cells and passages within a single batch of cells. Therefore, it

is essential that each experiment (i.e., co-culture plate) contains at least 2 naive control monolayers, which will allow for normalization of the data that can then be presented as the percentage of the control response and will allow suitable statistical analyses to be conducted.

12. A variety of physiological buffers can be used ranging from Ringer's solution to Hank's balanced salt solution. We use oxygenated Kreb's buffer. If small intestinal epithelium is being used, then mannitol can be used to replace glucose in the luminal buffer, since the inclusion of glucose here will support Na^+-glucose uptake, which will increase the Isc.

13. A number of strategies can be used to identify the ion species responsible for changes in Isc. Ussing chamber studies can be conducted with bathing buffers, in which specific ions have been removed and replaced with a similarly charged ion, to maintain the electrical balance (e.g., Cl^--free buffers) *(18)*. Also, experiments can be conducted in the presence of specific pharmacological blockers of ion channels or pumps (e.g., Cl^- or Na^+ channel blockers, inhibitors of the basolaterally located Na/Cl/K co-transporter). Using radiolabeled ions, such as $^{36}Cl^-$ (or ^{125}I), ^{22}Na or ^{86}Rb, and conducting bidirectional flux studies (*see* **Subheading 3.4.**) can unequivocally define the role of chloride, sodium, and potassium movements in any Isc change, respectively.

14. An additional approach to measuring the transepithelial electrical resistance is to use the differential pulse technique. The voltage clamp is set in the bipolar mode with voltage clamping at 1 mV (or more) for a 1-s duration at specified intervals (s to min). The current spike elicited by the automated jump from 0 to 1 mV allows for the calculation of resistance via Ohm's law. This method of measuring resistance is often preferred, as it is not dependent on the investigator manually changing the clamp from the voltage-clamp closed mode to the open-circuit position. The reading is more accurate and the timing is synchronized on all epithelia that are being examined in parallel Ussing chambers.

15. For flux experiments looking at the movement of radiolabeled ions or marker molecules, it is essential that the experiment be started with equal volumes on each side of the epithelial preparation and that this volume be maintained throughout the experiment. Loss of buffer caused by excessive bubbling or leaks from either buffer invalidates the data. Reduced volume in either buffer results in reduced counts and/or detection in the cold buffer giving an erroneously reduced flux rate. Silicon grease can be used to seal any leaks during the initial equilibrium period prior to addition of the probe to the designated hot buffer.

Acknowledgments

Studies cited from the authors' laboratories were funded by operating grants from the Medical Research Council of Canada, the Crohn's and Colitis Foundation of Canada (to D.M.M. and M.H.P.), and research support from Astra Draco/Pharma, Inc., Lund, Sweden (to M.H.P.).

References

1. Perdue, M. H. and McKay, D. M. (1994) Integrative immunophysiology in the intestinal mucosa. *Am. J. Physiol. (Gastrointest. Liver Physiol.)* **267,** G151–G165.
2. McKay, D. M. and Baird, A. W. (1999) Cytokine regulation of epithelial permeability and ion transport. *Gut* **44,** 283–289.
3. Sanders, S. E, Madara, J. L., McGuirk, D., Gelman, D., and Colgan, S. P. (1995) Assessment of inflammatory events in epithelial permeability: a rapid screening method using fluorescein dextrans. *Epithelial Cell Biol.* **4,** 25–34.
4. Yang, S.-K., Eckmann, L., Panja, A., and Kagnoff, M. F. (1997) Differential and regulated expression of C-X-C, C-C and C-chemokines by human colon epithelial cells. *Gastroenterology* **113,** 1214–1223.
5. Schmitz, H., Fromm, M., Bentzel, C. J., et al. (1999) Tumor necrosis factor-alpha (TNFα) regulates epithelial barrier in the human intestinal cell line HT-29/B6. *J. Cell Sci.* **112,** 137–146.
6. McKay, D. M., Croitoru, K., and Perdue, M. H. (1996) T cell-monocyte interactions regulate epithelial physiology in a co-culture model of inflammation. *Am. J. Physiol. (Cell Physiol.)* **270,** C418–C428.
7. Zareie, M. Z., McKay, D. M., Kovarik, G., and Perdue, M. H. (1998) Monocyte/ macrophages evoke epithelial dysfunction: indirect role of tumor necrosis factor α. *Am. J. Physiol. (Cell Physiol.)* **275,** C932–C939.
8. Madara, J. L., Patapoff, T., Gillece-Castro, B., Colgan, S. P., Parkos, C. A., Delp-Archer, C., and Mrsny, R. (1993) 5'-Adenosine monophosphate is the neutrophil derived paracrine factor that elicits chloride secretion from T84 intestinal epithelial cell monolayers. *J. Clin. Invest.* **91,** 2320–232
9. Resnick, M. B., Colgan, S. P., Patapoff, T., et al. (1993) Activated eosinophils evoke chloride secretion in model intestinal epithelia primarily via regulated release of 5'-AMP. *J. Immunol.* **151,** 5716–5723.
10. Baird, A. W., Cuthbert, A., and MacVinish, L. (1987) Type 1 hypersensitivity reactions in reconstructed tissues using syngeneic cell types. *Br. J. Pharmacol.* **91,** 857–869.
11. Taylor, C. T., Murphy, A., Keller, D., and Baird, A. W. (1997) Changes in barrier function of a model intestinal epithelium by intraepithelial lymphocytes requires new protein synthesis by epithelial cells. *Gut* **40,** 634–640.
12. Pang, G., Buret, A., O'Loughlin, E., Smith, A., Batey, R., and Clancy, R. (1996) Immunologic, functional, and morphological characterization of three new human small intestinal epithelial cell lines. *Gastroenterology* **111,** 8–18.
13. Coligon, J. E., Kruisbeek, A. M., Margulies, D. H., Shevach, E. M., and Strober, W. (1998) *Current protocols in immunology,* p. 3.19.0–1.19.11. John Wiley & Sons, New York.
14. McKay, D. M. and Singh, P. K. (1997) Superantigen-activation of immune cells evokes epithelial (T84) transport and barrier abnormalities via interferon-γ and tumour necrosis factor-α. Inhibition of increased permeability, but not diminished secretory responses by transforming growth factor β$_2$. *J. Immunol.* **159,** 2382–2390.

15. McKay, D. M., Brattsand, R., Wieslander, E., Fung, M., Croitoru, K., and Perdue, M. H. (1996) Budesonide inhibits T cell initiated epithelial pathophysiology in an *in vitro* model of inflammation. *J. Pharmacol. Exp. Ther.* **277,** 403–410

16. Karnaky, K. J.(Jr.) (1992) Electrophysiological assessment of epithelia, p. 257–273. In *Cell-cell interactions. A practical approach* (Stevenson, B. R., Gallin, W. J., and Paul, D. L., eds.). PIRL Press at Oxford University Press, Oxford.

17. Abraham, C., Scaglione-Sewell, B., Skaroski, S. F., Qin, W., Bissonnette, M., and Brasitius, T. A. (1998) Protein kinase Cα modulates growth and differentiation in Caco2 cells. *Gastroenterology* **114,** 503–509.

18. Saunders, P. R., Kosecka, U., McKay, D. M., and Perdue, M. H. (1994) Acute stressors stimulate ion secretion and increase epithelial permeability in the rat intestine. *Am. J. Physiol. (Gastrointest. Liver Physiol.)* **267,** G794–G799.

19. McKay, D. M., Philpott, D. J., and Perdue, M. H. (1997) In vitro models in inflammatory bowel disease research—a critical review. *Aliment. Pharmacol. Ther.* **(suppl. 3)11,** 70–80.

20. Zareie, M., Brattsand, R., Sherman, P., McKay, D. M., and Perdue, M. H. (1999) Improved effects of novel glucocorticosteroids on immune-induced epithelial pathophysiology. *J. Pharmacol. Exp. Ther.* **289,** 1245–1249.

30

Explant Cultures of Embryonic Epithelium

Analysis of Mesenchymal Signals

Carin Sahlberg, Tuija Mustonen, and Irma Thesleff

1. Introduction

The development of most organs is characterized by epithelial morphogenesis involving budding, branching, and folding of the epithelium, which is accompanied by growth and differentiation of the epithelial cells. Central mechanisms regulating this development are interactions between the epithelium and the underlying mesenchyme. Studies on the nature of such interactions require the separation of the interacting tissues from each other and the follow-up of their advancing development after various manipulations. The tissues can be either transplanted and their development followed in vivo, or they can be cultured as explants in vitro. Although transplantation methods offer certain advantages, including the correct physiological environment and the possibility for long-term follow-up, organ culture techniques are superior in many other aspects. The development of the tissues can be continuously monitored during in vitro culture. The tissue culture conditions are reproducible, and the composition of the medium is known exactly, and it can be modified. Most importantly, the tissues can be manipulated in multiple controlled ways. The isolated embryonic epithelium may be recombined with different tissues or cells, or it may be cultured on various extracellular matrices. In particular, the in vitro culture conditions allow analyses of the effects of the mesenchymal inductive signals, which can be added to the culture medium or introduced locally with beads or transfected cells.

Many types of organ culture systems have been used over the years for studies on embryonic organ development. The Trowell method *(1)* has been widely applied, and it has proven to be suitable for the analysis of the morphogenesis

From: *Methods in Molecular Biology, vol. 188: Epithelial Cell Culture Protocols*
Edited by: C. Wise © Humana Press Inc., Totowa, NJ

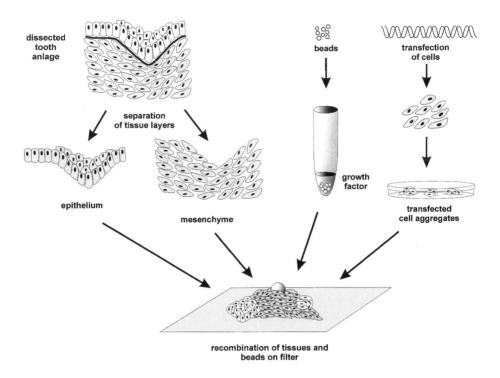

Fig. 1. Schematic representation of the method.

of many different organs *(2–7)*. In this system, the explants are cultured in vitro at the medium–gas interface on thin membrane filters that are supported by a metal grid. We have used the Trowell technique as modified by Saxén *(8)* for the analysis of the mechanisms of tissue interactions at various stages of embryonic tooth development *(9–16)*. The tooth is a typical example of an organ in which reciprocal epithelial–mesenchymal interactions regulate morphogenesis and cell differentiation. In this chapter, we describe the protocols for separation and culture of dental epithelial and mesenchymal tissues and for experiments in which the local effects of signaling molecules are analyzed by introducing them with beads or transfected cells (**Fig. 1**).

2. Materials

All solutions and equipment should be sterile. The glassware and metal instruments should be autoclaved and solutions filtered or autoclaved. All work should be done in a laminar flow hood; also the dissection microscope should be placed in the hood.

2.1. Reagents

1. Phosphate-buffered saline (PBS), pH 7.4.
2. Dulbecco's phosphate-buffered saline (D-PBS; Life Technologies) supplemented with penicillin–streptomycin (PS), 20 IU/mL (penicillin 10,000 IU/mL, streptomycin 10,000 µg/mL; Life Technologies).
3. Enzyme solution for tissue separation: trypsin (Difco, cat. no. 0152-15); pancreatin (Life Technologies, cat. no. 45720-018), stock solution of 1.25 g/mL. tyrode's solution: 8.0 g NaCl, 0.2 g KCl, 0.05 g NaH_2PO_4, 1.0 g glucose, 1.0 g $NaHCO_3$. Adjust pH to 7.2, make up to 1000 mL with distilled H_2O, and sterile-filter. Store at 4°C. Dissolve 0.225 g trypsin in 6 mL Tyrode's solution on ice, using a magnetic stirrer. Add 1 mL pancreatin and 20 µL PS. Adjust pH to 7.4 with NaOH. Make up to the final volume 10 mL with Tyrode's solution and sterile-filter. Aliquot 1 mL in Eppendorf tubes and store at –20°C. The enzyme solution can be stored at –20°C for 1 wk.
4. Medium for tissue dissection and culture: Dulbecco's modified Eagle medium with glutaMAX-1 (DMEM; Sigma, cat. no. D7777), supplemented with 10% heat-inactivated fetal calf serum (FCS) and PS (20 IU/ mL). Store at 4°C (*see* **Note 6**).
5. 0.1% Bovine serum albumin (BSA) in PBS.
6. Growth factors:
   a. 20 ng/µL Fibroblast growth factor (FGF)-4.
   b. 1 ng/µL Transforming growth factor β (TGFβ)-1.

2.2. Dissection and Culture

2.2.1. For Tissue Dissection

1. 10-cm Diameter plastic bacteriological Petri dishes.
2. 4- to 10-cm Diameter glass Petri dishes.
3. Small scissors.
4. Forceps.
5. Disposable 20- and 26-gauge needles attached to 1-mL plastic syringes (*see* **Note 1**).

2.2.2. For Cell Culture

1. Culture dishes: 3.5-cm diameter plastic Petri dishes (bacteriological or cell culture dishes).
2. Metal grids: prepared from stainless-steel mesh (corrosion-resistant, size of mesh 0.7 mm) by cutting approximately 3 cm diameter disks and bending the edges on a cutting form to give a 3 mm height (the height of the metal grids can be altered to allow the use of more or less culture media). Holes in the grid are produced either by nails in the cutting form or by punching. The holes facilitate the examination and photography of the explants (and they are handy when transfilter cultures are prepared) (*see* **Note 5**) (**Fig. 2**). There are commercially available organ culture dishes featuring a central well in which a metal grid (even without bent edges) can be placed (Falcon 3037; Becton Dickinson).

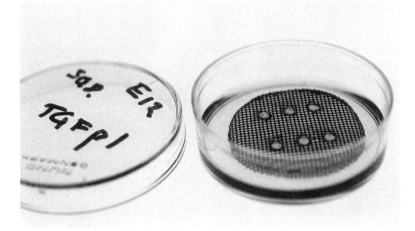

Fig. 2. The Trowell-type organ culture dish. The metal grid supports 6 pieces of filters. The cultured explants (like the one in the bottom of **Fig. 1**) are seen on the filters over the holes of the grid.

3. Filters: nuclepore polycarbonate filters (0.1 µm) (Nuclepore® Track-Etch membrane; Whatman , cat. no. 110 605). The pore size routinely used is 0.1 µm (*see* **Note 4**). The filters are cut in halves, washed in detergent, rinsed under running water for 2 h and 10 times in distilled water, and stored in 70% ethanol.

4. Matrigel (Collaborative Biomedical Products) is stored in the refrigerator and kept on ice in the laminar flow hood.

5. Glass Pasteur pipets for transferring tissues. They are siliconized (to prevent sticking of tissues), stuffed with cotton wool, and autoclaved. Before use, they are drawn by heating to adjust to the size of the tissues. Ideally, the diameter should be the minimal to allow free passage of the tissue. Alternatively, tissues can be transferred by watchmakers forceps or using pieces of Nuclepore filter.

6. Beads for growth factors: Affi-Gel Blue agarose beads (Bio-Rad) or heparin-coated acrylic beads (Sigma) are divided into aliquots and stored at 4°C.

3. Methods
3.1. Treatment of Beads

1. Pipet agarose beads or heparin-coated acrylic beads in a Petri dish containing PBS.
2. Count 100–200 beads under the microscope, and transfer to an Eppendorf tube.
3. Spin down the beads and remove PBS.
4. Add growth factors in a small volume (10–50 µL) of 0.1% BSA in PBS. In general, high concentrations of growth factors are used. We use FGF-4 at 20 ng/µL and TGFβ-1 at 1 ng/µL.
5. An equal amount of 0.1% BSA in PBS should be pipetted to control beads.

6. Incubate for 30 min at 37°C and store at 4°C. The beads can be used at least for 14 d (depending on the stability of the protein).

3.2. Preparation of Cell Aggregates

1. In order to aggregate the cells expressing the protein of interest, plate the cells in excess on a bacterial culture dish, e.g., the equivalent of half of a 75-cm^2 confluent culture flask into a 6-cm diameter Petri dish noncoated for cell culture.
2. Since the cells cannot adhere to the bottom of the plate, in 48 h they form clumps floating in the medium.
3. The aggregates can be moved by a pipet tip or a micropipet and grafted on the cultured tissue *(15,16)*.

3.3. Preparation of Tissue Culture Dishes

1. Take a sheet of Nuclepore filter from ethanol and rinse in a plastic 10-cm Petri dish containing PBS.
2. Cut the filter, using small scissors and watchmakers forceps, into approx 3 × 3 mm pieces and leave in PBS.
3. Place metal grids in 3.5-cm plastic culture dishes.
4. Add approximately 2 mL culture medium (DMEM plus 10% FCS; *see* **Note 6**) by pipeting through the grid. The surface of the medium should contact the plane of the grid, but not cover it (excess medium results in floating of the filters and tissues). No air bubbles should remain under the grid (if present, they can be sucked empty with a thin Pastour pipet).
5. Using forceps, transfer the Nuclepore filter pieces onto the grids placing them over the holes.
6. Pipet a drop of ice-cold Matrigel onto the filters.
7. Transfer the dishes to the incubator for 10 min to allow gelling of the Matrigel.
8. Place the tissue on Matrigel in the hood (*see* **Note 7**).

3.4. Dissection of Tissues

1. Place the mouse uterus (E12) in a 10-cm plastic Petri dish containing D-PBS, and cut open the uterine wall using small scissors and forceps. Continue the work under the stereomicroscope with transmitted light.
2. Remove the embryos from fetal membranes and transfer them to a fresh dish of D-PBS.
3. Cut off the heads using disposable needles as "knives". The needles are used during all subsequent steps of dissection.
4. Transfer the heads to a glass Petri dish containing D-PBS and dissect out the lower jaw.
5. Dissect out the tooth germs of the first mandibular molar with some surrounding tissue left in place (*see* **Notes 1** and **2**).
6. Transfer the tooth germs to a small culture dish.
7. Remove most of the liquid.
8. Thaw an aliquot of pancreatin-trypsin and add to the tooth germs.

9. Incubate for 2–10 min at room temperature or 37°C.
10. Remove most of the liquid and add culture medium, mix, and transfer the tooth germs to a glass Petri dish containing culture medium.
11. Leave the tissues for at least 30 min at room temperature.
12. Gently separate the epithelia from the mesenchymes using needles and remove excess surrounding nondental tissue (*see* **Note 3**).
13. Transfer the tissues to the Nuclepore filters in culture dishes that have been prepared in advance. Tissues can be lifted by a filter piece or by the capillary force between the tips of watchmakers forceps. If using glass pipet, avoid air bubbles in the pipet, and avoid sucking the tissue beyond the capillary part of the pipet. Ideally, the tissues should be placed directly in their final position, but if need be, they can be gently pushed with needles.
14. If you are using beads, rinse them quickly in PBS in a glass Petri dish (they tend to stick on plastic dishes).
15. Under the microscope, transfer the beads or transfected cell aggregates one at a time to the tissues.

3.5. Culture and Fixation

1. Culture the tissues in a standard incubator at 37°C, in an atmosphere of 5% CO_2 in air, and 90–95% humidity for 24 h.
2. Photograph the explants before fixation (the translucency is lost after fixation).
3. To avoid detachment of tissues from the filters, prefix the explants in ice-cold methanol on the grids as follows:
   a. Remove the culture medium by sucking, and then pipet methanol gently on the tissues.
   b. Leave for 5 min, and then transfer filters using watchmaker forceps to Eppendorf tubes for subsequent treatments (*see* **Notes 8** and **9**).
   c. Typical explants are shown in **Fig. 3**, (*see* **Note 10**).

4. Notes

1. For tissue dissection, disposable needles are superior to other instruments, such as scalpels or iris knives, because they need no sharpening or sterilization. The size of the needles can be chosen according to the sizes of tissues. The syringes need not be absolutely sterile and can be used many times. For best preservation of tissue vitality, dissecting should be done by determined cuts avoiding tearing. Glass Petri dishes are preferable to plastic ones during dissection of the tissues, because cutting with the needles tends to scrape the bottom of the plastic dish and loosen pieces of it.
2. The preparation and dissection of tissues should be done as quickly as possible to promote survival of the tissues. One uterus at a time should be prepared, and the rest stored in D-PBS at 4°C. The dissected tissues should not be stored for long periods of time (2–3 h maximum) before transferring to the culture dishes and incubator.

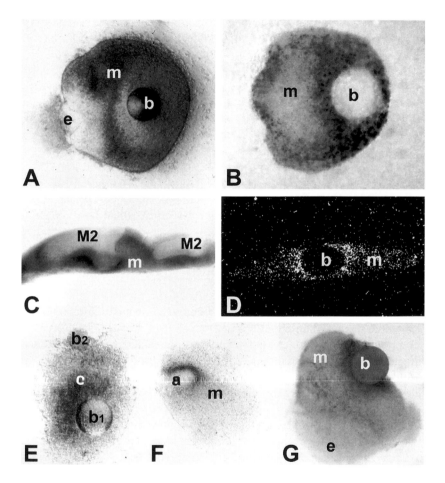

Fig. 3. Examples of the analysis of cultured explants. (**A**) Stereomicroscopical appearance of an explant in culture. The epithelium, as well as the FGF-4 releasing bead, have induced a translucent zone in dental mesenchyme. (**B**) Localization of cell proliferation with BrdU incorporation around an FGF-10 releasing bead. (**C**) A 400 μm thick vibratome section of cultured dental tissue stained in whole mount *in situ* using Runx2 probe. (**D**) In situ hybridization analysis of a paraffin section showing the induction of tenascin-C transcripts by a TGFβ-1 releasing bead (dark-field illumination). (**E**) Epithelium (E13) with FGF-4 releasing bead (b₁) inducing Lunatic Fringe transcripts and BMP-4 (bone morphogenic protein) releasing bead (b₂) not inducing. (**F**) Dental tissue (E12) cultured with wnt6, releasing cell aggregates, and stained by whole mount in situ using ectodysplasin probe. (**G**) Whole mount immunohistochemical staining showing stimulation of tenascin expression in the mesenchyme around an FGF-4 releasing bead. e, dental epithelium; m, dental mesenchyme; b, bead; M1, first molar; M2, second molar.

3. The dissection and culture techniques are basically similar when different organs or different developmental stages of tooth germs are studied. Separation of the epithelium and mesenchyme can be accomplished in young tissues, after enzyme treatment, even without dissection by briefly vortex mixing the tissues. On the other hand, more advanced tissues require a longer incubation in the enzyme solution (up to 10 min). The time needed for best separation depends also on the batches of enzymes, and therefore, the optimal time must always be checked for new batches of enzyme and for different tissues.

4. Different supporting materials can be used for the cultured explants. Lens paper may be used for large tissue pieces. The supporting material must allow good diffusion of the medium to the tissue, and therefore, Millipore filters of 100 µm thickness are not suitable. (The thickness of Nuclepore filters is approx 10 µm.) Different pore size Nuclepore filters may be used. Small pores (0.05–0.2 µm) allow better examination of the explants in the stereomicroscope using transmitted light, but the tissues tend to detach from these filters more readily during fixation and other treatments after culture. Therefore, larger pore sizes (up to 1 µm) may be preferable, depending on the experiment.

5. The Trowell-type organ culture can be used for a variety of other organ culture designs. One example is the transfilter culture, in which the interacting tissues are cultured on opposite sides of the filter *(4,9)*. The tissue to be grown below the filter is glued by heated 1% agar, after which the filter is turned upside down, and the other tissue is placed on top of the filter.

6. The composition of the optimal culture medium depends on the tissues. The medium in this protocol is good for a number of different organs at early stages of development, but during more advanced stages, different organs may have special requirements. Chemically defined media with varying compositions have been designed. For cultures of whole tooth germs, we routinely use chemically defined medium composed of DMEM and F12 (Ham's Nutrient Mixture; Life Technologies) 1:1, supplemented with 50 µg/mL transferrin (Sigma, cat. no. T-2252) (10 mg/mL, in 20-µL aliquots, and stored at –20°C). For more advanced stages of tooth development, ascorbic acid is added at 150 µg/mL to allow deposition of dentin collagen *(10)*. During prolonged culture, the medium should be changed at 2- to 3-d intervals.

7. Isolated epithelial tissue does not survive as well as the mesenchymal tissue when cultured alone. The growth of the dental epithelium (as well as epithelium from other organs) is significantly improved by culture on extracellular matrix material. Collagen has been used, but by far the best results are obtained with the basement membrane matrix, Matrigel, which also promotes epithelial morphogenesis *(17)*. Covering of the tissue with a drop of Matrigel further improves epithelial growth.

8. Some cell lines do not form aggregates as easily as others. They can be centrifuged in an Eppendorf tube at 2000*g* for 2 min, and then the big clump of cells can be transferred into a plate containing culture media and cut into smaller pieces using sterile needles.

9. Bromodeoxyuridine (BrdU) incorporation is commonly used for the analysis of cell proliferation (**Fig. 3B**). The explants are labeled by adding BrdU 0.5–3 h before fixation (we use cell proliferation kits from Amersham International or Boehringer-Mannheim). After fixation in ice-cold methanol, the explants are washed in PBS and immunostained as whole mounts using antibodies against BrdU *(12,15)*.

10. Usually, the tissues are analyzed after culture as whole mounts (**Fig. 3B–D**). After whole mount analysis, the explants may be embedded in gelatin–albumin and cut to thick sections (200 μm) by vibratome for examination of gross morphology (e.g., to differentiate between epithelial vs mesenchymal staining). For the examination of histological details, the explants should be paraffin-embedded and serially sectioned (**Fig. 3E, F**). For most purposes, they are fixed for 1 h in 4% paraformaldehyde (PFA) in PBS (after a 5-min prefixation in ice-cold methanol). PFA should be fairly freshly made (not more than 7 d old). The procedures used for whole mount immunostaining and for in situ hybridization have been described previously *(12,13,16)*.

References

1. Trowell, O. A. (1959) The culture of mature organs in a synthetic medium. *Exp. Cell Res.* **16,** 118–147.
2. Grobstein, C. (1953) Inductive epithelio-mesenchymal interaction in cultured organ rudiments of the mouse. *Science* **118,** 52–55.
3. Saxén, I. (1973) Effects of hydrocortisone on the development *in vitro* of the secondary palate in two inbred strains of mice. *Arch. Oral Biol.* **18,** 1469–1479.
4. Saxén, L., Lehtonen, E., Karkinen-Jääskeläinen, M., Nordling, S., and Wartiovaara, J. (1976) Morphogenetic tissue interactions: mediation by transmissible signal substances or through cell contacts? *Nature* **259,** 662,663.
5. Nogawa, H. and Takahashi, Y. (1991) Substitution for mesenchyme by basement-membrane-like substratum and epidermal growth factor in inducing branching morphogenesis of mouse salivary epithelium. *Development* **112,** 855–861.
6. Nogawa, H. and Ito, T. (1995) Branching morphogenesis of embryonic mouse lung epithelium in mesenchyme-free culture. *Development* **121,** 1015–1022.
7. Rice, P., Åberg, T., Chan, Y.-S., Kettunen, P., Pakarinen, L., Maxson, R. E., and Thesleff, I. (2000) Integration of FGF and TWIST in calvarial bone and suture development. *Development* **127,** 1845–1855.
8. Saxén, L. (1966) The effect of tetracycline on osteogenesis *in vitro*. *J. Exp. Zool.* **162,** 269–294.
9. Thesleff, I., Lehtonen, E., Wartiovaara, J., and Saxén, L. (1977) Interference of tooth differentiation with interposed filters. *Dev. Biol.* **58,** 197–203.
10. Partanen, A. M., Ekblom, P., and Thesleff, I. (1985) Epidermal growth factor inhibits tooth morphogenesis and differentiation. *Dev. Biol.* **111,** 84–94.
11. Vainio, S., Karavanova, I., Jowett, A., and Thesleff, I. (1993) Identification of BMP-4 as a signal mediating secondary induction between epithelial and mesenchymal tissues during early tooth development. *Cell* **75,** 45–58.

12. Jernvall, J., Aberg, T., Kettunen, P., Keranen, S., and Thesleff, I. (1998) The life history of an embryonic signaling center: BMP-4 induces p21 and is associated with apoptosis in the mouse tooth enamel knot. *Development* **125,** 161–169.

13. Vaahtokari, A., Åberg, T., and Thesleff, I. (1996) Apoptosis in the developing tooth: association with an embryonic signalling center and suppression by EGF and FGF-4. *Development* **122,** 121–129.

14. Mitsiadis, T., Muramatsu, T., Muramatsu, H., and Thesleff, I. (1995) Midkine (MK), a heparing-binding growth/differentiation factor, is regulated by retinoic acid and epithelial-mesenchymal interactions in the developing mouse tooth, and affects cell proliferation and morphogenesis. *J. Cell Biol.* **129,** 267–281.

15. Kettunen, P., Laurikkala, J., Itäranta, P., Vainio, S., Itoh, N., and Thesleff, I. (2000) Associations of FGF-3 and FGF-10 with signaling networks regulating tooth morphogenesis. *Dev. Dyn.,* **219,** 322–332.

16. Laurikkala, J., Mikkola, M., Mustonen, T., et al. (2001) TNF signaling via the ligand-receptor pair ectodysplasin and edar controls the function of epithelial signaling centers and is regulated by Wnt and activin during organogenesis, *Dev. Biol.* **229,** 443–455.

17. Gittes, G., Galante, P. E., Hanahan, D., Rutter, W. J., and Debas, H. T. (1996) Lineage-specific morphogenesis in the developing pancreas: role of mesenchymal factors. *Development* **122,** 439–447.

31

Bacterial Interactions with Host Epithelium In Vitro

Nicola Jones, Mary H. Perdue,
Philip M. Sherman, and Derek M. McKay

1. Introduction

During recent years there has been a resurgence of interest in the role that bacteria, both pathogenic and commensal, play in the pathogenesis and pathophysiology of disease. For example, antibiotics can be a useful therapy to relieve the symptomatology experienced by a cohort of patients with Crohn's disease, a major class of inflammatory bowel disease *(1)*. Traditionally, assessment of the impact of bacteria on the health status of an individual has focused on the role of their noxious products (e.g., lipopolysaccharide [endotoxin], exotoxins, and enterotoxins [e.g., cholera toxin, superantigens]) and recruitment and/or activation of immune cells. However, it is now clear that the direct interaction of bacteria with epithelial cells can mobilize intraepithelial signaling molecules, resulting in altered epithelial physiology. Studies using co-culture models of epithelial cell lines with bacteria have shown unequivocally that bacterial attachment to enterocytes affects a plethora of epithelial functions including vectorial ion transport, barrier function, and the production of immune mediators and chemokines; the latter response allowing participation in, and modulation of, mucosal immune reactions *(2–6)*. Indeed, awareness that bacteria can directly affect the host cells to which they attach has led to a new discipline in microbiology—namely, cellular microbiology *(7)*.

The aim of this chapter is to outline a methodology for the co-culture of bacteria with model epithelia and to describe some of the techniques that are used to examine bacterial–epithelial interaction in terms of bacterial attachment, effects on the enterocyte cytoskeleton (and tight junction-associated proteins) and concomitant changes in permeability, and epithelial cell apoptosis.

From: *Methods in Molecular Biology, vol. 188: Epithelial Cell Culture Protocols*
Edited by: C. Wise © Humana Press Inc., Totowa, NJ

The following description will refer exclusively to the effects of noninvasive bacteria (e.g., enteropathogenic *Escherichia coli* [EPEC], *Helicobacter pylori*) and not invasive species, such as *Salmonellae* and *Shigellae*, but clearly the same basic procedures and principals can be applied to an assessment of the impact of other bacterial species on epithelial form and function.

The hybrid science of cellular microbiology merges the disciplines of cell biology and microbiology *(7)*. A wealth of data have accumulated illustrating the direct effects of microbes and their products on epithelial intracellular signaling and, hence, physiology. Here, we have described a standard laboratory approach to juxtapose host epithelia with bacterial pathogens and outlined indices of epithelial function that can be used to define changes in epithelial function as a direct consequence of exposure to the bacterium, in the absence of other cell types *(2,13,29–32)*. The task facing the integrative physiologist or cellular microbiologist is to precisely define the cross-talk between the microflora (pathogen or commensal organism) and the host eukaryotic cell. Major advances are now being made in the study of cellular microbiology. The synthesis of the data being obtained undoubtedly will impact on our understanding of the regulation of cell function, pathophysiological mechanisms, and ultimately, highlight the way for novel therapies to combat infectious diseases.

We refer the reader to **Chapter 29**, which is complementary to this chapter.

2. Materials

2.1. Epithelial and Bacterial Culture

Initiation of an examination of the direct effects of bacteria on epithelial cells must be preceded by addressing two basic questions. First, what is the target host organ of interest, and hence, type of epithelium, and what is the pathogen or commensal strain of bacteria to be used? Second, what is the primary focus of the investigation? This latter question will influence the choice of model epithelium since, for example, only a limited number of cell lines form electrically tight monolayers that are suitable for examining vectorial ion transport, such as the human colon-derived T84 and Caco-2 transformed cell lines. A variety of epithelial cell lines are available that are representative of lung, kidney, urinary bladder, and gut epithelium, and these can be matched to bacterial species that will colonize or infect these tissues. For instance, co-culture studies can be conducted with *Pseudomonas aeruginosa* and airway epithelium (e.g., human A549 epithelia cell line) *(8)*, uropathogenic *E. coli* (strain Hu734) and urinary bladder epithelium (e.g., J82 or MDCK cell lines) *(9)*, or enteric bacteria pathogens with a variety of gut-derived epithelia (e.g., human T84, Caco-2, HT-29, Kato III or AGS) *(10)*.

Our laboratories have made extensive use of T84 cells (human colon-derived, crypt-like cell line), Kato III and AGS cells (human gastric cell lines), and HEp-2 cells (human laryngeal cell line) as model epithelia and have examined the direct effects of enteropathogenic *E. coli* (EPEC; prototype strain E2348/6, serotype O127:H6) or *H. pylori* (both clinical isolates and the murine adapted Sydney strain, SS-1). Appropriate controls for EPEC infection include the nonpathogenic laboratory strain HB101 (O:rough) and the isogenic *eaeA* (for *E. coli* attaching and effacing) deletion mutant of E2348/6, designated CVD206 *(2)*. Appropriate controls for *H. pylori*, which can be employed, include isogenic mutants of putative virulence factors, including *cagA*, *cagE*, and *Campylobacter jejuni (11)*.

2.1.1. Epithelial Culture

1. T84 Culture medium: 1:1 Dulbecco's modified Eagle's medium (DMEM):Ham's F12 supplemented with 10% (v/v) newborn calf serum, 1.5% (v/v) HEPES, 2% (v/v) penicillin–streptomycin.
2. Modified Eagle's medium for general cell culture.
3. RPMI for general cell culture.
4. 1% (v/v) Amphotericin B can be used as an additional antibiotic.
5. 200 M/L L-glutamine.
6. Sodium butyrate: 1–10 $\mu M/L$ added to culture medium to induce human colonic Caco-2 cells to differentiate from crypt-like to villus-like phenotype.
7. Trypsin-EDTA.
8. Phosphate-buffered saline (PBS), sterile, pH 7.4.
9. Additional growth factors may be required on a cell-specific basis (e.g., epidermal growth factor [EGF]).
10. Assorted plasticware: Petri dishes, 6- or 12-well plates, tissue culture flasks, Labtek chamber slides, pipet tips, 15- and 50-mL tubes.
11. Pasteur pipets.
12. Transwell plates with microporous filters (Costar). The size of the filter, filter pore size and filter composition will be determined by the nature of the investigation.

2.1.2. Bacterial Culture

1. EPEC: Columbia blood agar plates, Penassay broth, bile agar plates, and sterile 15-mL tubes.
2. *H. pylori*: Brucella broth (Difco): supplemented with 10% fetal calf serum (FCS), 10 μg/mL vancomycin, 5 μg/mL trimethoprim; Erlenmeyer flasks. For storage, 10% sterile glycerol is required.

2.1.3. Co-Cultures

1. *E. coli* antibiotic-free culture medium—culture medium is matched to the epithelial cell type of interest.

2. *H. pylori* culture medium—consists of medium appropriate for epithelial cell type being used supplemented with 10 μg/mL vancomycin, 5 μg/mL trimethoprim.

2.2. Analysis of Epithelial Form and Function

2.2.1. The Attaching and Effacing Lesion

1. 2% Glutaraldehyde in 0.1 *M* sodium cacoylate buffer (pH 7.4).
2. Graded alcohols (50, 70 and 100% ethanol).
3. Eponxy resin (Epon).
4. Uranyl acetate: saturated in ethanol.
5. Lead citrate: dissolve 1.33 g lead nitrate with 1.76 g of sodium citrate in 30 mL boiled water, add 8 mL of 1 *M* sodium hydroxide and 12 mL of boiled water (after Reynolds *[33]*).

2.2.2. Filamentous Actin

1. 10% Neutral-buffered formalin.
2. 0.1% (v/v) Triton-X 100 (Sigma) in PBS.
3. 2.5×10^{-6} *M* Fluorescein isothiocyanate (FITC)-phalloidin (Molecular Probes).
4. 1:1 Glycerol:PBS.
5. Methanol.
6. Bradford microassay (Bio-Rad).

2.2.3. Tight Junctions and Associated Proteins

1. Fixatives: methanol or 4% paraformaldehyde (PFA).
2. 1% (w/v) Bovine serum albumin (BSA)/0.1% (v/v) Triton X-100 in PBS.
3. Primary antibodies against tight junction-associated proteins (e.g., zona occludens 1 [ZO-1], occludin; can be obtained from a variety of commercial sources). For example, 1:200 anti-ZO-1 (Zymed Laboratories, San Francisco, CA).
4. Buffers for washing: PBS only or 0.1% Triton X-100 in PBS.
5. Complementary secondary antibodies conjugated to FITC, rhodamine (other flurochromes are available from Molecular Probes), or biotin.
6. 0.5 mg/mL 3,3'-Diaminobenzidine tetrahydrochoride (DAB).
7. Hydrogen peroxide:
    a. For quenching of endogenous peroxidase, use 10 mL of 30% H_2O_2 in 200 mL of 100% methanol plus 0.5 *M* HCl (incubate for 30 min at room temperature).
    b. For use in chromagen substrate add 10 μL of 30% H_2O_2 to 95 mL of chromagen.
8. Staining trays.
9. Pipets and tips.
10. Permount (Fisher Scientific) and Gel Mount™ (Biomedia, Foster City, CA).

2.2.4. Epithelial Calcium Mobilization

1. Flurochromes: Indo-1 acetoxymethyl (AM) esters, Furo-3 AM (Molecular Probes), 1–10 μ*M*, dissolved in dimethyl sulfoxide (DMSO) and diluted in cul-

ture medium. Manufacturer provides detailed analysis of the use and advantages of these and related compounds.

2. 10 µ*M* Calcium ionophore A23187, pharmacological agonist.
3. 100 µ*M* Carbachol, cholinergic agonist, physiological agonist.
4. Resuspension buffer: 140 m*M* NaCl, 3 m*M* KCl, 1 m*M* MgCl$_2$, 1.5 m*M* CaCl$_2$, 5 m*M* glucose, and 10 m*M* HEPES at pH 7.4.

2.2.5. Epithelial Monolayer Permeability

1. Ussing chambers (World Precision Instruments).
2. Assorted tubing.
3. Agar bridges (3% agar in 3 *M* KCl solution or a 1:1 solution of 3 *M* KCl:normal Kreb's saline).
4. Voltage clamp (model DVC-100; World Precision Instruments) and matched pre-amplifiers and calomel electrodes.
5. Heating pump.
6. Aeration regulator.
7. Chart recorder or computerized data acquisition system.
8. 5×10^{-5} *M* Horseradish peroxidase (HRP) (type II; mw, approx 44 kDa; Sigma).
9. PBS containing 0.003% (v/v) hydrogen peroxide and 80 µg/mL *o*-dianisidine (Sigma).
10. ^{3}H-mannitol (mw, 180 Da; 6.5 µCi/mL; 10 m*M* mannitol).
11. ^{51}Cr EDTA (mw, 360 Da; 2.5 µCi/mL; 8.5 µ*M* EDTA). Steps 8, 9, and 10 are all suitable marker molecules to assess epithelial barrier function (*see* **Note 1**).
12. 0.5 mg/mL DAB/0.01% (v/v) hydrogen peroxide in Tris Buffer.

2.3. Epithelial Cell Apoptosis

1. Commercial kits to examine apoptosis (e.g., terminal transferase-mediated dUTP nick end labeling [TUNEL] assay kit).

2.3.1. Morphological Assessment of Apoptosis by Transmission Electron Microscopy (TEM)

1. 2% Glutaraldehyde.

2.3.2. Determination of Apoptosis by Fluorescent Dye Staining

1. 100 µg/mL Acridine orange-ethidium bromide.
2. Aptex-coated slides (Fisher Scientific)—alternatively, other coated slides (for increasing adhesion of section to slide) can be substituted.

2.3.3. TUNEL

1. Sterile PBS.
2. Trypsin-EDTA.
3. Xylene.
4. Paraffin wax, for embedding.

5. 0.01% Hydrogen peroxide.
6. 0.01 M Citrate buffer.
7. 20 µg/mL Proteinase K (Boehringer Mannheim).
8. Terminal transferase buffer: 200 mM potassium cacodylate, 25 mM Tris-HCl, pH 6.6, 0.2 mM EDTA, 25 mg/mL BSA.
9. 1 mM Cobalt chloride.
10. 0.01 nM Biotin 16-dUTP.
11. 0.5 U/µL Terminal transferase (Boehringer Mannheim).
12. Stop solution: 300 mM sodium chloride, 30 mM sodium citrate.
13. Avidin-conjugated peroxidase.
14. Hematoxylin.

2.3.4. Cell Death Detection

1. Cell death detection enzyme-linked immunosorbent assay (ELISA)[plus] kit (Boehringer Mannheim).

2.4. Major Pieces of Apparatus

1. Centrifuge (bench top and microfuge).
2. Voltmeter and associated chopstick electrodes (Millicel-ERS; Millipore).
3. Sterile laminar flow hood.
4. Sterile cell culture incubator.
5. Incubator for bacterial growth.
6. Light microscope.
7. Inverted-light microscope.
8. Cytospin (Shanndon Scientific, Ltd., Cheshire).
9. Heated water bath.
10. Fluorescence spectrophotometer (model MPF-66; Perkin Elmer).
11. Radioactive scintillation counter.
12. Electron microscopy facilities.
13. Fluorescence microscopy facilities.

3. Methods

3.1. Growth of Epithelial Cells and Bacteria

3.1.1. Epithelia

1. Grow the epithelial cells on standard tissue culture plasticware. Culture media for different epithelia may differ slightly, and the reader should check the salient literature. For T84 cells, the predominant cell used in our laboratory, we use T84 culture medium
2. Plastic-grown T84 cells should be subcultured on a weekly basis, whereas faster growing cells (e.g., the murine gut cell line, IEC 4.1) need to be subcultured twice a week.
3. After seeding onto transwell filter supports (we use 10^6 cells/mL, although lower densities are also appropriate), the cells should be maintained under standard culture conditions (37°C; 5% CO_2).

4. Change the culture medium daily or every other day until the required degree of monolayer confluency has been obtained.
5. For plastic-grown preparations, the degree of monolayer confluence is determined by light or phase contrast microscopy.
6. A confluent filter-grown monolayer is typically defined by the transepithelial resistance. This is conveniently determined using a voltmeter fitted with asymmetrical chop-stick electrodes.
7. In the case of T84 monolayers, investigators often stipulate ≥800 Ω/cm^2 as a suitable control preparation, whereas lower resistance is the norm (250–400 Ω/cm^2) for the human colonic Caco-2 and HT-29 cell lines.

3.1.2. Bacterial Culture

3.1.2.1. EPEC

1. Twenty-four hours prior to experimentation, grow bacteria in Penassay broth at 37°C (*see* **Note 2**).
2. Pellet the bacteria by centrifugation at 2500*g* for 15 min.
3. Resuspend in sterile PBS to a concentration of approx 1×10^9 colony forming units (CFU)/mL.
4. Previously viable counts of EPEC should have been obtained by serial 10-fold dilutions plated onto bile agar plates.

3.1.2.2. *H. PYLORI*

1. Grow bacteria under micro-aerophilic conditions on Columbia blood agar plates for 72 h at 37°C (*see* **Note 2**).
2. For infection experiments, resuspend bacteria on plates in Brucella broth.
3. Grow overnight in an Erlenmeyer flask with shaking.
4. Pellet bacteria and resuspend in PBS at 1×10^9 CFU/mL.

3.1.3. Establishment of Co-Cultures

1. Rinse epithelial preparations (plastic or filter-grown) 3 times (10- to 20-s washes) with sterile antibiotic-free culture medium (medium matched to cell line being used in any particular study) if they are to be cultured with *E. coli*, or medium containing vancomycin and trimethoprim for *H. pylori* epithelial studies.
2. Add a 50-μL aliquot of the bacterial suspension (containing the desired number of CFUs) in 1 mL of culture medium (with or without the appropriate antibiotics) to the apical surface of the epithelium.
3. Agitate the plate gently for 10 s to enhance spreading of the bacterial inoculate over the epithelium.
4. Incubate the co-culture at 37°C for 3–24 h (*see* **Note 3**).
5. Remove nonadherent bacteria by gentle aspiration.
6. Rinse with appropriate cell culture medium and repeat 2 to 3 times.
7. Process the epithelium for further investigations (*see* **Subheading 3.2.**).

8. It is important to determine if any bacteria-induced change in epithelial function is due to bacterial attachment or products secreted from the bacteria. This can be tested by:
   a. Conducting co-culture experiments using dead bacteria.
   b. Exposing naive epithelium to bacterial homongenates or filtered (0.4 μm) medium from bacterial cultures that will include only the secreted bacterial products (*see* **Note 4**).
   c. Also, as noted in **Subheading 2.1.**, genetically altered strains of bacteria can be used that lack the ability to produce specific structures (e.g., adhesions) or products (e.g., toxins) *(11,12)*.

3.2. Analysis of Epithelial Form and Function

3.2.1. The Attaching and Effacing Lesion

EPEC attach closely to epithelial cells via a pedestal-type projection from the surface of the enterocyte that disrupts the usual pattern of the microvilli, which has been designated the attaching and effacing (A/E) lesion *(13,14)*. The induction of an A/E lesion can be readily identify using TEM.

Infect the epithelium with the bacteria for 6 h at 37°C:

1. Rinse the epithelium 4–6 times in PBS to remove nonadherent cells.
2. If the epithelium is plastic grown, gently scrape free with a rubber policeman and pellet at 1000*g* for 10 min.
3. Fix in 2% gluteraldehyde, followed by post-fixation in 2% osmium tetroxide (a standard EM procedure).
4. If epithelium is filter-grown, excise from the plastic basket support, and fix the epithelium as above (**step 2**).
5. Dehydrate through a graded series of alcohol (50–100%).
6. Embed preparations in eponxy resin (Epon).
7. Cut ultrathin sections (50–60 nm) and collect on mesh copper grids.
8. Stain with uranyl acetate and lead citrate, following the standard procedure for EM.
9. Grids can then be examined in a transmission electron microscope using an accelerating voltage of 60 kV *(14)*.
10. Alternatively, the epithelium can be processed for and examined by scanning electron microscopy (SEM)—again following routine procedures used in EM.

3.2.2. Filamentous Actin

The formation of the A/E lesion is accompanied by an accumulation of host cytoskeletal proteins directly beneath the lesion *(13)*. Tight junction-associated proteins are coupled to filamentous (F) actin, and it is postulated that actin-myosin contractions–relaxations will regulate paracellular permeability by pulling apart, or collapsing together, the tight junctions (*see* **Subheading 3.2.3.**). The fungal-deprived protein, phalloidin, binds to and caps F-actin, preventing further changes via the addition or removal of monomeric G actin. Thus, studies with FITC-phalloidin allow for identification of the distribution of F-actin *(2)*.

1. Fix epithelia for 20–30 min at room temperature with 10% neutral-buffered formalin.
2. Permeabilize by a 5-min incubation in 0.1% Triton X-100 in PBS.
3. Incubate the epithelium with FITC-phalloidin for 30 min, noting that the samples should be kept in the dark during this incubation.
4. Rinse the preparations 3 times in PBS.
5. Mount onto microscope slides in glycerol:PBS (1:1) and view under epifluoresence or by confocal scanning laser microscopy.
6. As an adjunct to this visualization technique, total cellular F-actin can also be quantified. Monolayers should be treated identically, except that following FITC-phalloidin treatment, they are extracted in the dark in 100% methanol for 1 h at 37°C.
7. The extract should be vigorously pipetted.
8. Collect into a cuvet and measure fluorescence in a spectrofluoremeter using an excitation wavelength of 465 nm and an emission wavelength of 535 nm (10-nm slit).
9. Record data as arbitrary units of fluorescence per milligram total cell protein, as determined by the Bradford protein microassay (*see* **Note 5**).

3.2.3. Tight Junction Associated Proteins

The epithelial tight junction regulates the paracellular permeability pathway. While the exact nature of the structure that represents the actual "seal" has been controversial, the current model of the tight junction is one of interlocking occludin and claudin proteins from adjacent cells, which are linked via cytoplasmic proteins (e.g., ZO-1 and others) to the enterocytic actin cytoskeleton *(15)*. The effect of bacterial attachment and bacterial products on the tight junction-associated proteins can be examined using commercial antibodies and indirect immunocytochemical detection methods *(2,12)*.

1. Grow monolayers on a filter support (sterile plasticware can also be used) with or without bacteria.
2. Rinse 3 times in PBS.
3. Fix in 100% cold methanol for 10–20 min (other fixatives such as 4% PFA can be used if specified as suitable by the manufacturer of the primary antibodies).
4. Rinse monolayers in PBS and incubate in PBS containing 1% BSA/0.1% Triton in PBS for 5 min.
5. Incubate for 1–4 h with the primary antibody diluted in 1% BSA/0.1% Triton in PBS (e.g., ZO-1, at, for example, 1:200 dilution).
6. After 3 buffer washes in 0.1% Triton in PBS, epithelial cell preparations should be incubated with the appropriate species-specific secondary antibody (diluted in buffer, for example, to 1:100), which is tagged with a fluorescent marker (e.g., FITC, rhodamine) or biotin for 1–4 h (*see* **Note 5**).
7. After a final series of 3 rinses 0.1% Triton in PBS, the epithelial monolayers should be excised from their plastic basket supports.
8. Mount onto slides in an aqueous mounting medium, such as Gel Mount™, and view by epifluoresence or confocal scanning laser microscopy *(2)*.

9. In the instance where a biotinylated secondary antibody has been used (note that this is considerably less common in the scientific literature), visualization of the tight junction protein of interest is by light microscopy following color development with avidin-conjugated peroxidase and reaction with DAB or other suitable chromagens following standard immunocytochemical protocols, as provided by manufacturers of the primary and/or secondary antibodies.

The basic immunocytochemical protocol given should be optimized for each specific investigation (*see* **Note 6**).

3.2.4. Epithelial Calcium Mobilization

A variety of literature can be accessed describing the ability of bacteria to elicit changes in epithelial intracellular signaling molecules such as inositol 1,4,5-triphosphate (IP_3), Ca^{2+}, protein kinase C, etc. (*16,17*). To assess $[Ca^{2+}]_i$ responsiveness, the epithelial cells are first loaded with a Ca^{2+}-selective fluorescence indicator, such as Indo-1 AM esters or Furo-3-AM. Cytosolic esterase hydrolysis of the indicators leads to their retention inside the cell.

1. Incubate cells with the cell-permeable form of the calcium indicator for 1 h at 37°C in the dark.
2. Rinse 3 times in fresh culture medium to remove nonincorporated fluorochrome.
3. After loading, the epithelial cells are scraped from culture dish and pelleted at 150*g* (1000 rpm) for 10 s.
4. Resuspend a known number of cells (e.g., 10^5 cells) in 1 mL resuspension buffer and place in cuvet.
5. Under constant stirring conditions at 37°C, fluorescence can be measured in a fluorescence spectrophotometer using an excitation wavelength of 340 nm and an emission wavelength of 410 nm.
6. In this manner, baseline Ca^{2+} is assessed and subsequent addition into the cuvet of the Ca^{2+} ionophore (A23187), or carbachol can be used to determine stimulated Ca^{2+} responses (*16*) (*see* **Note 7**).

3.2.5. Epithelial Monolayer Permeability

Antigens and other potentially noxious material can cross the epithelium via the paracellular pathway, negotiating the tight junctions and moving between adjacent cells or by the transcellular route, which involves passage directly through the cytosol. Epithelial paracellular and transcellular permeability can be measured by conducting flux studies (± localization studies) with selective marker molecules, which will preferentially use one or other pathway. For example, ^{51}Cr-EDTA and ^{3}H-mannitol are accepted markers of paracellular permeability, whereas transepithelial fluxes of large protein antigens, such as HRP, are, under normal circumstances, more reflective of transcellular transport (*18*). Assessment of epithelial permeability across T84 monolayers mounted in Ussing chambers is outlined in Chapter 29 (McKay and Perdue). Transepithelial fluxes of HRP can be conducted in Ussing chambers or performed directly in the culture transwell.

1. Add HRP (5×10^{-5} M) to the buffer or medium bathing the apical aspect of the epithelium.
2. Equilibrate for 30 min.
3. Take 500-μL aliquots from the serosal buffer at 30-min intervals over a 1-$^1/_2$-h period.
4. Replace with an equal volume of the original buffer.
5. Subsequently, mix 150 μL of the sample with 800 μL of phosphate buffer containing 0.003% H_2O_2 and 80 μg/mL o-dianisidine.
6. Transfer the solution to a cuvet and determine the HRP concentration by calculating the rate of increase in optical density at 460 nm over a 2-min period. The flux rate should be calculated and expressed as pmol·cm²·h (19). Data may also be expressed as percent recovery of initial amount of HRP added to apical aspect of the monolayer.
7. HRP is electron dense, and so transmission electron microscopy (**Subheading 3.3.1.**) can be used to trace the route by which it crosses the epithelium.
8. After monolayers have been exposed to HRP for 60 min or shorter time periods, fix, and process for DAB cytochemistry using 0.5 mg DAB/mL Tris buffer plus 0.01% (v/v) H_2O_2.
9. Dehydrate samples, embed in Epon, and stain ultrathin sections with uranyl acetate and lead citrate.
10. Observe preparations by transmission electron microscopy and photograph.
11. HRP in the paracellular space can be scored on a presence or absence basis and HRP-containing endosomes (number and area) can be determined in a specified area (e.g., complete single epithelial cell or 5×5 μm area apical to the nucleus) (19).

3.3. Epithelial Cell Apoptosis

Cell death can occur by necrosis or apoptosis, programmed cell death (20). A variety of stimuli induce apoptosis, with the apoptotic cell displaying characteristic plasmalemma blebbing with margination and condensation of nuclear chromatin (i.e., formation of apoptotic bodies). Direct visualization of cell and nuclear morphology (by TEM or fluorescent dye staining) complemented by techniques to identify chromatin fragmentation (e.g., the TUNEL assay, cell death ELISA) can be used to enumerate apoptotic epithelial cells grown on culture dishes and/or slides or as filter-grown monolayers (21–23).

3.3.1. Morphological Assessment of Apoptosis by TEM

1. Grow epithelial cells to confluence and then incubate with bacteria at different multiplicities of infection and for varying time periods (*see* **Note 8**).
2. Following infection, the epithelial cells should be trypsinized from their support and pelleted.

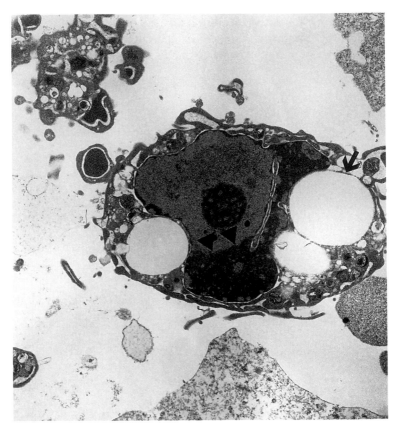

Fig. 1. Transmission electron photomicrograph of an apoptotic HEp-2 cell. The characteristic features of apoptosis, including cytoplasmic vacuolation (arrow) and condensation, as well as nuclear chromatin condensation (arrowheads) and margination, around the edge of the nuclear envelope are apparent (original magnification, ×12,000).

3. Fix in 2% gluteraldehyde and process for TEM.
4. Apoptotic cells are easily identified by their characteristic morphology (*see* **Note 9**) (**Fig. 1**).

3.3.2. Determination of Apoptosis by Fluorescent Dye Staining

1. After infection, tryspinize the epithelial cells from the plastic culture dishes or porous filter supports and resuspend in 1 mL of PBS, to which 100 µg/mL of acridine orange-ethidium bromide is added (this step should be performed under reduced light conditions).
2. After a 10- to 20-min incubation, cyto-spin (<100g [300 rpm]) a sample of cells (approx 1×10^5) for 2 min onto an aptex-coated slide.

3. Add a coverslip and examine by epifluoresence (*see* **Note 10**).
4. Green positivity identifies apoptotic cells that can be enumerated in a sample of 500 cells examined in randomly selected microscopic fields of view.

3.3.3. TUNEL

1. Prior to performing the TUNEL assay, the sample preparations differ depending on whether the co-culture was conducted with epithelium grown on plastic or as filter-grown monolayers.
2. In the former instance, after exposure to the bacteria, the epithelial cells should be rinsed in sterile cold (4°C) PBS.
3. Treat with trypsin-EDTA to remove the cells from the culture plates and count.
4. Cytospin 1×10^5 to 5×10^5 cells onto aptex-coated microscope slides.
5. Air-dry for 30 min at room temperature.
6. Fix with 10% neutral-buffered formalin for 10–20 min.
7. For filter-grown epithelial monolayers, fix the epithelium directly in situ in the Transwell after rinsing in PBS.
8. Dehydrate through graded alcohols.
9. Excise the monolayer and attendant filter support from the Transwell insert.
10. Clear in xylene, embed in paraffin wax, and section (3–10 µm).
11. Collect sections on aptex-coated slides.
12. The epithelial cell cytospins or sections of epithelial monolayers can then undergo the same steps in the TUNEL assay.
13. Rehyrdate preparations and block endogenous peroxidase by incubating for 30 min in 0.01% H_2O_2.
14. This should be followed by an antigen-retrieval step, in which the preparations are microwaved on the high setting in 0.01 *M* citrate buffer for 1 min (*see* **Note 11**).
15. Transfer sections to PBS containing proteinase K (20 µg/mL) for 15 min at room temperature.
16. Wash 3×2 min in distilled water.
17. Incubate in terminal transferase buffer for 5 min at room temperature.
18. Then incubate the preparations at 37°C for 60 min in transferase buffer with the addition of cobalt chloride, biotin 16-dUTP, and terminal transferase.
19. Subsequently, stop the reaction by transferring to stop solution.
20. Visualize via indirect immunocytochemistry using avidin-conjugated peroxidase and reaction with DAB *(24,25)*.
21. Counterstain preparations in hematoxylin and mount in Permount.
22. Apoptotic cells (i.e., positive brown stain) can be identified micoscopically and enumerated on a per monolayer basis, or in the case of cytospins, per 500 cells observed (*see* **Notes 5** and **6**).

3.3.4. Cell Death Detection by Immunoassay

The DNA fragmentation, which is characteristic of apoptosis, results in the formation of histone-complexed oligonucleosomes that can be quantified

(26,27). Methodology for using the cell death detection ELISA[plus] kit is outlined *(24)*.

1. Following epithelial infection, trypsinize the cells and lyse in the lysis buffer supplied by the manufacturer.
2. Pellet at 4000*g* (14,000 rpm) for 10 min.
3. T cells treated with high dose glucocorticoid *(28)* or HEp-2 cells treated with sorbitol (1 *M* for 2 h at 37°C *[24]*) can serve as positive controls. Cells that have undergone a freeze (–20°C for 1 h)-thaw cycle can act as a control for necrosis.
4. Add cell lysate supernatants in duplicate, in serial dilution (e.g., 1:4, 1:16, 1:64) to the streptavidin-coated microtiter wells in 96-well plates.
5. Following incubation, the presence of histone-complexed oligonuclosomes can be detected by the addition of biotinylated antihistone antibody and peroxisome-conjugated anti-DNA antibody followed by incubation with the peroxidase substrate, 2,2′-azino-di[3-ethylbenzthiazolin-sulfonate] (reagents provided in kit, or from kit manufacturer).
6. The histone–DNA complex supplied by the manufacturer is used to construct a standard curve.
7. Sample absorbance is measured spectrophotometrically.

By following the procedures outlined in **Subheading 3.2.**, we and others have shown that bacterial attachment to model gut epithelial results in altered epithelial Ca^{2+} handling, rearrangements in the epithelial F-actin cytoskeleton, disruption of the peri-junction distribution of ZO-1, decreased epithelial barrier function and induction of programmed cell death *(2,12,16,24,25)*.

4. Notes

1. A variety of other marker molecules or probes can be used including ^{3}H-met-leu-phe (bacterial tri-peptide), ^{14}C-polyethylene glycol (PEG) of various molecular weights, inulin, BSA, fluorescein-tagged dextrans (multiple sizes are available: Molecular Probes).
2. For more rapid induction of A/E lesions, EPEC can be grown in broth under optimal conditions for 3 h to produce a logarithmic growth culture *(11)*. If a micro-aerophilic incubator is not available, *H. pylori* can be grown in evacuation anaerobic jars. To obtain micro-aerophilic conditions within the jars, micro-aerophilic packs (e.g., "Campy packs" [BBL Microbiology Systems, Mississauga, ON, Canada]) can be employed. As an alternative, following evacuation the micro-aerophilic gas mixture is flushed into sealed jars. Before use, *H. pylori* in suspension should be assessed for motility of organisms under bright field microscopy and cultured on agar plates under aerobic conditions to exclude contaminants. Both EPEC and *H. pylori* can be stored long-term at –70°C by adding 10% sterile glycerol to the bacterial culture broth.
3. Care must be taken to avoid bacterial contamination of control epithelial preparations in the 12-well Transwell plate and, more importantly, of the stock epithelial

cell lines maintained in the laboratory. Accordingly, it is advisable to designate an incubator solely for studies that will use bacteria. An additional cautionary step uses a perspex isolation box (approx $12 \times 22 \times 28$ cm) fitted with a sealable inlet for the addition of CO_2/O_2, into which the transwell plate containing epithelial–bacteria co-cultures can be placed into the incubator. Once bacteria have been added to the apical surface of the designated epithelial preparations, care must be exercised in not cross-contaminating the control epithelia. Prior to experimentation (i.e., 3–24 h after infection), the investigator should ensure to check the control epithelial preparations for contamination by culturing spent medium on blood agar plates under aerobic conditions for 24 h at 37°C.

4. Bacteria-free culture supernatants can be obtained by centrifuging overnight broth cultures at $3000g$ for 15 min and then passing the supernatant through a 0.2-μm pore size filter *(12,29)*. Bacteria can be killed by γ-irradiation *(13)* or treatment with antibiotics such as kanamycin (10 μg/mL) for *E. coli (12,13)* or gentamicin (4 μg/mL) for *H. pylori (30)*, washed and resuspended in sterile PBS. To ensure the bacteria are nonviable, treated samples should be cultured under optimal grown conditions for the particular species of bacteria.

5. For immunohistochemistry, it is important to ensure that all the preparations are exposed to both primary and secondary antibodies for the same duration. Processing no more that 12 samples at a time is recommended (particularly for the novice immunohistochemist) to ensure that antibodies are added to all preparations within 1 min; this is particularly crucial for short incubations (i.e., 45–60 min). When examining filter-grown epithelia, clear polyester filter supports (Costar) are preferable. After excision from the basket support, the filters are mounted in an aqueous medium, covered with a coverslip, and the edges sealed with nail polish to prevent drying.

6. Optimization steps for immunohistochemical detection can include: (*i*) varying the antibody incubation times and number of washes; (*ii*) varying the dilution of either the primary or secondary antibodies; (*iii*) choice of fixative; (*iv*) antigen retrieval strategies, such as enzyme digests, heat retrieval in buffer or citrate-EDTA buffer; and (*v*) use of serum to block nonspecific binding.

7. The system described for trypsinized cells in suspension can also be adapted for monolayers grown on filter supports. Epithelial cells are grown on clear polyester filters (1.0 μm pore diameter) until confluent, infected with bacteria for the desired time, and then loaded with fluorochrome. Filters are then carefully cut from the plastic well support and placed in the cuvet containing physiological buffer and Ca^{2+} responses determined.

8. Cells grown in a monolayer tend to detach and float in suspension when undergoing apoptosis. Thus, the detached cells should be included in the sample; otherwise, the degree of apoptosis can be underestimated.

9. Nuclear changes are among the earliest detectable morphologic features of apoptosis *(21)*. Apoptotic cells have uniformly condensed and marginated chromatin along the inner surface of the nuclear envelope. Cytoplasmic condensation and vacuolation occurs in association with blebbing of the cell membrane. The

cytoplasmic organelles remain intact. Budding of the cell and nucleus into apoptotic bodies also can be observed. In vitro, apoptotic cells eventually undergo degradation with breakdown of the cell membrane and disruption of the organelles resembling necrosis. However, apoptotic cells undergoing secondary necrosis can be distinguished from "true" primary necrotic cells by the presence of the nuclear features described above.

10. Apoptotic cells can be identified by green fluorescence, reduced cell size, and condensed brightly fluorescent nuclei, with or without nuclear fragmentation *(24,25)*. By comparison, necrotic cells fluoresce orange and appear swollen with flocculation of the nuclear chromatin. Apoptotic cells that have undergone secondary necrosis will also fluoresce orange. However, condensation and fragmentation of the nucleus of these cells distinguishes them from those undergoing primary necrosis. Additional cell permeable and impermeable dyes, which can be used to distinguish apoptotic and necrotic cells, include DAPI, Hoescht reagent, and propidium iodide. As an alternative to cell enumeration by fluorescent microscopy, the degree of apoptosis can be determined by using flow cytometrical analysis of cells that have been treated with DNA intercalating dyes, such as propidium iodide.

11. Other retrieval techniques can be employed, including exposure to 0.05% (w/v) trypsin for 30 min at 37°C *(20)* or microwaving in 0.01 M sodium citrate buffer ($\pm$ 1 mM EDTA, pH 8.0) for 1 min on the high setting.

Acknowledgments

Studies cited from the authors' laboratories are funded by operating grants from the Canadian Institutes for Health Research (CIHR), the Canadian Association of Gastroenterology (CAG), the Crohn's and Colitis Foundation of Canada (CCFC), and the Canadian Digestive Disease Foundation (CDDF). N. L. J. is the recipient of a Research Scholar Award from the American Gastroenterology Association.

References

1. Peppercorn, M. A. (1997) Antibiotics are effective therapy for Crohn's disease. *Inflam. Bowel Dis.* **3,** 318–319.
2. Philpott, D. J., McKay, D. M., Sherman, P. M., and Perdue, M. H. (1996) Infection of T84 cells with enteropathogenic *Escherichia coli* alters barrier and transport functions. *Am. J. Physiol. (Gastrointest. Liver Physiol.)* **270,** G634–G645.
3. Collington, G. K., Booth, I. W., and Knutton, S. (1998) Rapid modulation of electrolyte transport in Caco-2 cell monolayers by enteropathogenic *Escherichia coli* (EPEC) infection. *Gut* **42,** 200–207.
4. Song, F., Ito K., Denniong, T. L., et al. (1999) Expression of the neutrophil chemokine KC in the colon of mice with enterocolitis and by intestinal epithelial cell lines: effects of flora and pro-inflammatory cytokines. *J. Immunol.* **162,** 2275–2280.

5. Kagnoff, M. F. and Eckmann, L. (1997) Epithelial cells as sensors for microbial infection. *J. Clin. Invest.* **100,** 6–10.
6. Weinrauch, Y. and Zychlinsky, A. (1999) The induction of apoptosis by bacterial pathogens. *Annu. Rev. Microbiol.* **53,** 155–187.
7. Cossart, P., Boquet, P., Normark, S., and Rappouli, R. (1996) Cellular microbiology emerging. *Science* **271,** 315–315.
8. Harder, J., Meyer-Hoffert, U., Teran, L. M., Schwichtenberg, L., Bartels, J., and Schroder, J. M. (2000) Mucoid *Pseudomonas aeruginosa*, TNFα, IL-1β, and IL-6 induce human β-defensin-2 in respiratory epithelia. *Am. J. Respir. Cell Mol. Biol.* **22,** 714–721.
9. Agace, W., Hedges, S., Andersson, U., Andersson, J., Ceska, M., and Svanborg, C. (1993) Selective cytokine production by epithelial cells following exposure to *Escherichia coli. Infect. Immun.* **61,** 602–609.
10. Jung, H. C., Echmann, L., Yang, S.-K., Panja, A., Fierer, J., Morzycka-Wroblewska, E., and Kagnoff, M. K. (1995) A distinct array of proinflammatory cytokines is expressed in human colon epithelial cells in response to bacterial invasion. *J. Clin. Invest.* **95,** 55–65.
11. Jones, N. L. and Sherman, P. M. (1999) *Helicobacter pylori*-epithelial cell interactions: from adhesion to apoptosis. *Can. J. Gastroenterol.* **13,** 563–566.
12. Philpott, D. J., McKay, D. M., Mak, W., Perdue, M. H., and Sherman, P. M. (1998) Signal transduction pathways involved in enterohemorrhagic *Escherichia coli*-induced alterations in T84 epithelial permeability. *Infect. Immun.* **66,** 1680–1687.
13. Rosenshine, I., Ruschowski, S., Stein, M., Reinschild, D. J., Mills, S. D., and Finlay, B. B. (1996) A pathogenic bacterium triggers epithelial signals to form a functional receptor that mediates actin pseudopod formation. *EMBO J.* **12,** 2613–2624.
14. Goosney, D. L., de Grado, M., and Finlay, B. B. (1999) Putting *E. coli* on a pedestal: a unique system to study signal transduction and the actin cytoskeleton. *Trends Cell Biol.* **9,** 11–14.
15. Tsukita, S., Furuse, M., and Ito,h M. (1999) Structural and signaling molecules come together at tight junctions. *Curr. Opin. Cell Biol.* **5,** 628–633.
16. Ismaili, A., Philpott, D. J., Dytoc, M. T., and Sherman, P. M. (1995) Signal transduction responses following adhesion of verocytotoxin producing *Escherichia coli. Infect. Immun.* **63,** 3316–3326.
17. Foubister, B., Rosenshine, I., and Finlay, B. B. (1994) A diarrheal pathogen, enteropathogenic *Escherichia coli* (EPEC), triggers a flux of inositol phosphates in infected epithelial cells. *J. Exp. Med.* **179,** 993–998.
18. Travis, S. and Menzies, I. (1992) Intestinal permeability: functional assessment and significance. *Clin. Sci.* **82,** 471–488.
19. Berin, M. C., Yang, P.-C., Ciok, L., Waserman, S., and Perdue, M. H. (1999) Role of IL-4 in macromolecular transport across intestinal epithelium. *Am. J. Physiol. (Cell Physiol.)* **276,** C1046–C1052.
20. Green, D. R. (2000) Apototic pathways: paper wraps stone blunts scissors. *Cell* **12,** 1–4.
21. Kerr, J. F. R., Gobe, G. C., Winterford, C. M., and Harmon, B. V. (1995) *Anatomical methods in cell death. Methods Cell Biol.* **46,** 1–26.

22. Ben-Sasson, S. A., Sherman, Y., and Garvrieli, Y. (1995) Identification of dying cells—*in situ* staining. *Methods Cell Biol.* **46,** 29–39.
23. Jones, N. L., Shannon, P. T., Cutz, E., Yeger, H., and Sherman, P. M. (1997) Increase in proliferation and apoptosis of gastric epithelial cells early in the natural history of *Helicobacter pylori* infection. *Am. J. Pathol.* **151,** 1695–1703.
24. Jones, N. L., Islur, A., Haq, R., et al. (2000) *Escherichia coli* Shiga toxins induce apoptosis in epithelial cells that is regulated by the Bcl-2 family. *Am. J. Physiol. (Gastrointest. Liver Physiol.)* **278,** G811–G819.
25. Jones, N. L., Day, A. S., Jennings, H., and Sherman, P. M. (1999) *Helicobacter pylori* induces gastric epithelial cell apoptosis in association with increased Fas receptor expression. *Infect. Immun.* **67,** 4237–4242 .
26. Nagata, S. (2000) Apoptotic DNA fragmentation. *Exp. Cell Res.* **256,** 12–18.
27. Aragene, Y., Kulms, D., Metze, D., Wilkes, G., Poppelmann, B., Luger, T. A., and Schwartz, T. (1998) Ultraviolet light induces apoptosis via direct activation of CD95 (FAS) independently of its ligand CD95L. *J. Cell Biol.* **140,** 171–182.
28. Ashwell, J. D., Lu, F. W., and Vacchio, M. S. (2000) Glucocorticoids in T cell development and function. *Annu. Rev. Immunol.* **18,** 309–345.
29. Philpott, D. J., Yamaoka, S., Israel, A., and Sansonetti, P. J. (2000) Invasive *Shigella flexneri* activates NF-κB through a lipopolysaccharide-dependent innate intracellular response and leads to IL-8 expression in epithelial cells. *J. Immunol.* **165,** 903–914.
30. Haeberle, H. A., Kubin, M., Bamford, K. B., et al. (1997) Differential stimulation of interleukin-12 (IL-12) and IL-10 by live and killed *Helicobacter pylori in vitro* and association of IL-12 production with γ-interferon producing T cells in human gastric mucosa. *Infect. Immun.* **65,** 4229–4235.
31. Ismaili, A., Philpott, D. J., McKay, D. M., Perdue, M. H., and Sherman, P. M. (1998) Epithelial cell responses to shiga toxin-producing *Escherichia coli* infection, p. 213–225. In *Excherichia coli 0157:H7 and other shiga toxin-producing E. coli strains. (*Kaper, J. B. and O'Brien, A. D., eds.). American Society for Microbiology, Washington, DC.
32. McKay, D. M. (1999) Intestinal inflammation and the gut microflora. *Can. J. Gastroenterol. 13,* 509–516
33. Reynolds, E. (1963) Preparation of material for electron mircoscopy. *J. Cell Biol.* **17,** 208–212.

Index

A

Actin, 390
Airway Cells, *see also* Tracheal cells
  human, 115
    applications, 118
    culture, 122, 128–131
    differentiation, 116
    isolation, 125–127
    media, 123, 124
  rabbit, 217
Alveolar Cells,
  human, 65, 66
  rabbit,
    culture, 221
    isolation, 221
    media, 219
  rat,
    culture, 67, 72
    isolation, 67, 70
    media, 70
Amphibian Cells,
  culture, 332
  media, 332
Annexin 5, 151
Apoptosis,
  analysis, 145
    adherent cultures, 147, 148
    detached cells, 149
    staining, 394
    TEM, 393
    TUNEL, 395

B

Bacteria, interaction with epithelia, 383
  culture, 389
  media, 385
Bax activity, 148, 151, 152
Beads, acrylic, 376
Bile Duct Cells, rat,
  culture, 46
  isolation, 42–49
  media, 38
Blood - Brain Barrier model,
  bovine, 85
  preparation, 94
Blood–CSF Barrier model, rat, 99
  preparation, 107
Bovine,
  aorta cells,
    culture, 351
    isolation, 351
    media, 348
  model of Blood-Brain Barrier, 85
Burn Wounds, *see* Wound Healing

C

Calcium,
  intracellular measurement, 352
  mobilisation, 392
Caspase 3, 148
Cell Lines,
  culture, 361, 388
  media, 360, 385
Cell Supports, 236–237

Chelex treatment, of Fetal Calf
    Serum, 140
Choroid Plexus Cells, rat,
  culture, 105
  isolation, 103
  media, 101
Caco-2 cells, 234
  culture, 241
  media, 238
Chemical Mutagens, *see* ENU
Co-cultures,
  bacteria and epithelial cells,
    preparation, 389
    media, 385
  endothelial cells and muscle,
    preparation, 351
  epithelial cells and immune cells,
    preparation, 362, 364
  hepatocytes and liver cells,
    media, 328
    preparation, 340
Collagen,
  coating, 10, 11, 12, 30, 40, 41,
    83, 94, 124, 135, 141, 279
Confluence, measurement of, 329
Confocal Microscopy, 173
Cryopreservation,
  Cultured Epithelium, 201
  Human Lens Cells, 4, 5
  Rat Liver Cells, 59
  Bovine Mammary Cells, 93
Cystic Fibrosis, 119, 122
Cytospinning, 149

D

Dermatological Disease, *see* wound
    healing
DNA synthesis, 296
Drug Transport,
  in cell lines, 233

  analysis, 254–266
  active transport, 252–254
  passive transport, 248–252
  sources of cells, 234
  in respiratory tract, 217
  model for uptake, 222
    analysis, 223
    preparation, 222

E

Endothelial Cells, bovine,
  culture, 90
  isolation, 89
  media, 86
ENU,
  effect on chromosomes, 297, 308
  induction of ovarian cancer,
    305, 307
  treatment of mammary cells, 294
  tumorgenicity, 298, 311
Electrical Resistance,
    transepithelial,
    assessment of, 243
Electrolyte Transport,
  human airway cells, 118
Embryonic Epithelia,
  culture, 378
  isolation, 377
  media, 375

F, G

Flow Cytometry, 174, 295, 308
Furan treatment, 40, 46, 48
Gastric Mucosal Cells,
  mouse,
    cell line, GSMO6, 22, 23
  rat,
    cell line, RGM1, 21
    culture, 20, 21
    isolation,
      adult, 20
      newborn, 19
    media, 19
Gene Transfer, 119

H

Hepatocytes, rat, 337
  isolation, 339
  media, 328
Human,
  Airway Cells, 115
  Alveolar Cells, 65
  Keratinocytes, 179
  Lens cells, 1
  Nasal cells, 284
  Prostate Cells, 77
  Thymic Cells, 27
  Tracheal cells, 7

I

Immune cells,
  conditioned media, 364
  isolation, 362
  media, 361
Immunocytochemistry,
  keratins, 161–163
Integrins, 169
  analysis of expression, 172
  detection of, 171
Ion transport, 366

K

Keratins, as markers, 157
  staining for, *see*
      immunohistochemistry
Keratinocytes,
  human,
    culture, 181
    differentiation, 181
    isolation, 180, 181
    media, 180
  mouse,
    culture, 142
    isolation, 141
    media, 141

L

Laminin, coating, 103
Lens Cells, Human,
  cryopreservation, 4,5
  culture, 3–4
  isolation, 3
  media, 1
  sources, 2
Liver Cells, Rat,
  cloning, 57
  cryopreservation, 59
  culture, 58, 341
  isolation,
    adult, 56
    newborn, 55
  media, 54

M

Mammary Cells,
  bovine,
    cryopreservation, 93
    culture, 93
    immunohistochemistry, 94
    isolation,
      ductal cells, 92
      secretory cells, 92
      teat sinus cells, 91
    media, 87
  rat,
    isolation, 293
    media, 292
Mannitol, ^{14}C, 241
  transport of, 244
Matrigel, 40, 242, 377
Membrane,
  capacitance, 315
    measurement, 321–324
  integrity, 246
  permeability, 392
  polarity, analysis of, 151

Migration,
of human epithelia, 213
culture, 215
isolation, 215
media, 215
Mitochondria, 151, 152
Mitomycin C, 81, 82, 199
Mouse,
Gastric mucosal cells, 22, 23
Keratinocytes, 139
Thymic cells, 27–36
Muscle cells, smooth, rat
culture, 350
isolation, 350
media, 348
Mutagenesis, chemical, 291

N–P

Nasal Cells, human, 284
N-ethyl-N-nitrosourea, *see* ENU
Nevi, *see* wound healing
Ovarian cancer, induction by ENU,
306, 307
Pharmaceuticals, models for testing,
121, 217
Phenol Red, 330, 333
Polymerase Chain Reaction (PCR),
102, 108
PrEGM media, 78, 79
Proliferation, 213
Prostate Cells, Human,
culture, 81
isolation, 80
media, 79
sources, 80
Pulmonary Cells, *see* Alveolar Cells

R

Rabbit,
alveolar cells, 221
tracheal cells, 217

Rat,
Alveolar Cells, 65
Blood–CSF Barrier Model, 99
Bile Duct Cells, 37
Gastric Mucosal Cells, 17
Hepatocytes, 337
Liver Cells, 53, 337
Mammary cells, 291
Muscle cells, 347
Ovarian cancer, 305
Respiratory Tract, *see* airway cells
and tracheal cells
RNA Extraction, 247
RT-PCR, *see* Polymerase Chain
Reaction

S

Sertoli cells,
culture, 307, 309
isolation, 307
media, 306
Shipment,
Human Lens Cells, 4
Skin Grafting, *see* wound healing
Spectroscopy, 329
Stomach, *see* Gastric Mucosa

T

Tight Junctions, 391
Titanium Grids, 282
Tracheal Cells, Human,
culture, 13, 14
isolation, 13
media, 10
Tracheal Cells, Rabbit,
culture, 220
isolation, 219
media, 219

Tracheal Submucosal Gland, Human
   culture, 14, 15
   isolation, 14
   media, 11
Transepithelial Resistance
   Measurement, 131
Thymic Cells,
   mouse,
      culture, 31–33
      isolation, 30, 31
      media, 28, 29
   human,
      culture, 33, 34
      isolation, 33
      media, 29,30
TUNEL, *see* Apoptosis

V–X

Vitrogen Gel,
   coating, *see* Collagen
Wound Healing,
   burns, 185
   clinical cases, 188, 201
   culture of grafts, 186, 200, 202
      cryopreservation, 201
      isolation, 199
      media, 198, 199
X-Ray analysis, 273
   cultured cells,279, 280
      cryosections, 279, 281
      media, 277